Managing Infectious Diseases

in Child Care and Schools

A Quick Reference Guide, 6th Edition

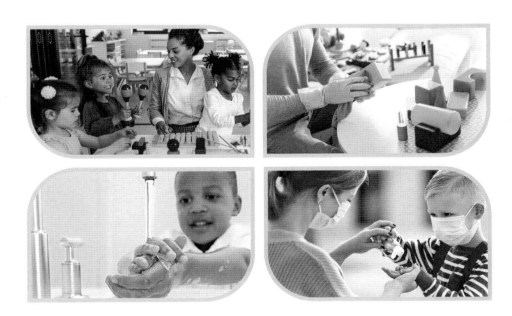

EDITORS

Timothy R. Shope, MD, MPH, FAAP   **Andrew N. Hashikawa, MD, MS, FAAP**

American Academy of Pediatrics

DEDICATED TO THE HEALTH OF ALL CHILDREN®

American Academy of Pediatrics Publishing Staff

Mary Lou White, *Chief Product and Services Officer/SVP, Membership, Marketing, and Publishing*

Mark Grimes, *Vice President, Publishing*

Sara Weissenborn, *Editor, Professional/Clinical Publishing*

Jason Crase, *Senior Manager, Production and Editorial Services*

Shannan Martin, *Production Manager, Consumer Publications*

Sara Hoerdeman, *Marketing and Acquisitions Manager, Consumer Products*

Published by the American Academy of Pediatrics

345 Park Blvd

Itasca, IL 60143

Telephone: 630/626-6000

Facsimile: 847/434-8000

www.aap.org

The American Academy of Pediatrics is an organization of 67,000 primary care pediatricians, pediatric medical subspecialists, and pediatric surgical specialists dedicated to the health, safety, and well-being of all infants, children, adolescents, and young adults.

The recommendations in this publication do not indicate an exclusive course of treatment or serve as a standard of medical care. Variations, taking into account individual circumstances, may be appropriate.

Statements and opinions expressed are those of the authors and not necessarily those of the American Academy of Pediatrics.

Any websites, brand names, products, or manufacturers are mentioned for informational and identification purposes only and do not imply an endorsement by the American Academy of Pediatrics (AAP). The AAP is not responsible for the content of external resources. Information was current at the time of publication.

The publishers have made every effort to trace the copyright holders for borrowed materials. If they have inadvertently overlooked any, they will be pleased to make the necessary arrangements at the first opportunity.

This publication has been developed by the American Academy of Pediatrics. The authors, editors, and contributors are expert authorities in the field of pediatrics. No commercial involvement of any kind has been solicited or accepted in the development of the content of this publication.

Every effort is made to keep Managing Infectious Diseases in Child Care and Schools: A Quick Reference Guide consistent with the most recent advice and information available from the American Academy of Pediatrics.

Please visit www.aap.org/errata for an up-to-date list of any applicable errata for this publication.

Special discounts are available for bulk purchases of this publication. Email Special Sales at nationalaccounts@aap.org for more information.

Printed in the United States of America

9-487

1 2 3 4 5 6 7 8 9 10

MA1080

ISBN: 978-1-61002-659-8

eBook: 978-1-61002-660-4

Cover and publication design by Peg Mulcahy

Library of Congress Control Number: 2022904006

Reviewers/Contributors

Editors

Timothy R. Shope, MD, MPH, FAAP

Andrew N. Hashikawa, MD, MS, FAAP

Technical Reviewers

Abbey Alkon, RN, PNP, MPH, PhD

Danette Glassy, MD, FAAP

American Academy of Pediatrics Committee on Infectious Diseases

American Academy of Pediatrics Council on Children and Disasters

American Academy of Pediatrics Council on Early Childhood

American Academy of Pediatrics Council on School Health

American Academy of Pediatrics Section on Oral Health

American Academy of Pediatrics Board of Directors Reviewer

Wendy S. Davis, MD, FAAP

American Academy of Pediatrics

Keisha Clark, *Program Manager, Early Childhood Initiatives*

Equity, Diversity, and Inclusion Statement

The American Academy of Pediatrics is committed to principles of equity, diversity, and inclusion in its publishing program. Editorial boards, author selections, and author transitions (publication succession plans) are designed to include diverse voices that reflect society as a whole. Editor and author teams are encouraged to actively seek out diverse authors and reviewers at all stages of the editorial process. Publishing staff are committed to promoting equity, diversity, and inclusion in all aspects of publication writing, review, and production.

Contents

Chapter 7 **Emergencies and Disasters: Infectious Disease Outbreaks,
Epidemics, Pandemics, and Bioterrorism**

Chapter 8 **Sample Letters, Forms, and Relevant Resources.**

Preface

In the United States, more than two-thirds of children younger than 6 years, and almost all children older than 6 years, spend significant time in early childhood education (ECE) settings, such as child care centers and family child care homes, religious-based programs, Head Start, and many others. Exposure to groups of children increases the risk of infectious diseases and has important personal, public health, economic, and social consequences. This book provides an easy-to-use reference for those responsible for preventing and managing infectious diseases in ECE programs and schools—educators, pediatric clinicians, public health professionals, and parents/legal guardians.

In this sixth edition of the book, new topics have been added at the request of enthusiastic users. Review of scientific evidence since the previous edition led to a few changes as well. The text was cross-checked and updated to be consistent with 2 other publications: the American Academy of Pediatrics (AAP) *Red Book®: 2021–2024 Report of the Committee on Infectious Diseases*, 32nd Edition, and the AAP, American Public Health Association, and National Resource Center for Health and Safety in Child Care and Early Education *Caring for Our Children: National Health and Safety Performance Standards; Guidelines for Early Care and Education Programs*, 4th Edition.

This edition will be the first for Dr Andrew Hashikawa, a pediatrician and emergency medicine specialist at the University of Michigan, who has many years of experience consulting with ECE programs, conducting research about the spread of infectious diseases in child care centers, and advocating for safe and healthy child care for young children. We would also like to pay tribute and sincerely thank Dr Susan Aronson for her previous contributions to the first through fifth editions. In 2000, Dr Aronson, along with Dr Shope and the AAP, first recognized the need to address the extreme variability, lack of evidence-based practices, and gaps in knowledge regarding the management of infectious diseases in children in ECE programs and schools, leading to the inception of this book. Dr Aronson's vision, and its practical application in the form of this book, started the transformation of practices and state policies. As of 2016, in an unpublished Centers for Disease Control and Prevention/AAP-sponsored survey of licensed US child care centers, *Managing Infectious Diseases in Child Care and Schools* was used by 73%. Dr Aronson's contributions to this publication are just one example of the tremendous efforts she has put forth over a long career as a pediatrician and fierce advocate for improving health and safety in ECE settings. She is truly a pioneer in this area—establishing the need to address specific public health issues in ECE, placing the responsibility to address that need in the pediatric health professional sphere of influence, and tirelessly working to address the need in practical ways that have provided actionable solutions for early childhood educators, parents, and pediatric health professionals.

Educators (including directors, teachers, and other education professionals from ECE and school settings) will find easy-to-read explanations for how infectious diseases spread, how to prepare for inevitable illness, and how to incorporate measures that limit illness in group activities. The Signs and Symptoms Chart (Chapter 5) will help educators have greater insight into what might cause various signs and symptoms. The Quick Reference Sheets (Chapter 6) describe infectious diseases in common terms, with guidance about spread and what may need to be done by educators, children, and families when someone has a disease. By using this book as a handy reference, educators can feel more confident in making decisions about the inclusion and exclusion of ill children. This book may prompt educators to seek advice from medical and public health professionals when necessary to reduce the burden of infectious diseases. Educators can send copies of the reference sheets home to parents.

Child Care Health Consultants (licensed health professionals with education, experience, and training in child and community health and health practices recommended for ECE programs) may find this book helpful in assisting programs and schools to create model policies and best practices for managing children with infectious diseases.

Pediatricians and other health professionals, including school and summer camp nurses, will find this book helpful as a reference that facilitates communication with educators. Pediatric health professionals can use the book's content to identify exclusion and inclusion recommendations, supplement their communications with educators about infectious diseases of patients, and augment their instructions for those involved in the child's care. They also can use the book to link educators with public health authorities when necessary.

Parents will benefit because the book's content provides a common means for communication among family members, pediatric health professionals, and educators based on the latest evidence and expert opinion about best practices. The Quick Reference Sheets describe a condition or infection affecting a child or a group of children. Parents can copy the Quick Reference Sheets to share with educators.

This book also addresses the subject of exclusion and return-to-care criteria. Educators, pediatric clinicians, public health professionals, and parents often disagree about which conditions require exclusion. There is no scientific evidence that exclusion reduces the spread of most common infectious diseases; however, this is a common requirement for most vaccine-preventable diseases. Exclusion and quarantine have been common requirements during the COVID-19 pandemic. Because children and adults can be contagious before they become ill, without ever becoming ill, and for days after becoming ill, the effectiveness and proper length of exclusion require more study. There is a tradeoff between the potential benefit of reducing the spread of an infectious disease against parental lost work, lost income for programs, and lack of continuity of education. Additionally, each state health department and licensing agency has unique rules or exclusion criteria for determining which symptoms, diseases, and conditions require exclusion from ECE programs or school.

For the sixth edition of *Managing Infectious Diseases in Child Care and Schools: A Quick Reference Guide*, we need to acknowledge the profound effects the COVID-19 pandemic has had on ECE programs, schools, children, parents, and educators. This edition is being produced amid a pandemic that has had many unpredictable twists and turns affecting everyone's lives and well-being. Current evidence shows that while COVID-19 spread can occur in ECE programs and schools, unlike other common respiratory viruses like influenza and respiratory syncytial virus, these settings do not seem to be accelerating community spread. COVID-19

transmission rates in these settings are much lower than in households. With this in mind, as well as increasing immunization and infection rates in the population and the vaccination of young children in ECE, we hope that a transition from pandemic (everyone in the world is vulnerable) to endemic (COVID-19 becomes a less-severe background infection similar to other respiratory viruses like seasonal influenza) is underway. For this reason, we have maintained the basic recommendations for exclusion and return-to-care for most infectious diseases, symptoms of infections, and infection control and prevention procedures and highlighted areas that are different due to the pandemic, pointing readers to the latest Centers for Disease Control and Prevention guidelines. We do acknowledge new variants on the horizon and humility in predicting what will happen next. For the first time, this edition includes a website where we can update COVID-19–related material as it becomes available: www.aap.org/midupdates.

The book's recommendations are based on the best available scientific evidence determined by AAP infectious diseases experts. Most of the practices suggested in this book can be followed without conflict with existing state or local rules or regulations. But in some cases, the recommendations in this book may differ from state or local regulations, guidance, or firmly held beliefs (whatever they may be). We hope this book can be a basis for change in these cases.

Timothy R. Shope, MD, MPH, FAAP

Andrew N. Hashikawa, MD, MS, FAAP

About This Book

Managing Infectious Diseases in Child Care and Schools: A Quick Reference Guide is a tool to encourage common understanding among educators, families, and health professionals about infectious diseases in ECE and schools for children. This book identifies

- The role of educators, families, public health officials, and health professionals in preventing and controlling the spread of communicable infections
- Common symptoms of infections in children in ECE programs and school
- How infections are spread (ie, routes of transmission)
- When to seek medical attention
- Inclusion and exclusion criteria
- Strategies and sample forms for communications involving administrators, directors, educators, parents/guardians, and health professionals
- Resources for professional development for directors and educators related to infectious diseases

The first 4 chapters of this book offer information to implement the specific guidelines found in the Signs and Symptoms Chart in Chapter 5 and Quick Reference Sheets in Chapter 6. Chapter 7 discusses infectious disease outbreaks, epidemics, pandemics, and bioterrorism. Chapter 8 provides many forms and links to websites with materials the reader may find helpful in implementing the recommended practices. The Glossary lists terms that may not be familiar or that have a special meaning in the fields of education and health. The Table of Contents at the front and the Index at the back of the book will help users find information quickly.

No permission is needed to make single copies of a Quick Reference Sheet for noncommercial, educational purposes. This book is intended to serve as a means of communication among educators, parents/ legal guardians, and health professionals. The Quick Reference Sheets in Chapter 6 are especially suited for this communication. Educators can share these Quick Reference Sheets with parents/legal guardians when children are affected by certain symptoms of infectious diseases. Pediatricians and other health professionals can communicate with families and educators by adding any relevant notes about the child's care to an appropriate Quick Reference Sheet, such as

- Any special care or follow-up required
- When a child who has been excluded from the ECE program can return

What Is New in This Edition?

- Text has been completely reviewed, updated, and consolidated to reflect the latest guidance and recommendations.
  - Relevant sections have been updated with COVID-19–related changes, recommendations, and links to the latest guidance from the Centers for Disease Control and Prevention.
  - Text has been cross-checked with *Red Book®: 2021–2024 Report of the Committee on Infectious Diseases*, 32nd Edition.
    - A designated website will feature COVID-related updates: www.aap.org/midupdates.
- A new COVID-19 Quick Reference Sheet has been added to Chapter 6.
- Chapter 7 includes updated information about pandemic preparedness.
- New links to online professional development materials have been added throughout the text.

CHAPTER 1

OVERVIEW OF
Managing
Infectious
Diseases
in Child Care and Schools

Overview of Managing Infectious Diseases in Child Care and Schools

Introduction

Keeping children and the adults who care for them healthy is a goal of educators, families, public health officials, and health professionals. One major challenge for staying healthy is that when children begin to participate with groups of other children in early childhood education (ECE) settings, they are exposed to more infectious diseases than when they were only at home. For many children, it may be their first exposure to some of the germs that cause common infections. It is a reality that children in ECE programs, such as child care centers or family child care homes, will transmit infectious diseases due to their normal developmental behaviors that include close contact with each other and exploration of the environment. Although it is not realistic to prevent all infectious illnesses in ECE programs, this book offers multiple strategies that, when used collectively, can mitigate the spread of mild and serious diseases so that children can remain healthy and reach their full potential.

Germ is a common term for a large variety of microbial agents that can grow in or on people. Infection occurs when a germ invades or multiplies in an abnormal manner. If this growth of germs causes symptoms, it results in disease. Germs include *viruses* (eg, influenza), *bacteria* (eg, streptococcus or "strep"), *fungi* (eg, thrush, ringworm), and *parasites* (eg, lice). Sometimes the common names for germs are misleading. For example, ringworm is a fungal infection and is not caused by a worm.

Generally, diseases caused by viruses are not treated with antibiotics, but there are some severe viruses for which treatment with antiviral medications is recommended (eg, influenza viruses in the first few days of symptoms; HIV, the virus that causes AIDS). Many bacterial infectious diseases are treated with antibiotics. Fungi are treated with antifungal medications. Parasites are treated with specific medications, creams, or shampoos along with environmental measures to prevent access of the parasite to human tissues. Many germs are present in the environment. Some germs are carried harmlessly by people who do not seem ill and, in some cases, treatment is not necessary. Others are in the soil and air around us. Still others are only present when someone has a disease that the specific germ causes.

While some germs can be harmful, others help to keep the harmful germs in check. That is why public health authorities urge avoiding unnecessary use of antibacterial soaps and medications that reduce the number of the helpful germs.

Immunity is a term used to describe the body's ability to fight an infection. Immunity to resist a specific infectious disease requires previously having the infection and/or having been immunized against it, in keeping with current national recommendations. Immunity often decreases over time, requiring booster vaccines to prevent reinfections. Groups that are most at risk for infection because of developing or impaired immunity are very young children, children and adults with ongoing chronic health conditions, and pregnant people. The developmental level and health status of children and adults in ECE settings also influence their risk of infection.

The term *immunization* describes the process of giving a vaccine that then induces the immune system to protect the individual if they are exposed to that infectious disease in the future. The terms *immunization* and *vaccines* can be used interchangeably. Immunizations are only developed for diseases that are considered severe enough to cause a major problem for public health. (See Immunization in the Glossary for more detail.) Each time someone is exposed to a new germ or to a substance that stimulates the body's immune system to respond to the specific germ, the immune system learns to recognize and defend against this type of germ in the future. People who have some immunity, from a prior exposure to a specific type of germ or a vaccine for that germ, may have their symptoms reduced or have no symptoms from the next exposure to that specific germ. If the immune system is not able to control the infection, the person becomes ill.

There are several circumstances that arise in ECE programs that may increase the frequency and/or severity of illness for children and EC educators in these settings.

- Infants and toddlers have many developmentally appropriate behaviors that make it easy for them to infect themselves and others. They explore what interests them in their environment by touching what they can reach. Then they put their hands in their noses and mouths. They put toys and other objects in their mouths. Germs can live on toys and objects for variable amounts of time. In this way, children can transfer germs to or receive germs from other children who touch and mouth these objects and toys.

- In the first year that young children participate in ECE programs, they are likely to have more infections than the same-aged children who are not in ECE programs because they are being exposed for the first time to large numbers of germs and need to develop immunity to them. However, when these children start preschool or elementary school, they are less likely to be sick when compared to those children who stayed at home only and are being exposed to different germs for the first time when they begin school.
- Many young children in ECE programs have not yet received enough doses of certain vaccines to have developed sufficient immunity to resist the infections that the vaccine can help prevent.
- Early childhood educators who work with groups of children also often have more infections in their first year of work than other adults who are not involved with caring for young children. The increased frequency of infections for children and adults usually improves significantly in the second year of ECE program participation.
- Children and adults with special health conditions may have more persistent symptoms when they are ill than others without these health problems. For example, children and adults with asthma may get more symptoms from respiratory infections.
- A pregnant EC educator may become infected with germs that young children commonly pass to others without having symptoms themselves. These germs, while mostly harmless to young children, can infect a pregnant person and can harm the fetus. Early childhood educators are at risk for occupational exposure to cytomegalovirus and parvovirus. See the Cytomegalovirus (CMV) Infection and Fifth Disease (Human Parvovirus B19) Quick Reference Sheets in Chapter 6 for more detail.

Common, minor illnesses sometimes have consequences and can cause short-term discomfort and missed school days for a child and lost work time for a family member staying home to care for the ill child. Adults who become ill with infections may not be able to work. If they work while ill, they may spread illnesses to others. Children are less likely to benefit from the educational program if they are absent for illness or ill when they are present. Educators are less likely to be able to implement a quality program if they themselves are ill. Family members who are infected by their children may not be productive at work or home. They may blame staff members for not doing enough to prevent their children from becoming ill.

The words *contagious*, *communicable*, and *infectious* all describe conditions in which a person is infected with a germ that may be passed to another person. Many germs are passed by children who do not appear ill. Educators and families should follow certain precautions to prevent the spread of germs all the time, whether they are in contact with a child who appears ill or not.

The *incubation period* is the time between when a person is exposed to a germ and when it causes symptoms.

Some practical measures help reduce the frequency and severity of common infections. The risk of spread of a particular infection among children, families, and educators is affected by the following factors:

- How common the germ is in the community at the time
- How many people are immune to the germ from previous infections or vaccination
- Whether there is close physical contact of people from different families and different groups
- Whether there is close physical contact of people who live in different parts of the community
- Whether the germ spreads easily, how many germs it takes to start an infection, how it spreads, and how hard or easy it is to kill the germ with certain chemicals (disinfectants), antibiotics, or environmental conditions, such as drying
- How often infection occurs in people who show no symptoms
- How carefully adults and children practice infection control and prevention measures, such as
  - Using hand hygiene at all appropriate times
  - Following food service sanitary routines
  - Using the proper method to catch a sneeze or cover a cough
  - Using recommended approaches for ventilation and fresh air
  - Using surface sanitation
  - Performing daily health checks of children at arrival and when symptoms appear (See Chapter 4 for more details.)
  - Limiting admission of new children to a group in the rare circumstance when this step is needed to control a serious, highly contagious infection
  - Limiting contact between children and certain disease-causing types of animals and their environments
  - Using cohorts to limit the mixing of children and adults from one room with another

Infection Spread by the Respiratory Route

Most germs that are spread by the respiratory route are caused by viruses and result in upper respiratory symptoms like cough, runny nose, congestion, and other cold symptoms. These are relatively harmless and usually resolve without treatment.

Infants in ECE programs have up to 12 common respiratory infections (colds) annually. As children grow older and have more group contact, they have fewer of these infections. Adults and children older than 3 years have an average of 4 common respiratory infections annually. The difference in number of infections is greatest between children in ECE programs and children who have no other children living in their home and do not participate in intermittent group gatherings of children such as drop-in care provided during parent fitness or religious organization activities. The increased number of infections is most troublesome for infants. Infants have small body structures and immature body systems that make them vulnerable to complications from common respiratory infections. For example, infants with common colds are more likely than older children to have feeding difficulties, a cough that lasts for 2 to 3 weeks, or ear infections. When a school-aged child has a cold, the symptoms are usually less bothersome and last a shorter time.

Most respiratory infections are spread by droplets or contact with surfaces. Droplets containing infectious material may be expelled into the air with a cough, sneeze, or talking and singing. If the germs in the droplets land on mucous membranes (on surfaces of the eyes or inside the nose or mouth) an infection can start. Most of the heavy droplets from a sneeze or cough fall from the air in the first 3 feet from the person who expelled them. For some infections, like measles, chickenpox, tuberculosis, and, to some extent, SARS-CoV-2 (the virus that causes COVID-19), the germ particles can float inside fine droplets that remain suspended in the air over longer distances (airborne). They can spread via air currents or ventilation systems to people in other rooms in a building.

Hands are another common way in which germs that cause respiratory infections are spread. Children with respiratory infections tend to contaminate their hands and other surfaces they touch with mucus from their noses, eyes, mouths, and throats. These contaminated surfaces easily spread germs to others.

To prevent the spread of respiratory infections, everyone should use recommended cough and sneeze etiquette. It is best to cover a cough or sneeze with a disposable tissue and then perform hand hygiene before touching anything else. This is not always possible. Few children and adults can get a disposable tissue to the right place quickly enough. Many fail to perform hand hygiene after using a tissue. It's best to teach children that if they don't have a tissue, they should catch a sudden cough or sneeze with an elbow or a shoulder. If visible secretions get on the elbow or shoulder, the secretions should be removed with a tissue and then, if possible, any soiled garment should be changed. Whoever might have touched the secretions should perform hand hygiene. Good hand hygiene requires an appropriate technique using soap and water or using an alcohol-based hand sanitizer as described in Chapter 2.

Infection Spread by the Fecal-Oral Route

Germs that spread by the fecal-oral route typically cause vomiting and diarrheal illnesses. For children at all ages, diarrhea and vomiting illnesses occur less often than common respiratory infections. However, nearly all young children get at least one episode of diarrhea or vomiting each year. As with respiratory infections, diarrhea and vomiting illnesses become less frequent and less severe as a child grows older. Some infectious diseases are caused by viruses that spread by both the respiratory and fecal-oral route, such as the enteroviruses that cause hand-foot-and-mouth disease.

Germs can spread by the fecal-oral route when germ-containing feces (poop or stool) from one person get into someone else's mouth. This happens when someone touches a surface contaminated by feces and does not perform correct hand hygiene to remove the germs. The germs can spread to many other people if this individual touches surfaces that are then touched by others, or if the individual prepares, serves, or feeds food to others.

Hands of young children become contaminated with feces when they either reach into their diapers or grab their bottoms or are learning to potty train and cannot consistently use proper hygiene. Early childhood educators also may contaminate their hands and nearby surfaces during diaper changing. With typical young children's toileting behaviors and diaper changing, hands, floors, toilet and faucet handles, diaper-changing areas, toys, and countertops are easily contaminated by feces.

To prevent the spread of germs that infect by the fecal-oral route, children and EC educators should practice proper hand hygiene and clean, sanitize, and disinfect surfaces as recommended in Chapter 2.

Infection Spread by Contact With People or Objects

A wide variety of respiratory and gastrointestinal illnesses can be spread by direct contact with contaminated surfaces. Because children in ECE programs play, eat, and sleep close together, they easily pass germs to each other. Infection can spread through direct contact with any substance or surface that has been contaminated with infectious material or, less commonly, contact with an infected area of someone's body, such as an open sore. For example, contaminated hands can mix germs into moist play materials, a runny nose can drip onto toys or objects that are subsequently mouthed or handled by others, and surfaces on or around the diaper-changing table can be touched by an EC educator's hands, soiled diapers, wipes or containers of wipes or other diapering supplies, or clothing that had contact with feces during the change.

Many objects can absorb, retain, and transport germs in ECE facilities and include the floors, activity and food tables, water tables, computer keyboards, diaper-changing tables, doorknobs/cabinet handles, toilet room surfaces, toys, and fabric objects. These objects and surfaces should be routinely cleaned and sanitized or disinfected. Eventually, after time, germs on surfaces lose their ability to infect others, so certain strategies, such as rotating difficult-to-clean toys and books in and out of circulation, can be an effective way to decrease the spread of germs. (See Glossary for definitions of and Chapter 2 for details about *clean*, *sanitize*, and *disinfect*.) Head-to-head touching can spread crawling lice, a parasite; shared hats and hairbrushes can spread ringworm, a fungal infection. Skin-to-skin or skin-to-bedding touching of someone with infected sores can spread impetigo (a bacterial infection). Mouth-to-mouth kissing can spread a variety of germs by transfer of saliva or infected mucus. (For more information about signs and symptoms of infection, see Chapter 5. For Quick Reference Sheets on specific types of infections, see Chapter 6.)

Infection Spread by Blood, Urine, and Saliva

Viruses such as HIV, hepatitis B, hepatitis C, and hepatitis D are the primary blood-borne infectious diseases; CMV can be spread in the saliva and urine. These viruses cause a wide variety of symptoms and diseases. Some of the viruses that are present in blood are spread during the birth process from mother to baby, or when blood is transferred from one person to another, or during intimate sexual contact. Biting is another potential way in which infection could spread, and many young children, particularly nonverbal toddlers, go through a phase of biting others. Spread of a blood-borne infection by biting could occur if the biter draws blood from an infected victim or if the biter has bleeding gums and breaks the skin of the victim, transferring blood to the victim. But bites usually do not break the skin or draw blood into the biter's mouth, and few children have bleeding gums. While theoretically possible, blood-borne infections (eg, HIV/AIDS, hepatitis B) are unlikely to spread by children who bite. There have been no reported cases of HIV transmitted through biting in ECE programs. Routine

infant and child immunization against the hepatitis B virus has virtually eliminated any risk of spread of hepatitis B through biting or care for bleeding wounds of immunized children. Children and adults may have some viruses in their blood, urine, and saliva for months to years without symptoms. Cytomegalovirus is one example of a virus spread by saliva and urine indefinitely.

To prevent infections spread by contact with body fluids, properly practice hand hygiene and clean, sanitize, or disinfect contaminated environmental surfaces as described in Chapter 2 with particular attention to the section on Standard Precautions for exposure to blood or body fluids. The basis of Standard Precautions is the assumption that all body fluids might be contaminated with germs that can cause diseases. Routine use of Standard Precautions and good hand hygiene protects everyone against the spread of illnesses by contact with saliva, urine, or blood.

Keeping Children and Adults in Educational Settings Healthy

The approach to keeping children, educators, and other adults who are involved with children in educational settings healthy involves 3 types of measures.
1. Strengthening individual child's and adult's resistance to infections
2. Infection control and prevention by structuring and managing routine practices as well as the environment to reduce the likelihood of contact between people and germs that might cause infectious diseases
3. Exclusion, when indicated

Strengthening Children's Resistance to Infections

Measures that foster health and well-being make people better able to resist infectious diseases.

Routine Health Assessments and Immunizations for Children

Educators see and interact with children and families much more often than pediatric health professionals. Children who are healthy are better able to learn. Education programs for children of all ages have opportunities to provide a safety net to ensure enrolled children have received recommended age- and condition-appropriate preventive health services. Despite the increased use of electronic medical records (EMRs) by health professionals, these software systems do not yet reliably track and alert parents/legal guardians, educators, and health professionals to ensure children have received recommended preventive health services. Many families use multiple health professionals. This makes tracking of a child's screenings and immunizations by any individual health professional difficult.

Some states have functioning immunization registries to which pediatric health care professionals report vaccines that children receive. Some of these registries will allow educators to access the vaccine records to check for up-to-date immunization status. Some states or cities have laws or regulations addressing required immunizations to attend an ECE program, and all states have laws addressing required immunizations for school. Early childhood education programs and schools should require up-to-date documentation from each child's source(s) of health care or an immunization registry that confirms the child has received the full schedule of routine preventive health services and health education for the child's age. Because it takes time to incorporate national vaccination recommendations into state or local government regulations, programs and schools should follow the most up-to-date national recommendations available from the Centers for Disease Control and Prevention (CDC) at www.cdc.gov/vaccines. To check whether a child's or an adult's immunizations are up to date, select the age group for the person whose vaccine record is to be checked.

Careful tracking is necessary to make sure children receive all recommended vaccines and screening assessments according to schedules that provide the best protection. The minimum age to receive a particular vaccine and the intervals between doses can be important to ensure immunity against certain infectious diseases. Simple dose counting does not address all the rules that make it most likely that immunity will be produced by the vaccine. For example, many states require repeating a vaccine dose if it was given more than 4 days before the recommended age that dose should have been given. Catch-up vaccine doses require a minimum interval between doses. A child who starts getting certain vaccines at a later age than recommended or does not keep up with the recommended vaccine schedule may require fewer doses. Early childhood education programs and schools could explore using software to track immunizations. WellCareTracker (www.wellcaretracker.org) is an example of one such program. But at a minimum, programs and schools should require documentation that a pediatric health professional has reviewed and documented the child's immunization status. In addition to immunizations, guidelines from the American Academy of Pediatrics (AAP), called the "Recommendations for Preventive Pediatric Health Care," outline services (eg, screening for vision and hearing problems, lead poisoning, and anemia) that should be done at each

health supervision visit. These recommendations are regularly updated as part of a national initiative of the AAP, supported in part by the US Department of Health and Human Services, known as Bright Futures (www.BrightFutures.org). The list of services begins with the prenatal visit of the parents and ends when the child reaches 21 years of age. The schedule is accessible at www.aap.org/periodicityschedule.

If the state provides an easily completed form, that form, or a printout from a pediatric health professional's EMR, may be used to collect information about the child's health care. The documentation should include the dates when the child received each of the recommended preventive health services. (An example of a Child Health Assessment Form is included in Chapter 8.) The information should identify any health problems that might make the child especially vulnerable to infectious diseases and any special care the child requires. If special care is required, the child's health professional should complete a Special Care Plan Form (see example in Chapter 8). If the child requires medication while participating in the program, educators should use the Medication Administration Packet (included in Chapter 8) to collect the necessary information to accommodate that special need. (Other special care forms are available in the AAP publication *Managing Chronic Health Needs in Child Care and Schools*.)

In preparation for subsequent routine health supervision visits, educators should share with families their assessment of how the child is doing physically, developmentally, and behaviorally. Written consent from parents/legal guardians for educators and pediatric health professionals to exchange information about a child is required if the information is not carried and presented by the family member to the professionals involved in the child's care. This information should be shared in writing with pediatric health professionals doing the child's checkup. The information can be attached to the education program's form for the pediatric health professional to document the child's preventive health services. The combined observations of educators who work with the child every day and pediatric health professionals during office visits helps to generate and coordinate better care of any child.

Routine Health Assessments and Immunizations for Adults Who Work in Early Childhood Education Programs

Adults who work in ECE facilities have specific occupational risks, which include exposure to infectious diseases commonly experienced by young children or by children who may have no symptoms of illness. This risk of exposure to infectious diseases is increased over what an adult normally experiences via interactions within their own families and in the community. As a result, educators in ECE programs and schools should receive the immunizations recommended by the CDC. Vaccines that are especially important for individuals working with young children include the tetanus, diphtheria, and acellular pertussis vaccine; measles-mumps-rubella (MMR); varicella (chickenpox); COVID vaccine series; and annual influenza vaccine. These vaccines reduce the risk of spread of these infectious diseases from adults to young children. Because these are vaccine-preventable and potentially life-threatening illnesses for children, it is essential that all workers receive these vaccines and all other routinely recommended adult vaccines.

The education program's records should document that EC educators have received all recommended vaccines for their age and routine screenings and other preventive health services that enable them to provide consistent, safe, and quality care for the children. (See Chapter 3 for more about the health of EC educators and other adults who work in the facility and Chapter 8, Letter to Staff About Occupational Health Risks and Staff Health Assessment Form.)

Vaccine Refusal

In 2011, the National Academy of Medicine (NAM), formerly known as the Institute of Medicine, reviewed evidence on the safety of 8 individual vaccines and, in 2013, the safety of the immunization schedule. Its conclusions were: (1) few health problems are caused by or clearly associated with individual vaccines; and (2) there is no evidence that the immunization schedule is unsafe. The NAM specifically found no links between the immunization schedule and autoimmune diseases, asthma, hypersensitivity, seizures, child developmental disorders, learning or developmental disorders, or attention-deficit or disruptive disorders. Additionally, use of nonstandard schedules is harmful because it increases the period of risk of acquiring vaccine-preventable diseases and increases the risk of incomplete immunization (*Red Book®: 2021–2024 Report of the Committee on Infectious Diseases;* pages 7–9).

Children and adult workers who have not received all recommended, age-appropriate immunizations should receive the vaccines they are missing as soon as possible. Some children and adults cannot receive certain vaccines because of a medical condition. Some states allow parents to refuse some or all vaccines for their children because of the parents' religious or philosophical beliefs. Common misconceptions about vac-

cines continue to be used to justify failing to follow the recommendations of national immunization experts.

Common myths about use of vaccines are described in Table 1.1, which was prepared by national immunization experts and published in the AAP *Red Book: 2021–2024 Report of the Committee on Infectious Diseases.*

Enrolling a child whose parents refuse some or all vaccines or allowing an under-immunized adult to work in an educational setting increases the risk of spread of certain infectious diseases. Under-immunized children and adults increase their own risk of having a vaccine-preventable illness. When they do become sick from a vaccine-preventable infection, these individuals pose a risk to others who have valid medical reasons for being unable to receive a specific vaccine or who are too young to have received enough doses of a vaccine to be protected. Additionally, if they are exposed to a vaccine-preventable disease they will be excluded from child care or work for a prolonged period.

Vaccine-preventable diseases still circulate in the United States and other countries. With worldwide travel, these infections are easily introduced into an insufficiently immunized population. Vaccine-preventable diseases can cause an illness that may range from mild to severe and life-threatening. There is no way to know how ill an individual who is under-immunized or un-immunized may become. For some infectious diseases, one case is enough to spread infection quickly, particularly in settings where many children are too young to receive certain vaccines.

Allowing participation of children or adults who do not have a licensed pediatric health professional confirmed medical reason to refuse vaccines may result in legal liability for the program if that action results in a preventable illness. Immunization laws and regulations differ from one state and even one city to another. Compliance with local legal immunization requirements may not meet national immunization recommendations. All EC educators must meet state licensing and federal Child Care and Development Fund requirements for documentation of up-to-date immunization of children in their care.

Administrators should consult an attorney about their liability in allowing participation of individuals who claim a nonmedical reason for refusing to use vaccines according to the schedules recommended by the CDC. The legal advice should address whether the program can reduce this liability by verbal review and subsequent signature of the parent/legal guardian or adult worker on a document that outlines the risks and procedures the program will use to limit adverse out-

Table 1.1. Common Misconceptions/Myths About Immunizations[a,b]

Claims	Facts
Natural methods of enhancing immunity are better than vaccinations.	The only "natural way" to be immune is to have the disease. Immunity from a preventive vaccine provides protection against disease when a person is exposed to it in the future. That immunity is usually similar to what is acquired from natural infection, although several doses of a vaccine may have to be administered for a child to develop an adequate immune response.
Giving multiple vaccines at the same time causes an "overload" of the immune system.	Vaccination does not overburden a child's immune system; the recommended vaccines use only a small portion of the immune system's "memory." Although the number of unique vaccines administered has risen over recent decades, the number of antigens administered has decreased because of changes in manufacturing. The NAM has concluded that there is no evidence that the immunization schedule is unsafe.[a]
Vaccines are ineffective.	Vaccines have spared millions of people the effects of devastating diseases.
Prior to the use of vaccinations, these diseases had begun to decline because of improved nutrition and hygiene.	In the 19th and 20th centuries, some infectious diseases began to be better controlled because of improvements in sanitation, clean water, pasteurized milk, and pest control. However, vaccine-preventable diseases decreased dramatically after the vaccines for those diseases were approved and were administered to large numbers of children.
Vaccines cause poorly understood illnesses or disorders, such as autism spectrum disorder, sudden infant death syndrome, immune dysfunction, diabetes, neurologic disorders, allergic rhinitis, eczema, and asthma.	These claims are false. Multiple, high-quality studies have failed to substantiate any link between vaccines and these health conditions. See NAM reports.
Vaccines weaken the immune system.	Vaccines actually strengthen the immune system. Vaccinated children have decreased risk of infections. Importantly, natural infections like influenza, measles, and chickenpox can weaken the immune system, increasing the risk of other infections.
Giving many vaccines at the same time is untested.	New vaccines are tested in concomitant use studies with existing vaccines that are administered on the same or overlapping schedule. These studies are performed to ensure that new vaccines do not affect the safety or effectiveness of existing vaccines administered at the same time and that existing vaccines administered at the same time do not affect the safety or effectiveness of new vaccines.
Vaccines can be delayed, separated, and spaced out without consequences.	Many vaccine-preventable diseases occur in early infancy. Optimal vaccine-induced immunity may require a series of vaccines over time. Any delay in receiving age-appropriate immunization increases the risk of diseases that vaccines are administered to prevent. Spacing out vaccines may also have psychological consequences, because many more office visits will be associated with injections.

Abbreviation: NAM, National Academy of Medicine.

[a] See National Academy of Medicine Reviews of Adverse Events After Immunization.

[b] Other common concerns and information addressing misconceptions are detailed online (https://www.cdc.gov/vaccinesafety/concerns/index.html, https://www.cdc.gov/vaccines/parents/why-vaccinate/vaccine-decision.html).

Adapted from Myers MG, Pineda D. *Do Vaccines Cause That? A Guide for Evaluating Vaccine Safety Concerns*. Immunizations for Public Health; 2008:79. Reprinted with permission from American Academy of Pediatrics. *Red Book: 2021–2024 Report of the Committee on Infectious Diseases*. Kimberlin DW, Barnett ED, Lynfield R, Sawyer MH, eds. 32nd ed. American Academy of Pediatrics; 2021:8–9.

comes of vaccine refusal. Further consideration should be given to whether the program is legally liable if it does not notify the families of other children in the facility about the risk to their children from participation of the under-immunized individual. (A sample Refusal to Vaccinate Form can be found in Chapter 8.)

More information about vaccines is available from the CDC at www.cdc.gov/vaccines.

Healthful Nutrition

Being well nourished helps support the body's immune system and resistance to infection. Encourage and support exclusive breastfeeding for infants through 6 months of age and continued breastfeeding (along with age-appropriate foods) as long as mutually desired by mother and child through at least 2 years of age. Human milk has components that decrease the infant's risk of infection from germs that cause respiratory illnesses, vomiting, and diarrhea. Beginning at about 6 months of age, or earlier if the child's health professional recommends it, infants should receive nutritious solid foods and human milk, or formula when human milk is not available. Thereafter, all children and adults who eat at the ECE facility should be offered recommended types and portions of food consistent with the recommendations of the US Department of Agriculture Child and Adult Care Food Program. These meal patterns are helpful guides for all facilities that serve children and for families to follow in feeding their children. They are accessible at www. fns.usda.gov/cacfp/meals-and-snacks. Although a well-balanced, nutritious diet is important to optimize the immune system's ability to fight infections, no supplements or foods specifically boost immunity or prevent infections. Vaccines are necessary to prevent specific harmful infections, according to the recommended schedule (www.cdc.gov/vaccines).

Sleep and Exercise

Getting enough sleep and exercise supports brain development and physical and social-emotional wellness. Sleep supports the body's immune system along with other body functions. Programs like Healthy Kids, Healthy Future at https://healthykidshealthyfuture.org and Active Schools at https://www.activeschoolsus.org help educators promote moderate to vigorous exercise to develop this key lifetime habit.

Safe Activities

Choosing safe activities is essential to prevent injury that can significantly impair an individual's quality of life. Injured tissues, such as skin, muscle, and bone, are easily infected. For example, EC educators of toddlers should be sure these children play on equipment appropriate for their size and skills. They should not play on equipment designed for use by school-aged children.

Care for Special Needs

Providing necessary care to individuals with special needs may help them resist infection. For example, children with asthma are more susceptible to infection when their airway is narrowed and filled with mucus during an asthma episode. Children with special medical needs (eg, asthma, seizures) are more severely affected by the influenza virus, so ensuring that they receive their yearly influenza vaccine is vital.

Health Education

Resources are available to help educators teach families and staff members about keeping healthy, practicing hygiene related to child development, and managing minor illnesses. These resources include the AAP website for parents, www.HealthyChildren.org; the current national health and safety performance standards in Caring for Our Children (https://nrckids.org/CFOC); and the section on physical health of the Head Start Early Childhood Learning & Knowledge Center (ECLKC), https://eclkc.ohs.acf.hhs.gov/physical-health. The ECLKC section on physical health has information that is relevant to prevention and management of infectious diseases.

Infection Control and Prevention by Structuring and Managing the Environment

See Chapter 2 for more details.

Space

Having enough indoor space for air to circulate among the children and adults in the room reduces the concentration of germs in the air and on surfaces. In ECE facilities, this should be no less than 42 to 54 square feet of indoor floor area per child, excluding the space occupied by furnishings or used only by adults. The recommended outdoor space is 75 square feet per child or a comparable indoor play area (Caring for Our Children, Standards 5.1.2.1, 6.1.0.1, and 6.1.0.2 [https://nrckids.org/CFOC]).

Group size should not exceed the specifications by age group stated in Caring for Our Children, Standards 1.1.1.2 (for centers and large group homes) and 1.1.1.1 (for small family child care homes) (https://nrckids.org/CFOC). Avoiding mixing groups of children (by using cohorts) will reduce the risk of transfer of infectious diseases from one group to another. Minimizing sharing of space and surfaces among groups reduces the sharing of germs.

Surfaces

Choose surfaces that can be easily cleaned and sanitized. The best are nonporous, smooth surfaces. Soft materials such as cloth and stuffed animals should be machine washable and washed often.

Toilets and Sinks

Provide enough flushing toilets and sinks so that each group of young children has easy access and preferably uses the ones that are assigned to their group. Schools should provide enough toilet facilities located where they serve students whose classrooms are nearby. Provide enough supplies (eg, liquid hand soap, paper towels, toilet paper) to meet the needs of users.

Changing Areas for Diapers, Disposable Training Pants, or Soiled Underwear

Do not use the floor to change diapers, disposable training pants, or soiled underwear, unless dealing with an emergency situation. Using the floor for these changes contaminates the floor and allows children who are crawling or walking in this area to spread germs around. See Caring for Our Children, Standards 3.2.1.4 and 3.2.1.5 (https://nrckids.org/CFOC), and Chapter 2 of this book for details about the procedure to follow when changing diapers, soiled disposable training pants, and soiled underwear.

Hand Hygiene

Hand hygiene removes germs from the skin. Germs on hands are often transferred by touching the hands to the mouth, nose, eyes, other body openings, or surfaces that other people touch. Some germs can live on surfaces for many hours. Frequent practice of hand hygiene with soap and water is a key tool to control infectious diseases.

Handwashing with soap and water is preferred over any other method. If washing with soap and water is not possible, use of alcohol-based hand sanitizers according to the manufacturer's directions is an allowable alternative if certain conditions are met. If adults or children use alcohol-based hand sanitizers, the supplies and procedure for use should be as specified in Caring for Our Children, Standard 3.2.2.5 (https://nrckids.org/CFOC) and summarized in Chapter 2.

Surface Hygiene

Surface hygiene removes germs from surfaces that are likely to be contaminated during routine use and contact with body fluids. Surfaces and objects that need routine cleaning, followed by sanitizing or disinfecting, include food preparation surfaces and equipment, mixed-use tables, eating utensils, drinking fountains, diaper-changing and toilet area surfaces, and handwashing sinks and faucets. Surfaces and objects that need routine cleaning, but not disinfection, are frequently touched toys and equipment; doorknobs and cabinet handles; computer keyboards and telephones; mouthed toys; shared art and writing tools; floors; mats and bedding; soft washable toys; and dress-up clothes, including hats and helmets. This routine cleaning must be supplemented with immediate cleaning and disinfection of these surfaces if they are contaminated with a body fluid. See Chapter 8 for a Routine Schedule for Cleaning, Sanitizing, and Disinfecting, as well as Selecting an Appropriate Sanitizer or Disinfectant. This information is in Caring for Our Children, Section 3.3 and appendixes J and K (https://nrckids.org/CFOC).

Standard Precautions

Mentioned earlier in this chapter, Standard Precautions is the term used to describe the special attention needed when there is a risk of direct contact or contact with a surface contaminated by body fluids. Common exposures occur when someone blows or wipes a nose, coughs or sneezes, has a cut or scrape, or puts feces anywhere other than in a flushing toilet.

Healthful Daily Practices

Following healthful practices, such as cough and sneeze etiquette, oral hygiene, and hand hygiene, reduces the risk of becoming infected with disease-causing germs.

Safe Food Preparation and Service

Foodborne illness caused by germs is a serious threat to health and a very common cause of infectious diseases. Illnesses associated with improper preparation, transport, storage, and serving of food are all risks that should be addressed by food safety procedures and education of staff, families, and children. Food preparation areas should be separate from any area used for another purpose. On-site visits by environmental health professionals can help identify potential trouble spots. For more information about safe food handling practices, go to www.foodsafety.gov.

Toothbrushing

Dental decay is an infectious disease. Bacteria in the mouth produce acid that erodes the enamel covering of the teeth. Once teeth come in, EC educators should clean every child's teeth at least once a day as part of the curriculum to learn and practice proper technique. This is in addition to any toothbrushing parents do for young children after breakfast and before bed at home. No harm will result from using toothpaste that contains fluoride if only a rice-sized amount of fluoride toothpaste (for those younger than 3 years) or pea-sized amount of fluoride toothpaste (for those 3 years and older) is applied, even if the child is not able to spit. School-aged children should be encouraged to brush their teeth after breakfast and before bed. See Chapter 2 for details about toothbrushing.

Healthful Environment

Heating, ventilation, and air-conditioning (HVAC) systems and maintenance routines should meet current national health standards. In ECE programs, as well as in schools, implement the recommendations of the US Environmental Protection Agency (EPA) for the facility. For guidance about how to maintain a healthful environment in schools, see www.epa.gov/schools. For ECE facilities, see the EPA standards at www.epa.gov/childcare. The EPA website has checklists and other tools, as well as information about a full range of environmental health issues. The Children's Environmental Health Network (https://cehn.org) offers an Eco-Healthy Child Care program. For air quality of the outdoor and indoor environment, follow *Caring for Our Children* Standards 5.2.1.1 through 5.2.1.15 (https://nrckids.org/CFOC). These standards include providing as much fresh outdoor air as possible in rooms occupied by children. The amount of outdoor air that should be supplied to each room ranges from 15 to 60 cubic feet (0.45–1.80 m³) per person per minute, depending on the activities that usually occur in the room. Other EPA standards specify room and water temperature, humidity, ventilation, allowable equipment and equipment maintenance, and use of chemicals that release toxic fumes, including those that might be used for cleaning, sanitizing, and disinfecting.

Qualified engineers can ensure HVAC systems are functioning properly and that applicable standards are being met. The American Society of Heating, Refrigerating, and Air-Conditioning Engineers (ASHRAE) website (https://www.ashrae.org) includes the qualifications required of its members and the location of local ASHRAE chapters. The contractor who services the ECE facility's HVAC system should provide evidence of successful completion of ASHRAE or comparable courses. Educators should understand enough about codes and standards to be sure the facility's building is a healthful place to be.

Integrated Pest Management

The CDC recommends using a science-based approach to pest management and if pests occur, using the safest and most effective methods to get rid of them (https://www.cdc.gov/nceh/ehs/Docs/Factsheets/What_Is_Integrated_Pest_Management.pdf). Common pests can spread infectious diseases. Insect bites may carry disease-causing germs into the body or make an itchy opening that can get infected with bacteria on the skin or other surfaces. Rodents and other vermin bring disease-causing germs into the facility, contaminating food and surfaces that people touch. Use the least toxic methods to avoid or control pests. Use methods to shut the pests out of the facility and keep food sources away from where they might attract pests. Especially in spaces used by children, if any pesticides are used, they should be chosen after careful review of the product Safety Data Sheets. Application of any toxic product should be supervised by educators to prevent careless application to areas and surfaces that can expose children and adults in the facility to risk. For further guidance, see the free California Childcare Health Program (CCHP) toolkits for integrated pest management in child care centers and for family child care homes, available in English and Spanish at https://cchp.ucsf.edu.

Exclusion

The following is an overview; please see chapters 4, 5, and 6 for details.

Exclusion of Children and Adults Who Are Ill

Sending home (*excluding*) those who are mildly ill is not an effective way to control the spread of most common germs. People may spread infections when they are developing an illness, before symptoms have begun, and when they have recovered from the major symptoms of illness, or when they have germs in their bodies but show no signs of illness. Most of the illnesses are respiratory infections, such as colds. Fewer infections involve the gastrointestinal system, causing symptoms such as abdominal discomfort, vomiting, and diarrhea.

Decisions about exclusion should be based on evidence-based written criteria that are shared with families at enrollment and that staff refer to when a decision about exclusion is needed. Written exclusion policies promote consistency and aid in diffusing disagreements between families and program or school staff members about the exclusion of children who are ill. Exclusion policies should be updated on an annual or as-needed basis (eg, before influenza season).

Staff members in ECE programs and schools must decide whether children are too ill to participate in planned activities or require more care than can reasonably be provided without compromising care of the others in the group. These are the 2 most likely reasons why children who are ill may need to be excluded. Early childhood educators who cannot provide care because of their own illness should be excluded from providing care for others. Family child care providers should have backup arrangements made in advance and used when the family child care provider is ill. In addition to the 2 most common reasons for exclusion, some specific symptoms or diagnoses require exclusion. Generally, the specific conditions or diagnoses recommended for exclusion meet all 3 of these criteria: They 1) are transmissible from one person to another, 2) are particularly harmful, and 3) have some evidence that exclusion might reduce the spread of illness. During the COVID-19 pandemic, exclusion was regularly used in ECE programs and schools because the first 2 criteria were certainly true—and possibly the third, as well. Programs must follow their state licensing or certification laws or codes related to exclusion even when these have not been updated to the most recent expert recommendations. The Quick Reference Sheets in Chapter 6 incorporate exclusion criteria from *Caring for Our Children*, Standard 3.6.1.1 (https://nrckids. org/CFOC), and provide reproducible handouts about each condition. It is usually best for the program director or school health professionals, rather than the educators, to make sure families are informed about exclusion policies at enrollment.

Roles of Families, Staff Members, and Health Professionals in Managing Infectious Diseases for Children in Early Childhood Education Programs and Schools

Three fact sheets on the Pennsylvania Chapters of the AAP (PA AAP) Early Childhood Education Linkage System (ECELS) website at https://ecels-healthychildcarepa.org outline the roles of families, staff members, and health professionals in managing infectious diseases in child care. On the ECELS home page, select the "Publications" tab at the top of the page and then "Fact Sheets" from the left pane. Scroll the alphabetically listed fact sheets to "Roles of Families, Staff Members and Health Professionals in Managing Infectious Diseases in Group Care." Then download each of the 3 fact sheets.

Information about serving as a school nurse is available from an AAP policy statement, "Role of the School Nurse in Providing School Health Services" (https:// doi.org/10.1542/peds.2016-0852).

Brief descriptions of the specific roles of the health advocate and Child Care Health Consultant (CCHC) who work with ECE programs follow:

Health Advocate

What Is the Role of the Health Advocate?

Every ECE program and school should identify a health advocate. The health advocate may have another primary role but should be present on a day-to-day basis to promote integration of best practices for health and safety into the program's planning and operations. Programs should choose someone to be the health advocate who is willing and accepted by others to fulfill this role. The health advocate systematically observes and ensures that everyone follows written policies and procedures that implement recommended national health and safety standards. Who performs these tasks for reducing the risk of infectious diseases will vary from setting to setting. In schools that have a school health professional on site or at least accessible every day to provide health consultation, this person could serve as the health advocate and CCHC.

What Are the Qualifications and Specific Responsibilities of the Health Advocate?

The qualifications and responsibilities of a health advocate in an ECE program are described in *Caring for Our Children*, Standard 1.3.2.7 (https://nrckids. org/CFOC). The health advocate should be able to foster collaboration among the individuals involved in achieving a safe and healthful program. Making sure best practices are understood and followed requires a combination of oversight by supervisors and peer-to-peer coaching, as well as an ongoing relationship with a health professional (CCHC or school health personnel) who visits the facility periodically to observe for hazards and risky practices and is available to respond to questions as needed.

How Does a Staff Member Learn to Perform the Health Advocate Role?

The staff member who accepts the responsibility of carrying out the role of health advocate can learn how to fulfill this role in a variety of ways. Here are 3 examples.
- *Health advocate workshop series:* The California Training Institute Curriculum for Child Care Health Advocates is a series of workshops in English

and Spanish and is accompanied by a companion instructor's guide. The curriculum includes lesson plans and readings for participants in the workshops. A health professional can use materials to teach health advocates about relevant topics. The curriculum can be accessed at no cost at https://cchp.ucsf.edu/content/california-training-institute-curriculum-child-care-health-advocates.

- *Child Care Health Advocate course:* Since 2007, Northampton Community College has offered an online 3-college-credit course that consists of 15 weeks of assignments, weekly participation by entering comments and responding to the comments of co-participants on a discussion board, and participating in the 7 live interactive sessions led by the instructor. The weekly assignments include readings, viewing audiovisual material and resources, implementing changes at the student's work site related to the course topics, and reporting the results of the work in a reflection journal. The course has been offered in the fall and again in the spring term each year. To learn more about this course, contact Northampton Community College Admissions at 610/861-5300 or adminfo@northampton.edu. Ask about EARL160.

- *Self-learning:* A health advocate can read about and implement desired changes in program operation by using the references in this and other readily available health and safety print and internet-accessible materials from credentialed sources such as

  – The ECLKC is funded for Head Start program use and provides information for all types of early learning programs. It has a section devoted to health and safety with many regularly updated resources. Access this section at https://eclkc.ohs.acf.hhs.gov.

  – The CDC (www.cdc.gov) has excellent explanations about infectious diseases and other health problems and prevention strategies. Select the search term "child care" to display the many topics with helpful information. This website has videos and downloadable handouts and posters.

  – *Healthy Young Children: A Manual for Programs,* 5th Edition, is a publication available from the National Association for the Education of Young Children. The content is aligned with *Caring for Our Children.* Pertinent information for EC educators about infectious diseases is in Chapter 2, Preventing Infections; Chapter 9, Staff Members and Consultants for Safe and Healthy Child Care; Chapter 10, Facility Design and Support Services for Safe and Healthy Early Care and Education; Chapter 11, Caring for Children with Short-Term or Chronic Health Needs or Disabilities; and the appendixes.

  – The PA AAP/ECELS website at https://ecels-healthychildcarepa.org is richly populated with many free materials, such as *Model Child Care Health Policies.*

  – The parent education website of the AAP, www.HealthyChildren.org, has content in English and Spanish for many child health issues.

Child Care Health Consultant

What Is a Child Care Health Consultant?

A CCHC is a licensed health professional with education, experience, and training in child and community health and in health practices recommended for ECE programs. A CCHC should know about resources and regulations that apply to ECE programs and be comfortable linking health resources with these programs. Every program that enrolls children should have an ongoing relationship with a health professional to provide advice about best practices. In schools, the CCHC is the health professional who implements the school health program.

The CCHC collaborates with EC educators and, as appropriate, serves as a bridge to community health professional resources for the staff and families. Many types of health professionals from a variety of health settings can function as CCHCs for education programs. Pediatricians, family practitioners, nurse practitioners, and nurses with pediatric experience are especially qualified to provide this service. Nurses and doctors usually provide school health advice and services in K–12 schools. Child Care Health Consultants and Head Start health managers provide consultative services and input into the health operations in other types of ECE programs for children.

Having a CCHC is a best practice for early childhood programs. Unfortunately, many ECE programs do not have a CCHC. It is best to have an ongoing relationship with a CCHC who makes periodic site visits and collaborates regularly with staff to make and carry out action plans. Child Care Health Consultants can also work with programs to review health protocols on how to conduct health checks. (See *Caring for Our Children,* Standard 1.6.0.1 [https://nrckids.org/CFOC], for the description of the role and knowledge of a CCHC.) As a minimum, it is essential to have a health professional who can be contacted about health concerns. Throughout this book, EC educators are advised when they should seek help or notify the program's CCHC. Several states have conducted studies to determine the effect of the use of CCHCs on child outcomes and program performance. The findings affirm that CCHCs help EC educators to improve health and safety in their programs. For a summary of these findings, go to https://ecels-healthychildcarepa.org/publications/

fact-sheets and select "Efficacy of Child Care Health Consultants-Research Findings."

What Are the Qualifications of a Child Care Health Consultant?

For ECE programs, the CCHC can be a pediatric health professional who works in the public or private sector. The CCHC should know or learn about the day-to-day operation of the program to be an effective collaborator in improving quality in that setting. Contractual and compensation arrangements for such work vary widely. In an ECE program housed in an elementary school, the CCHC might be employed by the school district as the school nurse or school physician. To perform some tasks, arrangements may need to be made for appropriate school personnel, such as dietary or maintenance personnel, to be involved.

For detailed information about the knowledge, skills, training, and functions of CCHCs and school physicians, see
- *Caring for Our Children*, Standards 1.6.0.1, 1.6.0.2, 3.6.2.7, 9.2.3.17, and 9.4.1.17 (https://nrckids.org/CFOC)
- Child Care Health Consultation: Skill-Building Modules at https://eclkc.ohs.acf.hhs.gov/health-services-management/article/child-care-health-consultation-skill-building-modules
- National Center on Health, Behavioral Health, and Safety at https://eclkc.ohs.acf.hhs.gov/about-us/article/national-center-health-behavioral-health-safety-nchbhs and https://eclkc.ohs.acf.hhs.gov/health-services-management/article/resources-child-care-health-consultants
- The PA AAP website at https://ecels-healthychildcarepa.org (search for "child care health consultant")
- The CCHP website at https://cchp.ucsf.edu/search/node/child%20care%20health%20consultant
- The AAP policy statement, "Role of the School Physician" (https://doi.org/10.1542/peds.2012-2995)

Where Can Early Childhood Education Programs Find a Child Care Health Consultant?

Some states have regulations that require programs to have a CCHC. Some have organized networks and registries of CCHCs. These registries may be maintained by resource and referral agencies, local and state health departments, licensing agencies, a state-based Healthy Child Care program, an Early Childhood Comprehensive Systems agency, or pediatric health professional organizations. Some CCHCs serve as volunteers; others will negotiate a fee for their services.

Contacting the following entities may help locate a health professional who is willing to be a CCHC:
- Local or state public health and regulatory agencies
- Local health clinics
- Children's hospitals
- Clinicians who care for children who are enrolled in the ECE program
- School nurses
- Nursing organizations, such as the National Association of Pediatric Nurse Practitioners (www.napnap.org)
- Early childhood education organizations, some of which have members who may be using a CCHC they can recommend
- A family member of an enrolled child who is a health professional (with appropriate limitations of access to confidential information about children and families in the program)
- Local child care resource and referral agencies (Contact information can be found through Child Care Aware of America at www.childcareaware.org.)

AAP Chapter Early Childhood Champions

The national AAP Council on Early Childhood has identified an Early Childhood Champion in many AAP chapters. Connecting with an AAP chapter Early Childhood Champion provides an opportunity to identify pediatric health professionals willing to serve as local CCHCs and to cultivate and connect with AAP leadership to provide input on early childhood issues across clinical, community, and policy settings. Learn more about the AAP Council on Early Childhood at https://www.aap.org/en/community/aap-councils/early-childhood/membership-criteria/why-should-i-join-coec. National AAP staff can identify the pediatrician who serves as the chapter Early Childhood Champion or contact the chapter president to ask for help to find a pediatrician or pediatric nurse practitioner to serve as a CCHC or work with state leadership to foster early education initiatives.

Planning and Policies

All ECE facilities and schools should have written policies and procedures dealing with control and prevention of infectious diseases.

The management of the educational health programming in ECE and K–12 school settings requires focused planning. All facilities need written health policies that clearly define the roles and responsibilities of each staff member and consultants, including determining who will communicate with families, children's health professionals, and others involved in caring for a particular child's illness. Health policies and procedures should be reviewed and updated routinely. Early childhood education programs and schools can review their policies with a CCHC, if available.

Some level of illness is inevitable and policies and procedures should be designed with that expectation in mind. For example, when their child is moderately or severely ill, parents/legal guardians should be asked to remind their child's health professional about the education settings where the child is enrolled and ask for specific information to share with the educators about the diagnosis and care of the child and whether the child's illness might pose a risk to other children and educators.

Health professionals are legally required to obtain the parent's/legal guardian's written consent before directly sharing any information about a child with anyone. Parents/legal guardians should authorize their child's health professional to call or email appropriate members of the child's education program about potentially communicable diseases or other conditions. (See the Sample Health Information Consent Form in Chapter 8.) Educators need firsthand information from the child's health professionals to provide appropriate care for the child and others in the child's group. Even if parents/legal guardians understand what a health professional tells them, the parents may not have the skills to accurately convey that information to others who care for the child.

Resources for Drafting Site-Specific Health Policies Relevant to Infectious Disease Control

Drafting policies and procedures can be a daunting task. The following resources are helpful tools:
- The content of this book.
- *Model Child Care Health Policies*, 5th Edition, is a publication of the AAP and PA AAP. This fill-in-the-blank, adaptable set of policies can focus discussion with staff and families as a starting point for development of site-specific consensus and guidance. *Model Child Care Health Policies* covers a broad range of health and safety in ECE. The publication is free to download from the ECELS website at https://ecels-healthychildcarepa.org/publications/manuals-pamphlets-policies/item/248-model-child-care-health-policies.html and available in paperback

and eBook formats at https://shop.aap.org. The sections in *Model Child Care Health Policies* that include topics that are most relevant to infectious disease control are sections 1, Admission/Enrollment/Attendance; 4, Nutrition, Food Handling, and Feeding; 6, Daytime Sleeping, Evening, Nighttime, and Drop-in Care; 7, Sanitation and Hygiene; 8, Environmental Health; 10, Health Plan; 11, Care of Children and Staff Members Who Are Acutely Ill or Injured; 13, Emergencies and Disasters; 16, Human Resources/Personnel Policies; 17, Design and Maintenance of the Physical Plant and Contents; and 18, Review and Revision of Policies, Plans, and Procedures, as well as appendixes A through J, L through N, Q, R, and U through AA.

Using Health Policies and Procedures to Evaluate Performance

Every program should have written health policies and procedures that are verbally shared with and made available in writing to all staff members and parents/legal guardians. These form the basis for orienting new staff and clarifying procedures and protocols staff can use for typical situations on a day-to-day basis and are a handy reference when unusual or more complex situations arise. In addition, these policies and procedures are a valuable tool to enable staff members and the program's CCHC to conduct an annual review of the policies to see whether events during the year suggest the need for a policy revision. This review refreshes everyone's memory and provides an opportunity to discuss the best approaches and needed updates. Program directors and administrators or their designees should routinely and directly observe substitutes and regular staff members to assess their adherence to the policies and procedures of the facility, especially those related to personal care routines, hygiene, and sanitation. In addition, planned peer-to-peer observations can be effective reinforcement for both parties involved. Discussing several hypothetical child illness scenarios (eg, a child with vomiting and diarrhea and what procedures need to be followed) with regular staff can be another way for program directors and administrators to reinforce the program's health policies and procedures. Personnel performance reviews should include an assessment of the individual's compliance with the program's health policies and procedures.

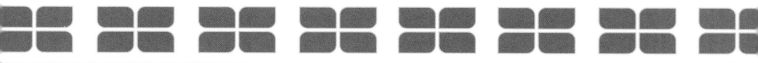

CHAPTER 2

Reduce the
Risk of
Infection
Practice Prevention

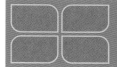

Reduce the Risk of Infection: Practice Prevention

Introduction

Children in early childhood education (ECE) settings learn desirable social interactions with other children. Children are naturally curious and frequently touch each other and environmental surfaces and place their hands in their mouths and noses. Children rely on EC educators to incorporate and teach them infection control and prevention measures such as setting up and maintaining a safe environment, containing coughs and sneezes, implementing frequent hand hygiene, and minimizing contamination during diaper changing and toileting.

Educators working in ECE programs and schools need regular advice from an expert about best practices to incorporate safe and healthy routines to reduce the risk of infectious diseases. An educator who serves as the program's designated health advocate systematically observes and ensures everyone follows appropriate written policies and procedures and is essential to reduce the risk of infectious diseases. The program's health advocate should also make sure best practices are understood and followed, calling attention to practices that need improvement. A program's Child Care Health Consultant, health services manager, or school health personnel should periodically observe performance of infection control measures and then collaborate with other staff members to implement acceptable and feasible changes. See Chapter 1 for an overview of the role, knowledge, skills, and preparation for health advocates and Child Care Health Consultants. For more details, see *Caring for Our Children*, Standards 1.3.2.7, 1.6.0.1, 1.6.0.2, 3.6.2.7, 9.2.3.17, and 9.4.1.17 (https://nrckids.org/CFOC).

During the COVID-19 pandemic, long-established conventions for reducing the spread of infectious diseases in ECE programs and schools were reevaluated. Due to the severity of the disease, previously untested or rarely practiced measures such as program and school closures, classroom closures, prolonged exclusion periods, masking, gowning, gloving, enhanced ventilation, daily temperature checks, cohorting, and others were implemented. Epidemiologists are still evaluating the relative benefit of these interventions. Some of these practices are still recommended (see the latest COVID-19 guidance from the Centers for Disease Control and Prevention [CDC] at https://www.cdc.gov/coronavirus/2019-ncov/community/schools-childcare/index.html) for COVID-19 at higher levels of community spread, and many may be part of a toolkit to use in future pandemics caused by other viruses that may spread in different ways.

Safe Food Preparation and Service

General Guidance

Most ECE programs for children are involved in food handling, even if it is only for food the children bring from home for meals and snacks. Programs should follow the general guidance to clean, separate, cook, and chill when handling any food.

- *Clean:* Wherever food is handled or prepared, clean the surfaces according to the recommended schedule in *Caring for Our Children*, Appendix W (https://nrckids.org/CFOC). (The Sample Food Service Cleaning Schedule has been reproduced in Chapter 8.) Always include tables, countertops, appliances, reusable food preparation utensils, plates, bowls, and trays in cleanup. Recommendations for selecting an appropriate sanitizer or disinfectant can also be found in *Caring for Our Children*, Appendix J (https://nrckids.org/CFOC), and Chapter 8, Selecting an Appropriate Sanitizer or Disinfectant.
- *Separate:* Be sure to separate foods that may carry disease-causing germs unless the foods are properly cooked (eg, uncooked meat, poultry, fish) from foods that are intended to be eaten without being cooked (eg, vegetables, fruits, dairy). In addition, do not allow potentially contaminated foods to touch other foods, surfaces, or utensils. Clean and sanitize all contaminated surfaces and utensils as soon as possible after use.
- *Cook:* Cook foods to recommended temperatures measured with a food thermometer placed in the center of the food. Inexpensive, easily read digital food thermometers are widely available. Foods that require cooking must be brought to safe temperatures prior to eating. Before serving, the temperature of the food should be dropped to no more than 120 °F (48.9 °C) so it does not cause burns. Foods that will not be eaten immediately should be quickly chilled and then kept below 40 °F (4.4 °C) until served. If foods are going to be kept warm prior to serving, the temperature should be maintained above 140 °F (60.0 °C) until ready to be cooled to safe eating temperature and served.
- *Chill:* Chill cooked foods quickly in shallow containers. Foods should be saved only if they have not been out of the safe food temperature zone. The unsafe food zone, between 40 °F and 140 °F (4.4 °C–60.0 °C), is the temperature range in which bacteria can grow quickly. Leftovers that have been handled or out of the safe temperature zone for longer than 2 hours must be discarded. Perishable cold foods must be held at temperatures below 40 °F (4.4 °C).

Surfaces

Food-handling areas should be separate from areas that are used for any other purpose. Make sure surfaces that are involved with food preparation (even those temporarily used for food containers) are as far away as possible from any surface involved with toileting or changing of diapers or soiled underwear. The only exception is that tables used for play may be used for eating if they are cleaned and sanitized immediately before and after being used for food preparation or eating. Even if plastic tablecloths are used to cover these tables, surfaces should still be cleaned and sanitized. Contact with the soiled table surface may make it difficult to keep a tablecloth clean and sanitary. All surfaces involved in any way with food should be cleaned and sanitized before contact with food, utensils, or containers with food in them. (See the Sanitation, Disinfection, and Maintenance section later in this chapter for the definition of the term *sanitize* and more details about how to sanitize surfaces.)

Food Handlers

Staff who handle food at any time should receive instruction from a nutrition consultant, such as a registered dietitian. Topics to discuss include selecting age-appropriate foods, food inspection and storage at the point of receipt from a supplier, food preparation, food holding and storage after preparation, and food service. Instructions should emphasize practices that prevent contamination by germs and their toxins that can cause illness. Education of food handlers should reinforce the importance of careful hand hygiene before any activity involving food.

The Child and Adult Care Food Program offers many food safety education resources for staff who work in ECE programs and schools. Search on the Food and Nutrition Service website of the US Department of Agriculture at https://www.fns.usda.gov/cacfp.

Food handlers in ECE settings may be called on to meet special challenges. For example, family-style meal service should be part of the curriculum to teach children how to make healthy food choices and serve themselves proper portions. This involves preparing food so it is easy for children to serve themselves without contaminating the food intended for others. Another example is safely handling food brought from home. Families may send food from home that requires refrigeration until served. A quick temperature check of perishable food brought from home with a digital food thermometer may be done before putting the food into the refrigerator until mealtime and can identify food that has not arrived at the facility at a safe temperature. Food should be at or below 40 °F (4.4 °C) and put immediately into the refrigerator. Food brought from home should be appropriately labeled so that it does not pose a risk to another child in the group who is food allergic. Policies and practices should be put in place to address these issues (eg, food allergies).

Staff members whose primary function is the preparation of food should not also change diapers, disposable training pants, or soiled underwear. If doing both tasks is unavoidable, to the extent possible, before doing any soiled diaper or underwear changing, the staff member involved should complete food preparation activities for the day. Staff members who do both tasks should be responsible for as few children as possible. Staff members who have symptoms of illness (eg, vomiting, diarrhea, infectious skin lesions that cannot be covered, nasal discharge that requires wiping while doing food-related activities) should not prepare food. Staff members who prepare food for children and have symptoms of vomiting and/or diarrhea or concern for norovirus should stay home for at least 48 hours after symptoms resolve to avoid spreading the virus in food. The CDC provides norovirus facts and tips for food handlers at https://www.cdc.gov/norovirus/downloads/foodhandlers.pdf.

Hand Hygiene

Hand hygiene with soap and water is preferred over any other method.

Fixtures and supplies for hand hygiene must be readily available, within the areas where children and adults can use them for the many times a day hand hygiene is necessary. Supplies should be within reach of the users where they are needed. For example, soap, paper towel dispensers, and hand lotion intended for use by children and adults should be within their reach while they are at the sink. Hand hygiene should be followed at all the times whenever germs need to be removed from the hands before and after specified activities.

Why Is Hand Hygiene Important?

Hand hygiene is a very effective means of reducing germs and infections in educational settings. Studies have shown that hands are primary carriers of infections. Lack of hand hygiene and poor hand-hygiene techniques contribute to outbreaks of diarrhea and respiratory infections among children and staff. Conversely, adherence to good hand-hygiene techniques has consistently demonstrated a reduction in disease transmission in educational settings.

Alcohol-based hand sanitizers have come into common use in most settings. For children and adults, closely supervised alcohol-based hand sanitizers are

When to Practice Hand Hygiene

All staff, volunteers, and children should follow the procedure in *Caring for Our Children*, Standard 3.2.2.1, for hand hygiene at the following times:

- On arrival for the day, after breaks, or when moving from one child care group to another
- Before and after the following:
  - Preparing food or beverages
  - Eating, handling food, or feeding a child
  - Giving medication or applying a medical ointment or cream in which a break in the skin (eg, sores, cuts, scrapes) may be encountered
  - Playing in water (including swimming) that is used by more than 1 person
- After the following:
  - Diaperinga
  - Using the toilet or helping a child use a toilet
  - Handling bodily fluid (eg, mucus, blood, vomit) from sneezing, wiping and blowing noses, mouths, or sores
  - Handling animals or cleaning up animal waste
  - Playing in sand, on wooden play sets, or outdoors
  - Cleaning or handling the garbage
  - Applying sunscreen and/or insect repellent
  - Touching face masks, if recommended during a pandemic (eg, COVID-19) or severe outbreak
- When children require assistance with brushing of their teeth, early childhood (EC) educators should wash their hands thoroughly between brushings for each child.

Situations or times that children and staff should perform hand hygiene should be posted in all food preparation, hand hygiene, diapering, and toileting areas. Also, if EC educators smoke off premises before starting work, they should wash their hands before caring for children to prevent children from receiving thirdhand smoke exposure.

a *After* diaper changing, hand hygiene must *always* be performed. Hand hygiene *before* changing diapers is required only if the staff member's hands have been contaminated since the last time the staff member practiced hand hygiene.

Adapted from *Caring for Our Children*, Standard 3.2.2.1 (https://nrckids.org/CFOC).

an acceptable alternative to handwashing with soap and running water *if there is no visible soil on the hands and soap-and-water washing is not practical.* Alcohol-based hand sanitizers do not kill all the germs that can cause illness. Hand hygiene practiced by children of any age, by any method, must be supervised to be sure it is being performed properly. Alcohol-based hand sanitizers should be kept out of reach of children.

Make Hand Hygiene Effective

Early childhood educators should avoid wearing elaborate jewelry or long or artificial nails because it can affect effective hand hygiene. Wearing hand or wrist jewelry may prevent proper handwashing. Long or artificial nails may harbor germs and dirt that are difficult to remove by handwashing alone. Instead, fingernails

should be kept short. Using hand lotion after hand hygiene to prevent chapping and cracking of skin is helpful because germs can get into chapped or cracked skin. The facility should arrange to monitor hand hygiene of adults and children with unannounced, regular direct observation.

Sinks for Routine Handwashing

A handwashing sink should be easily accessible to each indoor, infant, preschool, or school-age child care area. Handwashing sinks in infant, toddler, and preschool areas should not have barriers that limit access or visibility, such as partitions or doors. Handwashing sinks should not be used for food or formula preparation. Sinks should be located so the EC educators may visually supervise children while carrying out routine handwashing or having children wash their hands. Each sink should provide warm running water at least 60 °F (15.6 °C) and no hotter than 120 °F (48.9 °C), liquid soap, disposable paper towels or single-use cloth towels or a heated-air hand-drying device with heat guards, and whatever else is needed to facilitate frequent handwashing. Ideally, sinks should be placed at the child's height, or the child should have access to a safe step stool with slip-resistant steps for small children). The flow of water should be controlled by a foot pedal, electric eye, open, self-closing, slow-closing, or metering faucet that provides freely flowing water for at least 30 seconds without the need to reactivate the faucet. A hands-free faucet is best. Provide dispensers for liquid, foam, or other forms of soap that minimize contamination from one user to another. Provide a similar dispenser for liquid hand lotion to be used to prevent dry skin. These facility features should be adapted for programs that serve school-aged children.

Assisting Children With Handwashing

Encourage and teach children proper and safe handwashing practices. Children who are developmentally able to wash their own hands should be supervised to be sure they follow the proper procedure and wash at appropriate times. For infants who can be safely cradled in one arm, EC educators should wash the infant's hands at a sink. Washing infants' hands helps reduce the spread of infection. For children who can stand but not wash their hands by themselves, EC educators should provide assistance to complete the handwashing procedure correctly. For the child who is unable to stand and too heavy to hold at the sink to wash hands under running water, use separate disposable paper towels with the following 3-step method:

1. Wipe the child's hands with a wet paper towel on which there is a drop of liquid soap; lather for as close to 20 seconds as is feasible.

How to Wash Hands

Children and staff should wash hands using the following method, as outlined in *Caring for Our Children*, Standard 3.2.2.2:

Facility and Supplies

- Make sure a clean, disposable paper (or single-use cloth) towel or a safe warm-air hand-drying device is available.
- Have a source of clean, running water to rinse off any soil, provide moisture for a good lather, and rinse the skin thoroughly after lathering. As indicated in the Sinks for Routine Handwashing section of this chapter, the source of water should be adjusted to a safe and comfortable temperature (between 60 °F and 120 °F [15.6 °C and 48.9 °C]).
- Have liquid, foam, or other types of soap from a dispenser that does not touch the skin. Do not use antibacterial or bar soap or soap that contains fragrance.
  - Antibacterial soaps may kill some germs but leave those that are more resistant to the antibacterial ingredient in the soap, so they are not advised. Soaps that do not contain antibacterial ingredients clean hands just as well.
  - Although bar soap has not been shown to spread infectious disease, bar soaps sitting in water have been shown to be heavily contaminated with *Pseudomonas* and other bacteria. Many children do not have the dexterity to handle a bar of soap, and many adults do not take the time to rinse soil off bar soap before putting it down.
  - Fragrance may irritate or dry out the hands in some individuals with sensitive skin.

Procedure

- Moisten hands with running water. Then apply soap from the soap dispenser.
- With hands out of the water stream, rub hands together vigorously until soapy lather appears. Aim to continue lathering for 20 seconds; rub areas between fingers, around nail beds, under fingernails and jewelry, and on back of hands. ("Happy Birthday to You" and "Row, Row, Row Your Boat" each take about 10 seconds to sing. For 20 seconds, sing the song twice, or sing the A-B-C song from beginning to end once.) Keep handwashing interesting by using alternative lyrics such as these for "Row, Row, Row Your Boat": "Wash, wash, wash your hands. Play this handy game. Scrub and rub. Rub and scrub. Germs go down the drain!"
- Rinse hands under running water until free of soap and dirt. If the water does not automatically shut off, leave the water running while drying hands.
- Dry hands with a clean, disposable paper towel, single-use cloth towel, or safe warm-air hand-drying device.
- If taps did not turn off automatically, turn taps off with the disposable paper towel or single-use cloth towel used to dry the hands.
- If it is necessary to open a door to leave the handwashing area, use a disposable paper towel on the door handle.
- To dispose of towels
  - Throw disposable towel in lined trash container.
  - Place single-use cloth towel in laundry hamper.
- If desired, use hand lotion from a liquid lotion dispenser to prevent chapping.

Note: There is debate (and no studies to show) whether using a paper towel is necessary to turn off a faucet after washing hands. Using a paper towel might reduce the chance that clean hands would touch germs that were transferred to the faucet when it was turned on. Leaving the water running and using a paper towel to touch possibly soiled surfaces uses more water and paper towels. A hands-free faucet is the best solution.

Adapted from *Caring for Our Children*, Standard 3.2.2.2 (https://nrckids.org/CFOC).

2. Wipe the child's hands with clean paper towels wet with clean water until the child's hands have no dirt or soap on them.
3. Dry the child's hands with a clean paper towel.

Staff members should wash their own hands after assisting children with handwashing.

Premoistened cleansing towelettes (eg, diaper wipes, individually packaged wipes) do not effectively clean hands and may spread germs from one hand to another. However, cleaning towelettes may be used to remove visible soil before applying alcohol-based hand sanitizer when running water is not available (eg, during an outing). Another permissible use is after removing the soiled diaper, disposable training pants, or underwear and any gloves, but before putting on a clean diaper. The EC educator's hands (and, often, the child's hands too) may come in contact with feces or urine by touching soiled skin in the diaper area.

Stepping away from the diaper table to wash hands at a sink at this point is not practical. A reasonable compromise is to use a wipe to clean the EC educator's hands and then another wipe for the child's hands before putting on a clean diaper or underclothing. When cleaning a skin surface with the wipe is finished, the wipe should be put into the plastic-lined, hands-free container.

Using Alcohol-Based Hand Sanitizers

Proper use of alcohol-based hand sanitizers requires that the product contains at least 60% alcohol. The amount of product applied to the skin must be enough to keep all surfaces of the hands (not just the palms) wet with the solution for the length of time specified on the manufacturer's label (generally, 15 seconds). While alcohol-based hand sanitizers are convenient, they can be expensive, toxic if ingested, and flammable and are not effective against some germs that cause diarrhea (eg, *Giardia duodenalis*, *Cryptosporidium*, *Clostridioides difficile*, norovirus). Handwashing with soap and water is more effective to remove soil and germs.

All children who use alcohol-based hand sanitizers should have close staff supervision. If ingested in enough quantity, alcohol-based hand sanitizers can be toxic. If there is concern for ingestion of alcohol-based sanitizer, call the local Poison Control Center immediately (1-800-222-1222) and follow poisoning or ingestion protocols. To prevent contamination of the air, avoid aerosol dispensers. There is concern about the possibility that the fumes from aerosol-dispensed products might be harmful if inhaled.

Alcohol-based hand sanitizer dispensers in ECE facilities and schools must be placed according to specific guidelines for them. These guidelines establish the maximum volume each dispenser should hold, the maximum amount of alcohol-based sanitizer in a closed room (to minimize fire safety concerns), and the optimal spacing and placement of dispensers. Dispenser requirements and recommendations, adapted from *Caring for Our Children*, Standard 3.2.2.5 (https://nrckids.org/CFOC), are outlined as follows:
- The maximum individual dispenser fluid capacity
  – 0.32 gal (1.2 L) for dispensers in rooms, corridors, and areas open to corridors
  – 0.53 gal (2.0 L) for dispensers in suites of rooms
- Wall-mounted dispensers should be separated from each other by horizontal spacing of not less than 48 inches (1,220 mm).
- Wall-mounted dispensers should not be installed above or adjacent to ignition sources, such as electrical outlets.
- Wall-mounted dispensers installed directly over carpeted floors should be permitted only in ECE facilities protected by automatic sprinklers.

Remember that alcohol-based hand sanitizer products do not substitute for handwashing if there is visible soil on the hands. Any visible soil needs to be removed with soap and water. Although alternative hand sanitizers that do not contain alcohol are available, research is lacking to show these products are as effective as those that contain the required amount of alcohol. Hand sanitizers should contain at least 60% alcohol so that they are effective in killing germs. If the facility uses hand sanitizers, educators should
- Be sure hand hygiene using alcohol-based hand sanitizers conforms to the manufacturer's instructions and the location of the dispensers does not put people at risk of inhaling fumes.

- Apply the required volume of the product to the palm of one hand and rub both hands together; cover all surfaces of the hands and fingers until the hands are dry. The required volume should keep hand surfaces wet for the time indicated by the manufacturer, usually 15 seconds or longer.
- Check the dispenser systems for hand-hygiene products on a regular schedule to be sure they deliver the required volume of the product and do not clog or malfunction.
- Store supplies of alcohol-based hand rubs in cabinets or areas approved for flammable materials. *Caring for Our Children*, Standard 5.5.0.5 (https://nrckids.org/CFOC), requires storage of hand sanitizers in volume with other flammable materials in a separate building, in a locked area, away from high temperatures and ignition sources, and where they are inaccessible to children.

Respiratory Etiquette

When children or EC educators cough or sneeze, they should try to prevent the spread of droplets that might contain germs, which can land on other people or surfaces and spread infection. Learning how to reduce droplet spread is called *respiratory etiquette*. Early childhood educators and children should be taught to cover their mouths and noses with a tissue when they cough or sneeze. Staff members and children should also be taught to cough or sneeze into their inner elbow/upper sleeve and to avoid covering the nose or mouth with bare hands. Hand hygiene, as specified in *Caring for Our Children*, Standards 3.2.2.1 and 3.2.2.2, should follow a cough or sneeze that could result in the spread of respiratory droplets. At times during the COVID-19 pandemic, face masks were universally recommended for all people 2 years and older because they have been shown to reduce the transmission of COVID-19 illness in ECE programs and schools. Face masks, worn properly, still have a role during periods of high levels of COVID-19 community transmission (https://www.cdc.gov/coronavirus/2019-ncov/community/schools-childcare/k-12-childcare-guidance.html) and may have a role in reducing disease transmission in future pandemics or severe outbreaks of seasonal flu and other respiratory viruses. They may allow an earlier return to care after an infection and possibly avoid the need to quarantine an entire classroom after an exposure. Cloth masks that are obviously wet or soiled should be replaced and washed. Cloth masks should be washed at least once daily.

Changing Diapers, Soiled Disposable Training Pants, and Soiled Underwear

If EC educators are counted in the child to staff ratio while changing children, they must provide simultaneous supervision of the other children in the group. Position the changing table to allow the staff member doing the change to maintain sight and sound supervision of the other children. If possible, position the changing table to allow the staff person who is doing the changing to be seen by other adults during the diapering activity to avoid any presumption of inappropriate care during the change, including while cleaning the genital area during the diapering procedure.

There should be at least one changing area per infant, toddler, and preschool-age group to allow time for changing and performing sanitary procedures without spreading infectious diseases from group to group. When EC educators from different groups use the same changing surface and sinks, disease spreads easily from one group to another. Breaks in hygiene and sanitation can potentially involve more children if diapering/changing areas and equipment are shared. Changing tables should not be placed or shared between classrooms.

Early childhood educators should arrange the changing area to give the child visual stimulation. This avoids having to distract the child with objects that will add to the burden of cleaning and sanitation after the change. For example, mirrors on the wall or ceiling, mobiles, and laminated pictures on the walls or ceiling are interesting to children. They support verbal interaction between the EC educator and the child while the changing is done and distract the child, who might otherwise move around during the changing activity, while also fostering language and responsive relationships. Children who can help with the changing task can hold the bottom of their shirt or dress away from the area being cleaned, which serves to keep the child's hands away from the contaminated area. If the child holds a toy or similar object, that object must be considered contaminated and taken from the child to be cleaned and sanitized when the soiled diaper or clothing has been removed.

All staff members who will change children's diapers, soiled disposable training pants, or soiled underwear should undergo training and periodic assessment of diapering practices and proper sanitizing practices. Use the procedure as part of staff evaluation of EC educators who change children.

Components of a Changing Area and Table

As recommended in *Caring for Our Children*, Standards 3.2.1.4 and 5.4.2.5, areas used for changing diapers or other clothing soiled by urine or feces should

- Be designed to minimize contamination of surfaces during and as a result of the changing procedure.
- Be separated as much as possible from food preparation or service areas, entryways and activity areas, refrigerators, or areas where notes and logs are kept. Having these activities near changing surfaces might tempt someone to use the changing surface as a temporary place to put down articles unrelated to diapering and contaminate them.
- Contain surfaces made of moisture-proof, nonabsorbent, smooth materials without cracks or crevices that trap soil. The materials must not deteriorate when repeatedly cleaned and disinfected.
- Provide a sturdy changing surface at a convenient height (between 28 and 32 inches high) for use by EC educators. Surfaces should be equipped with railings or barriers that extend at least 6 inches above the changing surface to reduce the risk of the child rolling off.
- Changing surfaces should not have diaper supply containers, safety straps, or harnesses because they pose a challenge to cleaning and disinfecting after diaper changing and the straps and harnesses do not ensure safety of the child. Early childhood educators should have a hand on the child who is on the changing surface at all times to prevent falls and limit contamination of the environment where the changing is being done. If an emergency arises during the change, EC educators should bring any child on an elevated surface to the floor or take the child with them.
- Include a place for storing the containers with the changing supplies off but near the changing surface, so the supplies for a single change can be gathered easily and brought to the table without contaminating bulk supplies or their containers during the change. Bulk supplies should be stored so there are no barriers, such as cabinet doors, that would have to be handled to get to the supplies if an extra diaper or other supply is unexpectedly needed during the change.
- Be located within arm's reach (3 feet) from a sink. If the sink will be used for other purposes, it must be disinfected immediately after diaper changing is finished and before it is used for other purposes.
- Have tightly covered, hands-free receptacles within arm's reach for disposal of contaminated materials during the diaper change with the least risk of environmental contamination. Be sure the plastic-lined, lidded, hands-free container for disposable items is

big enough and in good working order so nobody needs to use hands to open it or push trash into it.

- Have the changing procedures posted in graphics that are large and clear enough to remind staff members and families who use the changing area to follow the steps of the procedure correctly. See Chapter 8 for a 3-page, reproducible Diapering Poster that can be taped together, laminated, and then hung over or next to a changing surface. The poster shows images and key words to prompt performance of the correct steps.

Sinks in Changing Areas

- Sinks in changing areas should be within arm's reach of EC educators so handwashing can be done before any other surfaces are touched and contaminated.
- At least 1 sink should be available for every 2 changing tables.
- Sinks and changing tables for infant and toddler groups should be assigned to one group of children.
- Sinks should meet the requirements for handwashing detailed in the How to Wash Hands box earlier in this chapter.
- Sinks should not be used for bathing or removing smeared fecal material.
- Drinking utensils and food should not be washed in sinks in changing areas.

Changing Procedure

The procedure for changing diapers, soiled disposable training pants, or soiled underwear is designed to reduce contamination of changing surfaces with other surfaces, such as hands, furnishings, and floors. Having the child lie down on a changing table reduces the likelihood of contamination of the environment and injury to the child and EC educator while making it easier to clean skin creases.

Staff members should use the following changing procedures for changing diapers and for changing soiled disposable training pants or soiled underwear as detailed in *Caring for Our Children*, Standard 3.2.1.4, for diaper changing and in Standard 3.2.1.5 for children's soiled underwear pull-ups and clothing (https://nrckids.org/CFOC). The diaper-changing procedure should be posted in the changing area and should be followed for all diaper changes and should also be part of the evaluation used for EC educators who change diapers. Signage should be simple and in multiple languages if EC educators who speak multiple languages are involved in diapering. All employees responsible for changing diapers or pull-ups should undergo training and periodic assessment of diaper-

ing practices. Remind EC educators that they should never leave a child unattended on a table or countertop, even for an instant. If an emergency arises, EC educators should bring any child on an elevated surface to the floor or take the child with them.

Step 1: Get organized.

Before bringing the child to the diaper-changing area, perform hand hygiene if hands have touched surfaces contaminated by body fluids, and then gather and bring the following supplies to the diaper-changing area:

- Nonabsorbent paper liner large enough to cover the changing surface from the child's shoulders to beyond the child's feet.
- Unused diaper, clean clothes (if you need them).
- Wipes, dampened cloths, or wet paper towels for cleaning the child's genitalia and buttocks.
- A plastic bag for any soiled clothes or cloth diapers.
- Disposable gloves, if you plan to use them. Put gloves on before handling soiled clothing or diapers and remove them before handling clean diapers and clothing.
- A thick application of any diaper cream (eg, zinc oxide ointment), when appropriate, removed from the container to a piece of disposable material such as facial or toilet tissue.

Step 2: Carry the child to the changing table, keeping soiled clothing away from you and away from any surfaces you cannot easily clean and sanitize after the change.

- Always keep a hand on the child.
- If the child's feet cannot be kept out of the diaper or from contact with soiled skin during the changing process, remove the child's shoes and socks so the child does not contaminate these surfaces with stool or urine.

Step 3: Clean the child's diaper area.

- Place the child on the diaper-changing surface and unfasten the diaper but leave the soiled diaper under the child.
- If safety pins are used, close each pin immediately once it is removed and keep pins out of the child's reach. (Never hold pins in your mouth.)
- Lift the child's legs as needed to use disposable wipes, a dampened cloth, or a wet paper towel to clean the skin on the child's genitalia and buttocks and prevent recontamination from a soiled diaper. Remove stool and urine from front to back and use a fresh wipe, dampened cloth, or wet paper towel each time you swipe. Put soiled wipes or paper towels into the soiled diaper or directly into a plastic-lined,

hands-free covered can. Reusable cloths should be stored in a washable, plastic-lined, tightly covered receptacle (within arm's reach of diaper-changing tables) until they can be laundered. The cover should not require touching with contaminated hands or objects.

Step 4: Remove the soiled diaper and clothing without contaminating any surface not already in contact with stool or urine. Do not dispose of any materials involved in diapering in the toilet.

- Fold the soiled surface of the diaper (or underwear) inward.
- Put soiled disposable diapers in a covered, plastic-lined, hands-free covered can. If a reusable cloth diaper or underwear was used, put it and its contents (without emptying or rinsing them) in a plastic bag or into a plastic-lined, hands-free covered can to give to parents/guardians or the laundry service.
- Check for spills under the child. If spills occur, use the corner of the liner paper to fold the paper that extends under the child's feet over the soiled area, so a fresh, unsoiled paper surface is now under the child's buttocks.
- If gloves were used, remove them using the proper technique (see *Caring for Our Children*, Appendix D [https://nrckids.org/CFOC]) and put them into a plastic-lined, hands-free covered can.
- Whether or not gloves were used, use a fresh wipe to wipe the hands of the EC educator and another fresh wipe to wipe the child's hands. Put the wipes into the plastic-lined, hands-free covered can.

> This is the end of the soiled portion of the changing procedure. Gloves should be off, hands should be wiped, and all soiled articles should be in the hands-free receptacle or bagged to be laundered at home.

Step 5: Put a clean diaper on the child and dress the child.

- Slide a fresh diaper under the child.
- Use a facial or toilet tissue or wear a clean, disposable glove to apply any necessary diaper creams, discarding the tissue or glove in a covered, plastic-lined, hands-free covered can.
- Note and plan to report any skin problems such as redness, cracks, or bleeding.
- Fasten the diaper; if pins are used, place your hand between the child and the diaper when inserting the pins.

Step 6: Wash the child's hands and return the child to a supervised area.

- Use soap and warm water, between 60 °F (15.6 °C) and 120 °F (48.9 °C), at a sink to wash the child's hands, if you can.

Step 7: Clean and disinfect the diaper-changing surface.

- Dispose of the disposable paper liner used on the diaper-changing surface in a plastic-lined, hands-free covered can.
- If clothing was soiled, securely tie the plastic bag used to store the clothing and send home.
- Remove any visible soil from the changing surface with a disposable paper towel saturated with water and detergent; rinse.
- Wet the entire changing surface with a disinfectant that is appropriate for the surface material you are treating. Follow the manufacturer's instructions for use.
- Put away the disinfectant. Some types of disinfectants require rinsing the change table surface with fresh water afterward.

Step 8: Perform hand hygiene according to the procedure in Caring for Our Children, Standard 3.2.2.2 (https://nrckids.org/CFOC), and record the diaper change in the child's daily log.

- In the daily log, record what was in the diaper and any problems (eg, loose stool, unusual odor, blood in the stool, skin irritation), and report as necessary.

Cleaning and Disinfecting the Changing Area

Use a fragrance-free product that is US Environmental Protection Agency (EPA) registered as a sanitizing or disinfecting solution. If other products are used for sanitizing or disinfecting, they should also be fragrance-free and EPA registered. All cleaning, sanitizing, and disinfecting solutions should be stored to be accessible to the EC educator but out of reach of any child. Refer to *Caring for Our Children*, Appendix J: Selection and Use of a Cleaning, Sanitizing, or Disinfecting Product and Appendix K: Routine Schedule for Cleaning, Sanitizing, and Disinfecting (https://nrckids.org/CFOC), and the corresponding sections in Chapter 8.

Preventive Oral Health

Good Dental Habits

Tooth decay is the most common preventable chronic disease or condition during childhood. By 2 years of age, 10% of children already have some tooth decay. Half of children by 5 years of age have at least 1 cavity. Decay of "baby teeth" can cause problems with a child's permanent teeth and lifelong oral health problems.

Dental decay is an infectious disease caused by bacteria that adults transfer to a child's mouth. These transfers occur when a child puts a hand into the adult's mouth and then, without handwashing, puts the hand and the germs it carries into the child's own mouth. Adults who kiss children on the lips, share spoons, or lick a dropped pacifier also transfer their decay-causing bacteria to the child.

The next step in tooth decay occurs when sugar in juice and high-sugar foods feeds the bacteria on the teeth. The bacteria use the sugar to make acid that damages the surface of the teeth. When children walk around carrying and drinking from sippy cups containing any beverage with sugar (including milk) for hours at a time, the saliva never has time to neutralize the acid produced by the bacteria feeding on the sugar.

Infants should not have juice or sticky foods because of their sugar content. For children between 1 and 3 years of age, juice without added sugar should be limited to no more than 4 oz per day. For children between 4 and 6 years of age, juice should be limited to 4 to 6 oz per day. Whole fruit should be served instead of other kinds of sweet desserts most of the time. Prevention of tooth decay focuses on avoiding sugar intake that feeds the bacteria in the mouth and on strengthening the surface of the teeth.

The first dental visit should occur within 6 months after the first tooth comes through the gum or by 12 months of age. The dental visit is an ideal time for planning when and how to do toothbrushing and for the first application of fluoride varnish. Fluoride varnish is a dental treatment that is applied to the tops and sides of the teeth to make them stronger and more resistant to cavities and may be done at the health supervision visits with the pediatric health professional. Children's teeth should be brushed at least twice a day with the right amount of fluoride toothpaste (see the following section), aiming to brush all surfaces. Most children are unable to do a good job of toothbrushing without adult supervision until they are 7 or 8 years old. It doesn't matter whether children brush sideways or up and down, as long as they brush all tooth surfaces.

Toothbrushing as Part of the Curriculum

Toothbrushing at least once a day should be part of the curriculum for toddlers and preschool-aged children. Children do not need to stand at a sink to brush their teeth. After a meal or snack, they can do toothbrushing as a group at the table where they ate.

- Give each child a small paper cup, a paper towel, and a labeled, soft-bristled, child-sized toothbrush.
- Put a small dab of fluoride toothpaste on the inside rim of each cup and have children use their toothbrushes to pick up the dabs of toothpaste. Use a smear of toothpaste no bigger than a grain of rice for children younger than 3 years and a pea-sized amount for those older than 3 years. Using the smear of toothpaste that is no bigger than a grain of rice is important to prevent dental caries (cavities) for infants and toddlers. Even if swallowed, this small amount of fluoride is not harmful.
- The EC educator can brush his or her teeth with the children or assist a different child each day with brushing correctly. Brush together for 2 minutes, using a timer or a song that lasts for about 2 minutes. Remind children to brush the insides, outsides, and chewing surface of their teeth.
- When 2 minutes are up, have the children spit any extra toothpaste into their cups or swallow what is left, then throw the small cups and paper towels away.
- Collect the toothbrushes without allowing the bristles of one brush to touch another child's toothbrush. Rinse and store the toothbrushes in cleanable cups or toothbrush racks to air-dry with their bristles up and not touching other brushes.
- Toothbrushes should be replaced every 3 to 4 months.

For more information about oral health, see the Dental Caries (Early Childhood Caries, Tooth Decay, or Cavities) Quick Reference Sheet in Chapter 6. Also visit HealthyChildren.org, the American Academy of Pediatrics website for parents, at https://www.healthychildren.org/english/healthy-living/oral-health/pages/default.aspx. Another good source is the American Dental Association website specifically related to dental health of children, www.mouthhealthy.org/en/babies-and-kids.

Standard Precautions

For spills of blood or body fluids, including urine, feces, saliva, vomit, nasal or eye discharge, and wound discharges, follow the specific guidelines for performance of Standard Precautions provided in *Caring for Our Children*, Standard 3.2.3.4 (https://nrckids.org/CFOC). The US Occupational Safety and Health Administration (OSHA) requires that employers provide training about use of Standard Precautions for all staff

Procedures for Standard Precautions

1. Surfaces that may come in contact with potentially infectious body fluids must be disposable or of a material that can be disinfected. Follow the manufacturer's instruction for preparation and use of disinfectant.
2. Staff members should use barriers and techniques that
   a. Minimize potential contact of mucous membranes or openings in skin to blood or other potentially infectious body fluids and tissue discharges.
   b. Reduce the spread of infectious material within the early childhood education facility. Such techniques include avoiding touching potentially contaminated surfaces unless those surfaces have been disinfected. (Using disposable gloves during cleanup of spills is required when anticipating contact with blood or blood-containing body fluids; otherwise, using disposable gloves is optional.)
3. When spills of body fluids, urine, feces, blood, saliva, nasal discharge, eye discharge, or injury or tissue discharge occur, these spills should be cleaned up immediately and further managed as follows:
   a. For spills of saliva, vomit, urine, and feces, all floors, walls, bathrooms, tabletops, toys, furnishings and play equipment, kitchen countertops, and diaper-changing tables should be cleaned and disinfected. The procedure is
      i. Remove any visible soil from the surface with a disposable paper towel saturated with water and detergent and then rinse with fresh, clean water.
      ii. Wet the entire changing surface with a disinfectant that is appropriate for the surface material being treated. Follow the manufacturer's instructions for use.
      iii. Put away the disinfectant where it is inaccessible to children. Most of these products have some level of toxicity. Many disinfectants may require rinsing the changing table surface with fresh water afterward.
   b. For spills of blood or other potentially infectious body fluids, including injury and tissue discharges, all surfaces in the area should be cleaned and disinfected as in item a. Care should be taken and eye protection used to avoid splashing any contaminated materials onto any mucous membrane (eg, eyes, nose, mouth).
   c. Blood-contaminated material and all soiled diapers, disposable training pants, or underwear should be disposed of in a plastic bag with a secure tie.
   d. Floors, rugs, and carpeting that have been contaminated by body fluids should be cleaned by blotting to remove the fluid as quickly as possible and then disinfected by spot-cleaning with a detergent-disinfectant. Additional cleaning by shampooing or steam cleaning the contaminated surface may be necessary. Educators should consult with local health departments or the Centers for Disease Control and Prevention for additional guidance on cleaning contaminated floors, rugs, and carpeting.
   e. If blood or body fluids come into contact with a mucous membrane (eg, eyes, nose, mouth), use the following procedure: Flush the exposed area thoroughly with water. The goal of washing or flushing is to reduce the number of germs to which an exposed individual has contact. The optimal length of time for washing or flushing an exposed area is not known. Standard practice for managing mucous membrane exposures to chemically toxic substances is to flush the affected area for at least 15 to 20 minutes. In the absence of data to support the effectiveness of shorter periods of flushing, it seems prudent to use the same 15- to 20-minute standard following exposure to blood-borne pathogens.

who might, in the course of their work, come in contact with blood. Anyone who might be expected to provide first aid, even for minor injuries, is included.

For practical guidelines for cleaning up spills of body fluids, see Cleaning Up Body Fluids in Chapter 8 and *Caring for Our Children*, Standard 3.2.3.4. Human (breast) milk is the only body fluid that does not require use of Standard Precautions. Using disposable gloves during cleanup of spills is required if there might be contact with blood or blood-containing body fluids; otherwise, using disposable gloves is often preferred but is optional. Unlike Standard Precautions in hospital settings, gowns and masks are not required when handling stool or vomitus in ECE facilities and schools. Moisture-resistant disposable diaper-table paper, disposable gloves, and eye protection are examples of barriers that could be used to prevent contact with body fluids. See Chapter 8 for a Gloving handout.

Educators should be taught about Standard Precautions to prevent transmission of blood-borne pathogens before beginning to work in an ECE facility and at least annually thereafter. This education must comply with US OSHA requirements.

Sanitation, Disinfection, and Maintenance

Routine housekeeping procedures can help reduce the spread of disease-causing germs in ECE and school settings. Use as few different products as possible. Minimizing the number of products will help staff members use them properly. The US OSHA requires that employers provide their workers with the Safety Data Sheet for any products employees are expected to use. Safety Data Sheets identify chemical type, intended use, and risks associated with using the chemical. *Caring for Our Children*, Appendix J and Chapter 8, Selecting an Appropriate Sanitizer or Disinfectant, contain detailed information about proper product selection, and *Caring for Our Children*, Appendix K and Chapter 8, Routine Schedule for Cleaning, Sanitizing, and Disinfecting, contain information about the suggested schedule of cleaning, sanitizing and disinfecting different surfaces (https://nrckids.org/CFOC).

While definitions and uses of *clean, sanitize,* and *disinfect* vary from one source to another, this book uses the definitions and notes for the terms as found in *Caring for Our Children*, Standard 3.3.0.1 (https://nrckids.org/CFOC) (Table 2.1).

Green Seal and ECOLOGO are nonprofit organizations that research and certify products that are biodegradable and that they consider to be environmentally friendly. Visit www.greenseal.org,

Table 2.1. Definitions of *Clean, Sanitize,* and *Disinfect*

Task	Purpose
Clean	To remove dirt and debris by scrubbing and washing with a detergent solution and rinsing with water. The friction of cleaning removes most germs and exposes any remaining germs to the effects of a sanitizer or disinfectant used later.
Sanitize[a]	To reduce germs on inanimate surfaces to levels considered safe by public health codes or regulations.
Disinfect[a]	To destroy or inactivate most germs on any inanimate object, but not bacterial spores.

Note: The term *germs* refers to bacteria, viruses, fungi, and molds that may cause infectious diseases. Bacterial spores are dormant bacteria that have formed a protective shell, enabling them to survive extreme conditions for years. The spores reactivate after entry into a host (eg, a person), where conditions are favorable for them to live and reproduce.

Only US Environmental Protection Agency (EPA)-registered products that have an EPA registration number on the label can make public health claims that can be relied on for reducing or destroying germs. The EPA registration label will also describe the product as a *cleaner, sanitizer,* or *disinfectant.* In addition, some manufacturers of *cleaning* products have developed "green cleaning products." As new environmentally friendly cleaning products appear in the market, check to see if they are third-party certified by Green Seal (http://www.greenseal.org), UL/ECOLOGO (https://www.ul.com/services/ecologo-certification), and/or EPA Safer Choice (http://www.epa.gov/saferchoice). Use fragrance-free bleach that is EPA-registered as a sanitizing or disinfecting solution. If other products are used for sanitizing or disinfecting, they should also be fragrance-free and EPA-registered. All products must be used according to manufacturer's instructions. See *Caring for Our Children*, Appendix J: Selection and Use of a Cleaning, Sanitizing, or Disinfecting Product (https://nrckids.org/CFOC), and Chapter 8, Selecting an Appropriate Sanitizer or Disinfectant, for updated information on green cleaning.

[a] See *Caring for Our Children*, Appendix K (https://nrckids.org/CFOC), and Chapter 8, Routine Schedule for Cleaning, Sanitizing, and Disinfecting, for guidance on use of sanitizers versus disinfectants.

https://www.ul.com/resources/ecologo-certification-program, and the EPA Safer Choice website, https://www.epa.gov/saferchoice, to look for environmentally safer products to use. Avoid homemade recipes for sanitizing and disinfecting, such as vinegar and baking soda, as they have not been tested for effectiveness in settings comparable to ECE programs.

Cleaning

Look for a cleaning product that is EPA labeled as a detergent. The instruction on the product label should indicate that it is safe and effective for cleaning. Most detergent labels say to rinse the detergent off with water. Be sure to do the rinse step before applying any other chemical. Sanitizers and disinfectants work on visibly clean surfaces. They may be applied without a pre-cleaning step if the surface is visibly clean. If in doubt about whether a surface needs the pre-cleaning step, wipe the surface with a clean paper towel and rinse the paper towel in cold rinse water. If the surface is clean, no residue will appear in the rinse water.

Sanitizers and Disinfectants

Many products specify contact with surfaces for a specific amount of time. Be sure to follow the manufacturer's instructions for contact time with a disinfectant or a sanitizer. Unless the product label specifies otherwise, apply a sanitizer or disinfectant by pouring or spraying the product onto the object's surface rather than dipping a rag, paper towel, mop, or object itself into the solution. Dipping into a solution adds germs to the solution, making the solution less effective than when it was freshly made. Pouring or spraying the solution onto the surfaces avoids this problem. Many solutions are applied using a spray dispenser that should be adjusted so that the spray wets the surface but does not make fine mist that disperses the solution into the air that people breathe.

Level of Cleaning, Sanitizing, or Disinfecting

Whether an area needs to be cleaned, sanitized, or disinfected depends on what the area is used for and the frequency it may be touched, as described in *Caring for Our Children*, Appendix K, and Chapter 8, Routine Schedule for Cleaning, Sanitizing, and Disinfecting. In food preparation and meal service areas, surfaces need to cleaned and sanitized. This applies to food preparation surfaces and equipment, eating utensils and dishes, bottle-feeding equipment, mixed-use tables, and high chair trays. Child care and classroom areas generally need only cleaning (pacifiers, mouthed toys, washable cloth toys, classroom toys, play activity centers, counters and shelves, mixed-use tables for activities, washable dress-up clothes, floors and carpets, bedding and pillows, and cribs/cots/mats) except for drinking fountains, water tables and water equipment, and animal areas (feeders, fish tanks or animal cages), which require disinfecting after cleaning. High touch areas like doorknobs, handles, light switches, shared computer keyboards and phones need only cleaning except in the case of an outbreak where sanitizing or disinfecting may be advised by local health authorities. Cleaning and disinfecting is required for toileting/diapering areas (changing tables, diaper pails, toilets, sinks and faucets, countertops, and floors). Follow the instructions on the product label for the acceptable places to use and how to use the product. Some sanitizers can be used as disinfectants but have different instructions for use on the label.

Many different types of sanitizing and disinfecting solutions are available. Choose only those that are registered by the EPA. These will have an EPA registration number on their label. The EPA calls all such products "pesticides." Federal regulations require that manufacturers of EPA-registered products use the 3-signal word system to warn consumers about potential toxicity. The most toxic products are labeled with the word "Danger," followed in sequence for those of lesser toxicity labeled with the word "Warning"; those even less toxic are labeled with the signal word "Caution." Nontoxic EPA-registered products do not need to have any signal word on their label. Products that are a potential poisoning risk for children must bear the words, "Keep out of the reach of children," in addition to the signal word. In general, except in an outbreak situation, any EPA-registered sanitizer or disinfectant product that has a "Caution" label is suitable for use in ECE facilities and schools. Be certain to look for and be vigilant about storing or using any product with a label that says, "Keep out of the reach of children." For example, shaving cream that many programs use for children to finger paint on a table is labeled, "Keep out of the reach of children," and should not be used in ECE programs. Products with such a label that are stored for adults to use them should be put where they are inaccessible to children.

Products that are registered with the EPA as *detergent-disinfectant* or *hospital-grade* germicides may be used for sanitizing also. Some products are specifically listed as effective against different types of infectious agents. Disinfecting strength is usually greater for the same chemicals than the strength that is used for sanitizing. Surfaces that must be disinfected in ECE facilities include those used for diaper changing, doorknobs and cabinet handles, drinking fountains, handwashing sinks and faucets, toilet and diapering area countertops, toilets, diaper pails, floors in toilet and diapering areas, and any surface that has been contaminated by body fluids such as blood, feces, or secretions from the nose or sores.

All EPA-registered sanitizing and disinfecting solutions must be used according to the directions on the label of the product. The dwell time is the amount of time a solution must be in contact with a visibly clean surface to kill the germs on that surface. Dwell times indicated on the product label must be followed. For some products, the dwell times are too long to make the use of the product feasible in ECE settings. Be cautious about using industrial products advertised as "having germicidal action" or "killing germs." They may not have the same effectiveness as EPA-approved, hospital-grade germicides or a properly made disinfectant or sanitizing solution.

Frequency of Cleaning, Sanitizing, and Disinfecting

The baseline routine frequency of cleaning, sanitizing, and disinfecting (see Routine Schedule for Cleaning, Sanitizing, and Disinfecting in Chapter 8 and *Caring for Our Children*, Appendix K) should be followed every day. Staff members should be more vigilant about practicing the routines when
* There are outbreaks of illness in a particular classroom or the whole facility or in the community (eg, influenza, which usually produces outbreaks every winter).
* There is known contamination of surfaces by contact with body fluids like mucus, fecal material, wound or eye discharge, or blood.
* There is visible soil.
* There are recommendations by the health department or the CDC about the need to be more vigilant to control certain infectious diseases. Health officials may recommend a more frequent cleaning schedule than usual or products to use in certain areas to address a specific problem.

General Guidelines for Surfaces and Equipment

* Carpets, porous fabrics, other surfaces that trap soil, and potentially contaminated materials should not be used in toilet rooms, changing areas, and food preparation areas.
* Walls, ceilings, floors, furnishings, equipment, and other surfaces should be smooth and nonporous wherever possible. All surfaces should be maintained in good repair and kept clean.
* Because children will touch any reachable surface (including floors), assume all surfaces can spread germs that cause infectious diseases and should be routinely cleaned.
* Respiratory tract secretions (eg, nasal discharge, drool, eye secretions) may contaminate surfaces. These secretions may contain viruses that remain infectious for hours to days, making it possible to

acquire an infection by touching contaminated surfaces. Children usually have respiratory tract secretions on their hands and may have viruses in their respiratory tract before and after they seem sick. That is why any surface that might have been in contact with a child's hands must be cleaned and sanitized or disinfected.

- All surfaces, furnishings, and equipment that are not in good repair or have been contaminated by body fluids should not be used until repaired, cleaned, and, if needed, sanitized or disinfected effectively. Have a way to take out of service any surfaces or furnishings that cannot be cleaned or repaired right away (eg, ripped or cracked mattress). For example, use a plastic bin labeled "Dirty—to be washed" for soiled toys and yellow plastic tape or crepe paper streamers to rope off areas that must be temporarily put out of use.
- Adhere to appropriate hand and personal hygiene for children and staff. (See Hand Hygiene section earlier in this chapter.)
- Try to use toys that can be washed safely in a dishwasher or washing machine. Toys that are only surface washable must have surfaces that can be thoroughly cleaned. If they were mouthed, they must be able to be sanitized.
- Make sure all staff members and volunteers follow the routine cleaning, sanitizing, and disinfecting schedule to keep surfaces from spreading disease within the group. Children can help with cleaning under supervision and in situations in which their participation in this life skill learning doesn't lead to increased risk to them.
- Use caution when shampooing rugs used by children who are crawling. Cleaning with potentially hazardous chemicals should be scheduled to minimize exposure to children.

Cleaning Equipment

- Single-use disposable or utility gloves and equipment designated for cleaning and disinfecting toilets should be used. Disposable gloves are commonly made of latex or vinyl. If individuals sensitive to latex are present in the facility, use only vinyl disposable gloves. After each use, discard disposable gloves. If reusable utility gloves are used, wash them with soapy water, and then let them air-dry.
- Disposable towels are better than reusable rags for cleaning. After use, disposable towels should be placed in a plastic-lined container until removed to outside garbage. Avoid reusable rags or sponges because they hold material that allows germs to grow in them, which can be spread on future use. If reusable rags or microfiber cloths are used, place

them in a closed, foot-operated receptacle after each use. Keep them there until they can be laundered and sanitized. Reusable rags should be laundered and sanitized at the end of the same day they were used.

- Mops should be assumed to be contaminated because they are used to remove contamination from floors and other soiled surfaces. Be sure they are cleaned and sanitized after each use and by the end of the same day they were used.

Waste Receptacles

Waste receptacles in toilet rooms should be kept clean, lined with plastic bags, and in good repair, and emptied daily. Those receptacles that receive materials with body fluids should be of the hands-free type, such as a foot-operated or electric-eye receptacle. All other waste receptacles should be kept clean and emptied daily.

Toys

- Toys can spread disease. Toys become contaminated when children touch them or put them into their mouths. If other children play with or mouth the same toy, those children can get the germs left by others on their hands and mucous membranes.
- Toys that cannot be washed and, if mouthed, cannot be sanitized should not be used.
- A dishwasher that can sanitize dishes can be used to clean and sanitize hard-surfaced toys.
- Mouthed toys or toys contaminated by body secretions or excretions should be removed from the play area until they are washed with water and detergent, rinsed, sanitized, and air-dried or washed in a mechanical dishwasher that meets local health codes. Small, hard-surfaced toys can be precleaned by soaking them in a dish pan that contains soapy water, kept in the child care area that is labeled "Soiled toys." Soaking until they can be properly cleaned will help remove some of the soil. Alternately, the soiled toys can be placed in a dry labeled container and then brought to a toy-cleaning area later in the day.
- Machine-washable cloth toys should be used only by one child until these toys are laundered.
- Indoor toys should not be shared between groups of infants or toddlers unless they are washed and sanitized before being moved from one group to another.
- Have more than one set of toys on hand so that one set can be used while the other is cleaned. For toys that are difficult to clean, they may be rotated out of use for a week, which is long enough for viruses on the surface to die.

Mouthed Objects

- Thermometers, teething toys, and similar objects should be cleaned, and reusable parts should be sanitized between uses.
- Pacifiers should be cleaned and not shared. Pacifiers should never be placed in an EC educator's mouth.

Bedding, Personal Clothing, and Cribs

- Sleep equipment and bedding should be used only by one child and washed before use by another child. Equipment used by one child should be stored separately from that used by others. Any bedding (eg, sheets, pillows, blankets, sleeping bags) should be removed before individual sleep equipment, such as cots or mats, is stored in a stack. All bedding should be washable. Bedding that touches the child's skin should be laundered weekly.
- Select, space, and maintain equipment for children to sleep (eg, cribs, cots, mats) so that there are at least 3 feet between children. Use and maintenance should be as required by *Caring for Our Children*, Standard 5.4.5.1 (https://nrckids.org/CFOC). Alternating children head to toe increases the spacing, thereby increasing the chance that large coughed-out or sneezed droplets will fall to the floor rather than onto another child's sleeping space.
- Cribs should meet the current standards for safety of the US Consumer Product Safety Commission. The crib structure and mattress should have a nonporous, easy-to-wipe surface. Nothing should be in the crib other than the child positioned on their back and a tightly fitted sheet over a firm and flat sleep surface. (See https://safetosleep.nichd.nih.gov/safesleepbasics/risk/reduce.)
- If possible, keep bedding material, jackets with hoods, and hats used by different children separate, so they do not touch. Lice infestation and ringworm are common problems in ECE and school settings. Although no evidence exists to show that lice are transmitted except by head-to-head contact, some skin diseases such as ringworm have been shown to spread if bedding materials, jackets with hoods, and hats used by various children are stored so they touch each other.

Toilets and Non-flushing Toilets (Potty Chairs)

- Equip toilets with toilet-paper dispensers within reach of the toilet users. The toilets should be sized for the children who use them or have steps and modified toilet seats to make them appropriate for the size of the children.

- Remove anything that interferes with visual supervision by an EC educator to ensure children follow proper toileting behaviors. Privacy for toileting should not be offered until most of the children in the group become capable of independent and proper toileting procedures, generally between 5 and 6 years of age. Younger children who request privacy and have well-established appropriate toileting behaviors may be allowed to use separate, private toileting facilities (see *Caring for Our Children*, Standard 5.4.1.2 [https://nrckids.org/CFOC]).
- Non-flushing toilet (potty chair) use is not recommended and should be strongly discouraged. Flushable child-size toilets with fitted seats are preferable. If non-flushing toilets (potty chairs) are used, they should be made with a surface that is easily cleaned and sanitized. Their use should be limited to a bathroom area where they are used over a surface that will not be damaged by moisture. Each potty chair should be out of reach of toilets or other potty chairs. Urine and feces in a potty chair should be emptied into a toilet immediately after each use, and promptly thereafter the contaminated surfaces of the potty chair and the area where the potty chair was used should be cleaned using cleaning equipment and a sink that is only for cleaning and disinfecting potty chairs.

Animals—Pets and Pests

- Choose pets that do not have a high risk of spreading infection. Certain animals should not be allowed in ECE programs. The animals not allowed include reptiles (turtles, snakes, and lizards), amphibians (frogs, toads, salamanders, and newts), live poultry (chicks, ducklings, and goslings), and ferrets. For more details, go to https://www.cdc.gov/healthy-pets/specific-groups/schools.html and https://www.cdc.gov/healthypets/pets.
- To prevent animal and insect access, cover sandboxes when they are not in use. Open sandboxes are frequently contaminated by cat and raccoon feces.
- Ensure pets are appropriately enclosed and their enclosures are kept clean of waste.
- Ensure staff members practice hand hygiene before and after contact with any animal and after handling animal waste, cages, or bedding (including fish tanks).
- For pest control, observe where and what any contractor does to control pests. Staff members cannot rely on pest control contractors to know where children use rooms and surfaces and refrain from application of toxic pesticides anywhere that might lead to exposure of children to them.

- Use methods to shut pests out of the facility and keep food and water sources away from where they might attract pests. Contractors should agree to follow the principles of Integrated Pest Management (IPM), an approach that uses the least toxic method to control pests. To learn how to hire a pest management professional who does IPM, see the recommendations in the IPM curriculum of the California Childcare Health Program on page 28 at https://cchp.ucsf.edu/sites/g/files/tkssra181/f/Curriculum_FINAL%2010.2010.pdf. Learn more about the principles of IPM and how to apply them at https://www.epa.gov/childcare/managing-pests-child-care-centers-using-integrated-pest-management-ipm-module-4-ipm-child.
- See Infections Caused by Interactions of Humans With Pets and Wild Animals in Chapter 8 for more information.

Staff Education

At least annually, and more frequently if needed, provide training for staff members who are responsible for cleaning, sanitizing, and disinfecting, including
- How to handle, mix, and store solutions.
- Proper use of protective barriers (eg, use of disposable gloves) and when and how to follow Standard Precautions. Remember to practice hand hygiene even if gloves were used.
- Proper handling and disposal of contaminated materials, such as soiled diapers or bandages that are contaminated with blood or body fluids.
- Information required by OSHA about the use of any chemical agents. Be sure staff members have read and understand the Safety Data Sheets for any products they use.

- If custodial services are provided under a contract with an outside service organization, be sure an assigned staff member supervises routine cleaning of the facility according to the facility's schedule and procedures.

Heating, Ventilation, and Air-conditioning

Air quality and circulation of fresh outdoor air are key factors in reducing the spread of infectious diseases. Maintain heating, ventilation, and air-conditioning systems so they meet current health standards. Have these systems checked by a contractor who is certified by the American Society of Heating, Refrigerating, and Air-Conditioning Engineers to ensure fresh air circulates and the equipment prevents buildup of germs in the air that people will breathe. Replace or clean air filters as recommended by the equipment manufacturer. For more detail about how to improve air quality in ECE and school facilities, see *Caring for Our Children*, Section 5.2 (https://nrckids.org/CFOC); the EPA Creating Healthy Indoor Air Quality in Schools website at www.epa.gov/iaq-schools; and Head Start Early Childhood Learning & Knowledge Center information about working with a ventilation consultant at https://eclkc.ohs.acf.hhs.gov/publication/tips-working-ventilation-consultant. Much has been learned about ventilation during the COVID-19 pandemic. Additionally, use of air fresheners, incense, or sanitizers (both artificial and natural, such as essential oils) should be avoided, as noted in *Caring for Our Children*, Standard 5.2.9.11.

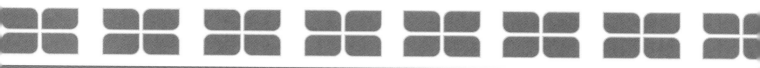

CHAPTER 3

Health of
Educators
and Other Staff Members

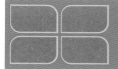

Health of Educators and Other Staff Members

Introduction

Staff member health is a key component of successful operation of early childhood education (ECE) programs and schools. Educators and those who provide administrative and maintenance functions are also essential for healthy and safe operations. Working with children is physically, mentally, and emotionally demanding. To perform their roles well, all the adults who work in the program must be physically and emotionally fit for their tasks. Adults who work in ECE programs and schools should be protected from job-related exposure to illness and injury to the extent that such prevention is reasonable and possible.

Preemployment Requirements and Ongoing Adult Health Appraisals and Immunizations

Health appraisals for paid and volunteer staff members should include aspects of their well-being that are likely to directly affect job performance. Relevant health problems should be revealed by the following procedures to be performed by the staff member's health professional(s):

a. Review of health history.
b. Physical examination.
c. Dental examination.
d. Vision and hearing screening.
e. Tuberculosis (TB) screening using the tuberculin skin test (TST) or interferon-gamma release assay (IGRA), with appropriate follow-up results. The IGRA is a blood test that is the preferred TB screening for individuals who have received BCG vaccine because the BCG vaccine may make the TST give a false-positive result. BCG vaccine is commonly given in many countries where TB is still prevalent. Low-risk, otherwise healthy staff members with previously negative TB screening test results do not routinely need repeated testing unless required by the local or state health department or after a new high-risk exposure. Because children usually become infected with TB by exposure to adults who have active TB, any adult at high risk for TB and who resides, works, or has regular contact with children should have completed TB screening as specified in *Caring for Our Children*, Standard 7.3.10.1 (https://nrckids. org/CFOC). People at high risk for TB include health care workers, people born in or formerly residents of countries with a high rate of TB, residents of homeless shelters or correctional facilities, and those who use illicit drugs, are HIV infected, or have contact with someone who has active TB. Adults who test positive for TB need to undergo further testing, including a chest radiograph, before being cleared to work with children or having contact with children in ECE facilities.

f. A review and certification of up-to-date immune status per the current recommended adult immunization schedule from the Centers for Disease Control and Prevention (CDC), including annual influenza, COVID-19, and up-to-date tetanus, diphtheria, acellular pertussis (Tdap); measles, mumps, rubella (MMR); and varicella vaccinations.

g. A review of occupational health concerns based on the essential functions of the job.

As specified in *Caring for Our Children*, Standard 1.7.0.1 (https://nrckids.org/CFOC), all paid and volunteer staff members who care for children or are involved in other functions in ECE and school facilities should have a preemployment health appraisal (checkup) performed by a health professional who provides primary care for adults. Unless the role or health status of the staff member changes, subsequent health appraisals should be performed as frequently as recommended by the health professional. As a minimum, the health appraisal should assess the adult worker's ability to perform job functions and should address relevant occupational health risks and preventive measures.

The health professional who conducts this assessment needs to be informed about the worker's expected job functions. Job descriptions should explicitly state the expected work performance and the abilities required to do these tasks. While reasonable accommodation of workers with disabilities is required by federal law, the worker must be able to perform specific duties with these accommodations. For example, EC educators for infants and toddlers must have adequate vision and hearing to observe and interact with children in their care, read children's books to them, and lift at least 20 pounds to perform required functions of an EC educator for this age group, including lifting children to the diaper-changing surface.

Health professionals may not have enough experience with work roles in ECE programs and schools to identify the aspects of a person's health status that could affect the worker's performance. The ECE program's and school's request for a report of the results of a health professional's review of a worker's health status should include specific details about the occupational risks and performance expectations. Putting those details explicitly in the request or on the form will help focus the health professional's assessment. This request can be on a form that identifies pertinent details to look for in the adult's health history, in relevant screenings, and in evaluation of physical abilities required to perform the intended role in the program, accompanied by a list of known occupational health hazards in ECE and school settings. (See Letter to Staff About Occupational Health Risks and a sample Staff Health Assessment Form in Chapter 8.) The health professional's documentation of the health assessment should include findings related to these details based on a review of the worker's health history, the results of screening tests, and a physical examination. Health assessments should include a review of the adult worker's vaccine history, highlighting gaps in immunization that the health professional provided or arranged to be provided based on current recommendations from the CDC. Up-to-date immunization status is especially important for individuals who have contact with young children. Specific concerns that may be included in the health assessment request are

- Frequent hand hygiene. An adult who has a skin problem that would be worsened by frequent hand hygiene may need to take additional precautions but should not decrease necessary hand hygiene.
- Any condition that might result in the adult's need to be absent from work for illness more often than the typical adult. Frequent absence for illness interferes with providing continuity of caregiving relationships for children who are enrolled in the program and maintenance of preventive measures. For staff members who provide support services, frequent absence makes it difficult for the program to carry out the necessary functions for quality care. For example, adults with conditions associated with decreased immunity or a condition that increases susceptibility to the infections that commonly occur among infants, toddlers, and preschool-aged children might be absent too frequently to qualify for a position where these exposures occur.
- Women of childbearing age who might become or who are pregnant and who are exposed to young children in their job setting may acquire cytomegalovirus (CMV) or parvovirus infections from contact with urine, saliva, blood, and other secretions of young children, which could damage their developing fetus. Up to 70% of children aged 1 to 3 years who are in ECE settings excrete CMV. The American

Academy of Pediatrics (AAP) *Red Book®: 2021–2024 Report of the Committee on Infectious Diseases* recommends: "Female child care workers in child care centers should be aware of CMV and its potential risks and should have access to appropriate hand hygiene measures to minimize occupationally acquired infection" (page 300). Women of childbearing age should receive counseling to educate them about the risk of exposure to CMV so they can decide whether they want to accept this risk and, if so, reliably practice steps to minimize the risk.

The essential elements the health professional should assess and document in the report to the ECE facility are listed on the Staff Health Assessment Form in Chapter 8.

Improved access to low-cost health insurance is necessary to reduce financial barriers to getting preventive health care for staff. Many EC educators are paid little more than minimum wage and do not have employer funding for health benefits. When staff members do not have health insurance that covers health supervision, arrangements should be made for the worker to use community health service resources, such as federally qualified health centers and public health clinics.

Adults who work in ECE facilities need to learn about and practice ways to minimize the risk of illness and injury and promote wellness for children and themselves. The program can offer this professional development via face-to-face or distance learning opportunities. Staff members need to learn what to do and why to do it. Identifying what concepts staff members need to learn involves having staff members welcome and participate in evaluations of performance of health and safety policies and procedures, so what they are taught is what they need to know.

Immunization With Recommended Vaccines

Caring for Our Children, Standard 7.2.0.3 (https://nrckids.org/CFOC), refers to the current recommended adult immunization schedule at www.cdc.gov/vaccines/schedules. This schedule is updated each year. Adults can use the Adult Vaccine Assessment Tool on the CDC website (https://www2a.cdc.gov/nip/adultimmsched) to identify any gaps in their immunization status. Someone in the facility should track this for all staff members and any volunteers or helpers who work in the ECE facility. Many programs have volunteers or teenaged helpers working alongside staff. The program should have a policy about what to do to be sure staff members, volunteers, and helpers have all the recommended vaccines. These vaccines include the Tdap vaccine, COVID-19 vaccine, annual influenza vaccine, and routine childhood vaccines missed in the staff member's childhood and should be reviewed with the individual's health professional. Anyone who works in the facility who does not have a record of receiving all recommended vaccines, evidence of immunity, or a medical reason that precludes getting a specific vaccine should be required to get all missing vaccines. This chapter briefly describes some infections that are prevented by recommended vaccines. For more details about these infections, see the Quick Reference Sheets for these infections in Chapter 6.

Tetanus, Diphtheria, Acellular Pertussis

Infants younger than 6 months are too young to receive enough doses of diphtheria, tetanus, and acellular pertussis vaccine to give them immunity with protective levels of antibody against whooping cough (pertussis). Pertussis in young infants can be severe, causing hospitalization and death. Pertussis in adults and teens is often mild but with symptoms that may persist for a long time. It can, therefore, be spread to vulnerable infants and young children, which is why it is essential to immunize teens and adults who spend time in close proximity to young infants.

The CDC recommends 1 dose of Tdap vaccine for all adults, boosted every 10 years, and 1 dose for women with each pregnancy. Making sure adults receive this vaccine helps protect the adult from a nuisance cough and young children from whooping cough.

Measles, Mumps, Rubella and Varicella Vaccines

Adults should also ensure that they are completely up to date on their MMR and varicella (chickenpox) vaccines. Infants do not receive their first measles and varicella vaccines until 12 months of age and can become ill if exposed before then. These highly contagious viruses can cause outbreaks and lead to significant absences.

Hepatitis A Vaccine

Hepatitis A vaccine is not a requirement for adults who work in ECE or schools. However, it should be considered for several reasons. Outbreaks can occur in these settings, hepatitis A is more common in other countries from which some people in ECE and schools may have recently immigrated, and there are some uncommon risk factors which may necessitate immunization (see https://www.cdc.gov/vaccines/schedules/downloads/adult/adult-combined-schedule.pdf). Young children who are infected with hepatitis A often seem well. However, adults who become infected with hepatitis A can be very ill. Universal use of hepatitis A vaccine for children in the United States has reduced, but not eliminated, this risk of exposure of adults who have not received hepatitis A vaccine.

Influenza Vaccine

Adults should receive the influenza vaccine each year no earlier than September to ensure immunity lasts through the flu season. Influenza can be unpredictably severe and lethal for otherwise young and healthy people. However, influenza is most severe in the very young, the very old, and those with underlying medical conditions. See the Quick Reference Sheet for Influenza in Chapter 6 for a list of these conditions. Contact with adults and children who are in ECE and school is a common way that influenza spreads to family and community members. Approximately 2 weeks are required after receiving the vaccine to build sufficient immunity to prevent severe infection. The vaccine protects adults, children in their care, and others that the adults and children in child care contact in the community.

COVID-19 Vaccine

As of summer 2022, COVID-19 vaccines are recommended for all people 6 months and older. Depending on the order in which the vaccines were developed, they may have CDC authorization within the scope of the Emergency Use Authorization or full US Food and Drug Administration licensure. Vaccine development and boosting schedules are evolving as the SARS-CoV-2 virus evolves, so see the latest recommendations from the CDC at https://www.cdc.gov/vaccines/covid-19/clinical-considerations/covid-19-vaccines-us.html. COVID-19 has caused extremely high hospitalization and death rates in older adults and people with underlying medical conditions. Although COVID-19 is generally less severe in young children compared with adults, children can become severely ill and, throughout the pandemic, have experienced hospitalization and death rates significantly higher than those seen in a severe influenza season. Because infants and children between ages 6 months and 5 years and school-aged children still have low vaccination rates, it is essential for the adults who teach and care for them to be immunized.

Pneumococcal, Meningococcal, and Hepatitis B Vaccines

Pneumococcal vaccine is a routine vaccine for all young children (through 5 years of age), all adults 65 years or older, and people 2 through 64 years old with certain medical conditions. The CDC recommends vaccination with a meningococcal conjugate vaccine for all preteens and teens at 11 to 12 years old, with a booster dose at 16 years old. Immunization records of teen helpers in ECE programs should show that they have received all recommended vaccines for their age.

Like hepatitis A, hepatitis B vaccine is a routine immunization series for young children in the United States. The Advisory Committee on Immunization Practices has recommended that all adults aged 19 to 59 years should receive hepatitis B vaccines. The US Occupational Safety and Health Administration (OSHA) requires that employers offer hepatitis B vaccine at the time of employment at no cost to the employee if the worker may be exposed to blood. Many employees in ECE programs and schools are called on to provide first aid for split lips, scrapes, and cuts. Responding to children with these injuries, even briefly, may include exposure to blood. If a worker refuses the vaccine when first employed, the employer must offer hepatitis B vaccine immediately after a blood exposure.

Oral Health Practices in Early Childhood Education Settings

Oral health examinations for adults should include special attention to detection and management of tooth decay. As was discussed in Chapter 2, early childhood caries (tooth decay or cavities) is a preventable infectious disease caused by a type of bacteria that can be spread from an EC educator to a child early in the child's life. Infants often put their hands into the mouth of their EC educators. When babies put their (unwashed) hands back in their own mouths, they spread the cavity-causing bacteria to themselves. Some adults taste an infant's heated cereal or other heated foods for safe temperature and then use the same spoon to feed the infant. These practices are not recommended, and such potential transfers of bacteria should be avoided. Kissing babies on their heads is a common and acceptable expression of affection. However, adults should not kiss babies on or around their lips or allow children to put their hands into the adult's mouth.

For adults and children, brushing teeth and tongue twice daily are essential prevention measures. Encourage staff to have oral health examinations and tooth cleanings by a dental health professional every 6 months to control caries-causing bacteria. See the Dental Caries (Early Childhood Caries, Tooth Decay, or Cavities) Quick Reference Sheet in Chapter 6.

Health Limitations for Staff Members
Task Assignments and Occupational Risks

As mentioned in other chapters, staff members in ECE programs and schools should review and reduce known occupational hazards, including exposure to infectious diseases from close interactions with groups of children and adults and provision of personal care for children. Some are mentioned in this chapter. See *Caring for Our Children*, Standard 1.7.0.4 and Appendix B (https://nrckids.org/CFOC), which lists the specific infectious diseases and organisms that are considered occupational hazards, and the Letter to Staff About Occupational Health Risks in Chapter 8 of this book.

Food Handling

Some tasks in ECE settings pose special risks for spreading infectious diseases. For example, people involved in food handling tasks of storing, preparing, or serving food should not be allowed to continue their duties if they are ill with vomiting, diarrhea, or respiratory symptoms; have open sores on parts of their bodies that cannot be covered; or have skin sores on their hands (even if hands can be covered with gloves). Everyone should use utensils to handle food. However, using utensils is insufficient to prevent contamination of food by someone who is ill with an infectious disease.

See the Food Handlers section in Chapter 2 for more discussion about limiting opportunities for staff members to transfer disease-causing germs via preparing or handling food.

Exposure to Chemicals

Many staff members use chemicals to maintain environmental hygiene—cleaning, sanitizing, and disinfecting. Some products have ingredients that can cause health problems for sensitive individuals. Employers are required by OSHA to provide Safety Data Sheets (formerly known as Material Safety Data Sheets) to staff members that give the user information about the toxicity and risk of using specific products.

Program directors should minimize the number of products used in the facility and choose the least toxic but effective products for the required tasks. As was emphasized in Chapter 2, select products that have a US Environmental Protection Agency (EPA) registration number on the label and an indication that the product is intended for sanitizing or disinfecting the surface where the program will use it. Federal law requires that users of an EPA-registered product must follow the instructions on the product label. Violations are subject to heavy fines.

Products regulated by the EPA must carry signal words that indicate the level of toxicity. The law requires manufacturers to label their products according to the level of risk. Among toxic products, 1 of 3 signal words must be on the label. Those labeled "Caution" are safer than those labeled "Warning," which, in turn, are safer than those labeled "Danger." For more information, visit the EPA Safer Choice website at https://www.epa.gov/saferchoice.

Risk to the Fetus of a Pregnant Staff Member

Many staff members in ECE programs are women in their childbearing years. Some of these women who work with young children will become pregnant and deliver their babies during their teaching careers. Special risks to the health of the pregnant staff member or developing fetus may exist when the pregnant woman is exposed to certain infectious diseases, such as CMV and parvovirus B19 (fifth disease), which are commonly spread by young children. Exposure to CMV occurs at a higher rate in ECE programs than in the community. Employers of women in their childbearing years should explain to them how their exposure can cause harm to their fetus if they become pregnant. All female staff of childbearing age should be urged to discuss with their health professional their exposure to these risks during their work and, if pregnant or intending to become pregnant, how to minimize these risks by using Standard Precautions and meticulous hand hygiene or choosing roles that do not involve exposure to body fluids of young children.

Stress

Staff wellness should be a top priority because poorly managed stress can affect staff performance and increase risk of infection and injury. Staff members require regular breaks, places to refuel themselves away from children during the day, paid vacation, and sick leave to manage stress. Many educators have low wages and few benefits, which make it difficult for them to seek and pay for health maintenance services and health care for illness. Early childhood education programs and schools must recognize the negative effects of stress, attempt to reduce stress if possible, and help staff members to manage unavoidable stress. These measures can help prevent negative effects on the performance of the workforce and their susceptibility to infection. See *Caring for Our Children*, Standard 1.7.0.5 (https://nrckids.org/CFOC), for more details about stress, resources, and measures to lessen stress.

Temporary Exclusion of Staff Members for Illness

The administrator or director or their designate should be responsible for observing all adults in the facility for signs of illness; this is analogous to the daily health check for children. Daily health checks should be performed as adults arrive and periodically throughout the day. When a staff member develops signs of illness, the administrator or director must evaluate the situation to see if this person needs to leave the facility or can stay with some accommodation.

All ECE programs, but especially family child care settings, should have an emergency backup plan for times when staff become ill while working or are absent due to illness.

Certain conditions warrant temporary exclusion of ill staff members from working in the facility. These conditions are similar to the reasons for exclusion of children from ECE programs. Staff members should be excluded from the program if they are unable to participate or perform the functions required to carry out their role or if their illness is considered to be a harmful communicable disease by their health professional or the local health department. Refer to the CDC for the most current information about exclusion for staff members during the COVID-19 pandemic (https://www.cdc.gov/coronavirus/2019-ncov/community/schools-childcare/index.html).

Especially during their first year or so of contact with young children, adults who work in ECE programs or schools may have more symptomatic infectious illnesses than those who have worked in ECE programs for multiple years. Usually, the frequency of infectious illnesses decreases as adult workers develop immunity. Staff members, substitutes, and volunteers should be expected to report their own health problems to a supervisor if they are aware that their condition might affect their ability to perform their role or the health and safety of the children. Unfortunately, many educators come to work when they are too ill to work because they are concerned about the burden their absence puts on other staff or they lack sufficient paid time off. Working while ill may lengthen the time to recover. If the illness is a harmful communicable disease, working while ill may put others (children and coworkers) at risk. This has been especially true during the COVID-19 pandemic.

Understandably, ill staff members may be reluctant to stay home or leave work to go home if it affects their income or places a significant burden on the program to maintain child to staff ratios, provide quality care, and arrange for a substitute educator. The facility must have a contingency plan for worker illness. Authorized paid staff sick leave is important for the program and may minimize spread of harmful communicable diseases. Benefits of sick leave may include the promotion of full recovery of the worker from illness and improve job performance.

When Staff Members Who Have Been Excluded for an Infectious Disease May Return

When a staff member must leave for illness, the program administrator/director and staff members need to know when the ill person should return. *Caring for Our Children*, Standard 1.7.0.3 (https://nrckids.org/CFOC), specifies circumstances when staff members and volunteers should have return-to-work documentation from their health care professional. Early childhood education programs should require documentation when educators have experienced a health condition that might affect the person's performance of assigned tasks, when the person's condition might risk causing illness in others, or when someone is returning after a prolonged absence for illness or injury.

The following conditions require exclusion of staff. The Quick Reference Sheets in Chapter 6 discuss these in more detail, including when the staff may return to work.

a. Chickenpox, until all lesions have dried and crusted, which usually occurs by 6 days after the first lesions appear or in immunized people without crusts, until no new lesions appear in a 24-hour period.

b. Shingles; only exclude the worker if the lesions cannot be covered by clothing or a dressing. If the worker has been excluded, return to work is allowed when all the lesions have crusted.

c. Rash with fever or joint pain, until diagnosed not to be measles or rubella.

d. Measles, until 4 days after onset of the rash (if the staff member or substitute has a normal immune response and a normal recovery).

e. Mumps, until 5 days after onset of facial gland swelling (if the staff member or substitute has a normal immune response and normal recovery).

f. Rubella, until 7 days after onset of the rash.

g. Diarrheal illness, if stool frequency exceeds 2 or more stools above normal for that individual or there is blood in stools, until diarrhea resolves, or until a health professional determines that the diarrhea is not caused by a germ that can be spread to others in the facility.
For all cases of bloody diarrhea and diarrhea caused by Shiga toxin–producing *Escherichia coli* (STEC), *Shigella*, or *Salmonella* serotype Typhi I, exclusion must continue until the person is cleared to return by a health professional. Exclusion is warranted for STEC, until results of 2 stool cul-

tures are negative (at least 48 hours after antibiotic treatment is complete [if prescribed]); for *Shigella* species, until at least 1 stool culture is negative (varies by state); and for S Typhi, until 3 stool cultures are negative. Stool samples need to be collected at least 48 hours after antibiotic treatment is complete. Other types of *Salmonella* do not require negative test results from stool cultures.

h. Vomiting illness, 2 or more episodes of vomiting during the previous 24 hours, until vomiting resolves or is determined to result from noninfectious conditions.

i. Hepatitis A virus, until 1 week after symptom onset or as directed by the local health department.

j. Pertussis, until after 5 days of appropriate antibiotic therapy are completed or until 21 days after the onset of cough if the person is not treated with antibiotics.

k. Skin infection, such as impetigo, until treatment has been initiated; exclusion should continue if the lesion is draining and cannot be covered.

l. Tuberculosis, until noninfectious and cleared by a health department official or a health professional.

m. Strep throat or other streptococcal infection, until 12 hours after initial antibiotic treatment and end of fever.

n. Head lice, from the end of the day of discovery until after the first treatment. Exclusion is not necessary if nits are still present after treatment. The nits are unlikely to contain live lice.

o. Scabies, until after treatment has been completed (usually overnight).

p. *Haemophilus influenzae* type b, until cleared by a health professional.

q. Meningococcal infection, until cleared by a health professional.

r. Respiratory illness, if the illness limits the staff member's ability to provide an acceptable level of child care, the illness compromises the health and safety of the children, or the staff person is unable to manage respiratory secretions using cough and sneeze etiquette into a tissue or elbow/upper arm and hand hygiene.

s. COVID-19, as described by the CDC guidelines at https://www.cdc.gov/coronavirus/2019-ncov/community/schools-childcare/index.html.

Educators who have herpes cold sores should not be excluded from EC programs and schools, but they should

a. Not touch their lesions and cover them if possible. (If lesions are touched, hand hygiene must be performed immediately.)

b. Carefully observe hand hygiene policies.

c. Not kiss any children.

Policies and Procedures Related to Caring for Staff and Children Who Are Ill

Chapter 1 gave an overview of health policy development and use. Sections in *Model Child Care Health Policies* that include topics related to the overall prevention and control of infectious diseases are listed in Chapter 1 also. *Model Child Care Health Policies* is a joint publication of the national AAP and the Pennsylvania Chapter of the AAP. The joint publication is recommended as a source of adaptable, fill-in-the-blank policies and is available, at no cost, online at https://ecels-healthychildcarepa.org.

Caring for Our Children, Standard 9.2.3.2 (https://nrckids.org/CFOC), describes what all ECE facilities should have in their written policies and procedures. The program's Child Care Health Consultant should be involved in providing technical assistance and collaboration in the preparation of these policies and procedures, monitoring of intended practices, and periodic updates. In addition to policies and procedures to ensure all staff have recommended immunizations to minimize the occurrence and severity of vaccine-preventable illnesses, programs should have the following policies related to the care of staff and children who are ill:

a. Policies and procedures for urgent and emergency care
b. Admission, inclusion/exclusion, and reentry policies for children
c. A description of illnesses common to children in ECE, their management, and precautions to address the needs and behavior of the child who is ill, as well as to protect the health of other children and staff
d. A procedure to obtain and maintain updated individual care plans for children and staff with special health care needs
e. A procedure for documenting the name of person affected, date and time of illness, a description of symptoms, the response of the educator or other staff to these symptoms, who was notified (eg, parent/guardian, primary health professional, nurse, physician, health department), and the response
f. Medication administration policies
g. Seasonal and pandemic influenza policy
h. Staff illness guidelines for exclusion and reentry

In educational settings for children, the priority of the policy should be to meet the needs of a child or staff member who is ill and the children in the facility. The policy should address the circumstances under which separation of the affected individual (child or staff member) from the group is required; the circumstances under which the staff, parents/guardians, or other designated persons need to be informed; and the

procedures to be followed in these cases. The policy should take into consideration

a. The physical limitations of the facility.
b. The number and qualifications of the facility's personnel.
c. How the ECE program or school makes sure substitute educators perform competently. Although many adults have experience caring for children, health and safety routines in ECE programs and schools differ from what many people do in their homes. *Caring for Our Children*, Standard 1.5.0.2 (https://nrckids.org/CFOC), requires that programs orient substitutes to the policies and procedures for the tasks assigned to them. As a minimum, substitutes should be able to demonstrate the necessary knowledge and skills for nutrition, hand hygiene and sanitation, diaper- and soiled underwear-changing routines, emergency care, and medical procedures that children might require.
d. That children do become ill frequently and that both staff and children become ill at unpredictable times.
e. That adults may be on staff with known health problems (which do not preclude meeting requirements specified in their job descriptions when hired but require accommodation) or that staff members may develop health problems over time that need to be addressed if these problems affect their work.
f. That children and their families may experience negative consequences when educators are given leave for illness if it results in frequent disruption of continuous warm, positive staff/child/family relationships.
g. The delegation to (specified) staff of decisions about
   • The amount of care an ill child requires if the child remains in the program
   • Whether the ill child can participate in the activities planned for the child's group
   • Whether staff can devote the time for caring of a child who is ill without compromising the care of the other children
   • Whether the child has an illness on the list of specific conditions that require exclusion

Staff Learn, Teach, and Practice Minimizing Infectious Diseases

Staff members should participate in preservice training mandated by federal funding to states under the Child Care and Development Block Grant that includes infectious disease prevention and management, as well as ongoing education about health and safety. Professional development and training should include explanations of what must be done, why it is required, and any skills that must be performed correctly. The focus should be about how to integrate health and safety with other components of the program. Training should include physical, oral, cognitive, social-emotional, and nutritional health concepts and practices; prevention and management of infections and injuries; health promotion, including detection of adverse childhood experiences such as child abuse; and emergency/disaster preparedness. Staff need to learn about how to teach these topics to children and to practice as role models and protectors. *Caring for Our Children*, Standard 2.4.1.1 (https://nrckids.org/CFOC), lists specific topics staff members should learn about and teach to children. Among the many areas to be covered are some key behaviors for infection control, including hand hygiene, masking and gloving when necessary, wiping bottoms, flushing toilets, cough and sneezing etiquette, wiping noses, toothbrushing, and handling food safely. Educators can creatively integrate teaching recommended infection control measures with math, language, and science in the existing curriculum. Benefits may be realized for children and adults in the program and in fewer illnesses brought home to families.

Staff members in ECE facilities should participate in at least 24 hours of health-related professional development annually. The objective of this education is to renew and update staff members about current concepts and improve skills appropriate to their roles. This education should be in the form that works best for the learner. It can include workshops taught by subject experts, internet-based and printed self-learning modules, expert mentoring, and peer-to-peer coaching. In collaboration with staff members, a Child Care Health Consultant can help plan, provide, or arrange for needed education. Public health agencies, emergency medical services, school health programs, home nursing agencies, clinics, and private health professionals in the community may be able to contribute some instruction. In addition to topics to be taught to children, education of staff members should address the topics listed in *Caring for Our Children*, Standard 10.6.1.2 (https://nrckids.org/CFOC). Many of these topics are related to prevention and management of infectious diseases.

Topics for Staff Education About Infectious Diseases That Might Be Provided by Community Health Agencies or Health Consultants

Public health departments, other state departments charged with professional development for early childhood educators, and emergency medical services agencies should provide training, written information, and consultation in at least the following subject areas or referral to other community resources (eg, Child Care Health Consultants; licensing personnel; health care professionals, including school nurses) who can provide such training in these areas:

a. Immunization
b. Reporting, preventing, and managing of infectious diseases
c. Techniques for the prevention and control of infectious diseases, including Standard Precautions
d. Exclusion and inclusion guidelines and care of children who are acutely ill
e. General hygiene and sanitation
f. Food service, nutrition, and infant and child feeding
g. Care of children with special health care needs (eg, chronic illnesses, physical and developmental disabilities, behavior problems)
h. Prevention and management of injury
i. Preparation and planning for emergencies and natural or man-made disasters
j. Oral health
k. Environmental health
l. Health promotion, including routine health supervision and the importance of a medical or health home for all children and adults, and detection of adverse childhood experiences and sources of behavioral health services that families may need
m. Health insurance, including Medicaid and the Children's Health Insurance Program
n. Strategies for preparing for and responding to infectious disease outbreaks, such as the role of and indications for personal protective equipment like masking, gloving, and gowning in a pandemic; knowing when it is or is not necessary to exclude a child with an infection from the usual early childhood education program
o. Age-appropriate physical activity
p. Sudden unexplained infant death (SUID) and safe sleep practices
q. Shaken baby syndrome or abusive head trauma
r. Injury prevention

Adapted from *Caring for Our Children*, Standard 10.6.1.2 (https://nrckids.org/CFOC).

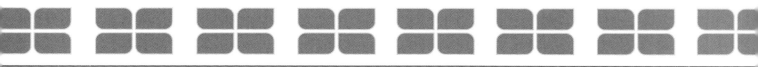

CHAPTER 4

Recognizing the Ill Child

Inclusion/Exclusion Criteria

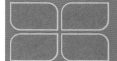

Recognizing the Ill Child: Inclusion/Exclusion Criteria

Health Check

Educators in an early childhood education (ECE) program or school who are familiar with the behavior and appearance of the enrolled children can assess each child's health status when the child arrives and periodically throughout the day. Health status assessments involve a warm, relaxed, respectful greeting of the child and accompanying caregiver. During the greeting, the EC educator should observe and interact with the child and should ask the caregiver if there are any symptoms of illness or injury or any change in the child's status from the last time the child participated in the program. A Child Care Health Consultant (CCHC) or school health professional can explain and demonstrate how to conduct a health check. Doing the daily health check and keeping a daily record of symptoms routinely are good ways for EC educators to monitor trends and watch for signs of an infectious disease outbreak or epidemic. An example of a daily health check poster can be found on the California Childcare Health Program website at https://cchp.ucsf.edu/content/daily-health-check.

The Symptom Record Form in Chapter 8 can be used by families or educators to document symptoms a child experiences while at home or at the ECE facility or school. The Enrollment/Attendance/Symptom Record in Chapter 8 can be used by educators to record attendance and document symptoms for individual and groups of children to potentially recognize patterns of illness and detect outbreaks.

Information to Observe and Gather

The following symptoms and conditions should be observed and supplemented by information shared by the family or other staff members who have been with the child:

Symptoms
* Changes in behavior or appearance, such as sleepiness or fatigue and decreased playfulness or appetite
* Any runny nose, cough, or breathing trouble (fast breathing, flaring nostrils, belly breathing)
* Any new skin rashes or itchy skin or scalp
* Any new bumps or bruises
* Any open sores or weeping skin rashes
* Signs of fever, such as flushed appearance or shivering (Checking a child's temperature in the absence of behavior change is not recommended.)
* Increased irritability; symptoms of pain or not feeling well

* Vomiting, diarrhea, or stomachache
* Any irritation or drainage from the eye(s)
* Severe mouth pain while eating or napping that prevents child from eating, napping, or engaging in usual activities.

Conditions
* Whether the child has received any medication at home or needs any special care during the day
* Whether the family reveals that the child or the child's family member has been exposed to a harmful communicable disease

Routinely sharing this information with the child's EC educator and the child's family helps everyone remain on the lookout for signs and symptoms of illness. Program staff can use the information from this health check to decide whether the child is well enough to participate in the daily planned activities or whether the child needs special attention or more attention than the staff can responsibly provide. If the child seems well enough to stay, the information and observations from the health check enable the staff to plan how to meet the needs of the child and what to observe for during the day. The Signs and Symptoms Chart in Chapter 5 lists conditions that require exclusion from ECE programs and school. The chart is organized by symptoms so that educators can use this information to determine the possible causes and when it is appropriate to notify the program's CCHC. Pediatric health professionals can use this chart to discuss with educators what signs and symptoms of illness require a health care visit. The Quick Reference Sheets in Chapter 6 review the information about each type of infection in more detail and identify common causes, signs and symptoms, required notifications, the role of parents and educators, exclusion guidelines, and when to readmit the child if they are excluded for illness.

Situations That Require Medical Attention Right Away

Educators in ECE programs and schools must be able to recognize and respond to situations that are medical emergencies and distinguish those from others that require urgent, but not emergency, action. Preparation for such circumstances includes that staff members will
* Know how to access emergency medical services (EMS) in the area where the program is located. In most communities, calling 911 works. Some commu-

nities still lack the 911 system. Some facilities have phone systems that are unique or depend on staff always having a mobile phone available. Procedure and emergency numbers to call should be posted in every occupied location in the facility and staff should be trained in the proper procedure.

- Know how to call Poison Help at 1-800-222-1222. Calling this number automatically connects the caller with the local poison center. This number should be posted in every occupied location in the facility. Staff should be trained in the proper procedures when there are concerns for child-related ingestions or poisonings.

Call Emergency Medical Services (EMS) (911) Immediately If

- The child's life seems to be at risk or there is a risk of permanent injury.
- The child is acting strangely, much less alert, or much more withdrawn than usual.
- The child has difficulty breathing or is unable to speak.
- The child's skin or lips look blue, purple, or gray.
- The child has rapidly spreading raised red skin areas with throat-closing, tongue swelling, trouble breathing or wheezing, or decreased consciousness (severe allergic reaction—anaphylaxis).
- The child has rhythmic jerking of arms and legs and loss of consciousness (seizure).
- The child is unconscious.
- The child is becoming less responsive or increasingly confused.
- After a head injury, the child has any of the following signs or symptoms: decrease in level of alertness, confusion, headache, vomiting, irritability, difficulty walking.
- The child has increasing or severe pain anywhere.
- The child has a cut or burn that is large or deep or won't stop bleeding.
- The child is vomiting blood.
- The child has a severe stiff neck, headache, and fever.
- The child is significantly dehydrated (eg, sunken eyes, lethargic, not making tears, not urinating).
- Multiple children are affected by injury or serious illness at the same time.
- When in doubt about whether to call EMS (911), make the call.
- After calling EMS (911), call the child's parent/legal guardian.

- Educate all staff members about recognizing an emergency medical situation (see "Call Emergency Medical Services [EMS] [911] Immediately If" and "Get Medical Attention Within 1 Hour" boxes). **When in doubt, always call EMS.**
- Know how to contact each child's parent/legal guardian at any time when the child is in the ECE facility (See the Child Emergency Information Form in Chapter 8). If the parent/legal guardian doesn't carry a cell phone or has a schedule that may interfere with being available, have contact information for someone who will be able to reach the parent or temporarily take responsibility at any time. Health professionals may delay providing care if the situation is not life-threatening and the parent/legal guardian is unavailable to give consent for care. It's a good idea to ask parents and guardians to update their contact information and backup person and phone numbers every 6 months. Creating an automated text-based or email system to collect this information may be helpful.
- For children with special needs, make plans with the family and the usual source of health care for handling any special types of emergencies that may affect these children. Make sure all who care for these children understand the special circumstances and have a copy of the health plan or emergency care plan for emergency medical services if called.
- Document what happened in an emergency—day, date, and time, along with observed symptoms and actions taken.
- Put into family and staff handbooks and prominently post in all rooms the 2 lists of situations that require medical attention right away: those that require calling EMS (911), and those that require getting medical attention within an hour (see Situations That Require Medical Attention Right Away in Chapter 8 for this content).

Get Medical Attention Within 1 Hour

Some children may have urgent situations that do not necessarily require emergency medical services (EMS) (911) for ambulance transport but still need medical attention without delay. For the following conditions, the educator may first call the parent/legal guardian. If the parent/guardian is immediately available to pick up the child and take the child to a source of urgent pediatric health care within an hour, the parent/legal guardian should be instructed to do so. EMS (911) should be called to bring the child to a pediatric health professional if the parent/legal guardian cannot do so. When EMS is transporting the child, if possible, a staff member who knows the child should accompany the child until the parent/legal guardian can be present to provide information and reassure the child. Program policies should be clear about how such situations will be handled given local resources. Staff should develop contingency plans for emergencies or disaster situations when it may not be possible or feasible to follow standard or previously agreed on emergency procedures. The situations that require medical attention within an hour are

- Any infant or child older than 2 months who looks more than mildly ill with a temperature above 101 °F (38.3 °C) taken by any method (Note: Rectal temperatures in early childhood education programs or schools should be taken only by persons with specific health training in performing this procedure and with permission by parents/guardians. Never "correct" for an axillary temperature by adding 0.5 or 1 degree.)
- Temperature above 100.4 °F (38.0 °C) by any method in an infant younger than 2 months (8 weeks)
- A quickly spreading purple or red rash or a rapidly spreading rash that raises concern for an allergic reaction (eg, hives)
- A large volume of blood in stools
- A cut that may require stitches
- Any medical condition specifically outlined in a child's care plan that requires immediate action and/or notification of the child's parent/legal guardian

Conditions That Do Not Require Exclusion to Control Spread of Disease to Others

(During a pandemic, follow the Centers for Disease Control and Prevention [CDC] or local health department recommendations.)

- Common colds, runny noses (regardless of color or consistency of nasal discharge), and coughs.
- Yellow, white, or watery eye discharge without fever, eye pain, or eyelid redness.
- Pinkeye (bacterial conjunctivitis), without fever or behavior changes, usually associated with pink or red conjunctiva (ie, "whites of the eyes") with white or yellow/green eye mucus drainage; often also associated with matted eyelids after sleep. (See the Pinkeye [Conjunctivitis] Quick Reference Sheet.)

- Fever (for this purpose, defined as temperature above 101 °F [38.3 °C] by any method) without any signs or symptoms of illness in infants and children who are older than 4 months. (See the Fever Quick Reference Sheet). Devices to measure body temperatures include thermometers intended for use in the mouth, armpit, ear canal, rectum, or skin that overlies an artery next to the outside corner of the eye. To read more about how to take a child's temperature and the special issues associated with each method, go to https://www.healthychildren.org/English/health-issues/conditions/fever/Pages/How-to-Take-a-Childs-Temperature.aspx (available in English and Spanish). **Note:** Do not adjust the reading for the location in which the temperature was taken. Simply record the temperature and the location where it was taken.
- Rash without fever and without behavioral changes. Exception: a child with a new, rapidly spreading rash characterized by bruising or small red or purple "blood" spots under the skin. In that case, EMS (911) should be called.
- Hand-foot-and-mouth disease. No exclusion needed unless the child has mouth sores with constant drooling or meets other exclusion criteria (eg, fever, requiring too much care). In some cases, the local health department may require children with hand-foot-and-mouth disease to stay home to control an outbreak.
- Impetigo. Lesions should be covered, but treatment may be delayed until the end of the day. As long as treatment is started before return the next day, no exclusion is needed.
- Lice or nits without lice. Treatment may be delayed until the end of the day. As long as treatment is started before return the next day, no exclusion is needed, even if nits are still present after treatment.
- Ringworm. Treatment may be delayed until the end of the day. As long as treatment is started before return the next day, no exclusion is needed.
- Scabies. Treatment may be delayed until the end of the day. As long as treatment is started before return the next day, no exclusion is needed.
- Thrush (ie, white spots or patches in the mouth).
- Fifth disease (slapped cheek disease, parvovirus B19) in someone with a typical immune system and without an underlying blood disorder like sickle cell disease.
- Staphylococcal colonization or carrier state in children without an illness that would otherwise require exclusion (see Boil/Abscess/Cellulitis and *Staphylococcus aureus* [Methicillin-Resistant (MRSA) and Methicillin-Sensitive (MSSA)] Quick Reference Sheets).
- Molluscum contagiosum. Exclusion or covering of lesions is not required.
- Cytomegalovirus infection.

- Chronic hepatitis B virus infection.
- HIV infection.
- Children who have no symptoms but are known to have a germ in their stools that causes disease do not need to be excluded, except when they have an infection with a Shiga toxin–producing *Escherichia coli* (STEC), *Shigella*, or *Salmonella* serotype Typhi. In these cases, exclusion is warranted as follows: for STEC, until results of 2 stool cultures are negative; for *Shigella* species, until at least 1 stool culture is negative (varies by state); and for S Typhi, until 3 stool cultures are negative. Other types of *Salmonella* do not require negative test results from stool cultures.

Note: During an outbreak of a harmful infectious disease (eg, *Shigella*) or vaccine-preventable disease (eg, measles), children determined to be contributing to the spread of the illness or who are unvaccinated may be excluded until the risk of spread is no longer present or the unvaccinated child receives the necessary vaccine. This is usually determined by the local health department. The guidance in this chapter may change during a pandemic.

Conditions Requiring Temporary Exclusion

Three Key Criteria for Exclusion of Children Who Are Ill

When a child becomes ill but does not require immediate medical help, a determination must be made about whether the child should be sent home (ie, should be temporarily excluded from the early childhood education program or school). Most illnesses do not require exclusion. A designated staff member should determine whether the child's illness meets the following criteria for exclusion:

- Prevents the child from participating comfortably in activities as determined by staff members of the early childhood education program or school
- Results in a need for care that is greater than staff members can provide without compromising the health and safety of other children
- Poses a risk of spread of harmful disease to others based on the list of specific excludable conditions

If any of these criteria are met, the child should be excluded, regardless of the type of illness, unless a pediatric health professional determines the child's condition does not require exclusion.

Specific Excludable Conditions

Exclude if the child has

- A severely ill appearance. Symptoms could include lethargy or lack of responsiveness, irritability, persistent crying, difficulty breathing, or having a quickly spreading rash.
- Fever with behavior change or other signs and symptoms. (See the Fever Quick Reference Sheet in Chapter 6 for more detail.)
- Diarrhea. *Diarrhea* is defined by stool that is occurring more frequently or is less formed in consistency than usual in the child and is not associated with changes of diet. Exclusion is required for all diapered children whose stool is not contained in the diaper and toilet-trained children if the diarrhea is causing "accidents." Exclude children whose stool frequency exceeds 2 stools above typical for that child while the child is in the program or whose stool contains more than a drop of blood or mucus. For diapered children, the increased frequency of stool may cause too much work for the EC educator and thereby challenge the EC educator's ability to maintain sanitary diaper-changing techniques. For toilet-trained children, this greater frequency of having bowel movements poses a significant risk for accidents and contamination of toilet facilities. Readmission after onset of diarrhea can occur when all the following conditions are met:
  - Diapered children have their stool contained by the diaper (even if the stools remain loose).
  - Toilet-trained children do not have toileting accidents.
  - The frequency of passage of stool is no more than 2 stools above what was typical for that child during the time the child was in the program, before the diarrhea began.
  - A pediatric health professional has cleared the child for readmission for all cases of bloody diarrhea and diarrhea caused by *Shigella*, S Typhi, and STEC. See Quick Reference Sheets in Chapter 6 for specific guidelines for these uncommon types of diarrhea. State laws may govern exclusion for these conditions and should be followed by the pediatric health professional who is clearing the child for readmission.
- Vomiting 2 or more times in the previous 24 hours, unless the vomiting is determined by a pediatric health professional to be caused by a noncommunicable or noninfectious condition (eg, healthy infants with reflux).
- Abdominal pain that continues for more than 2 hours or intermittent abdominal pain associated with fever or other signs or symptoms (eg, incessant crying).
- Mouth sores with drooling that the child cannot control unless the child's primary health professional or local health department authority states the child is noninfectious.

Temperature Tips

When taking a child's temperature, remember

- Only digital thermometers, not mercury thermometers, should be used. Ear thermometers should not be used in infants younger than 6 months.
- Higher body temperatures do not necessarily indicate a more severe infection. The child's activity level and sense of well-being are far more important than the temperature reading. A child who is smiling and running around is generally not a concern; a child who is listless and not responsive is always a concern, even if the child's temperature is normal.
- If a child has been in a very hot environment and heatstroke (hot, dry, red skin with lethargy) is suspected, a higher temperature is more serious.
- The method chosen to take a child's temperature depends on the need for accuracy, available equipment, the skill of the person taking the temperature, and the ability of the child to assist in the procedure. See this American Academy of Pediatrics link for more details: https://www.healthychildren.org/English/health-issues/conditions/fever/Pages/How-to-Take-a-Childs-Temperature.aspx.
- Oral temperatures usually are not reliable for children younger than 4 years.
- Rectal temperatures should be taken only by persons with specific health training in performing this procedure.
- Axillary (armpit) temperatures are accurate only when the thermometer remains within the closed armpit for the period recommended by the manufacturer of the device.
- Any device used improperly may give inaccurate results (eg, temporal or forehead thermometers, ear thermometers).

- Rash with fever or behavioral changes, until a primary health professional has determined the illness is not a communicable disease.
- Skin sores that are weeping fluid and are on an exposed body surface that cannot be covered with a waterproof dressing.
- Other conditions with specific diagnoses as follows:
  - Streptococcal pharyngitis (ie, strep throat or other streptococcal infection): exclusion until the child has received an appropriate antibiotic for 12 hours.
  - Head lice: only if child has not been treated after notifying family at the end of the prior program day. (**Note:** Exclusion is not necessary before the end of the program day.)
  - Scabies: only if child has not been treated after notifying family at the end of the prior program day. (**Note:** Exclusion is not necessary before the end of the program day.)

- Ringworm: only if child has not been treated after notifying family at the end of the prior program day. (**Note:** Exclusion is not necessary before the end of the program day.)
- Impetigo: only if child has not been treated after notifying family at the end of the prior program day. (**Note:** Exclusion is not necessary before the end of the program day as long as lesions are covered.)
- Chickenpox (varicella): until all lesions have dried or crusted (usually 6 days after onset of rash) and no new lesions have appeared for at least 24 hours.
- Rubella: 7 days after the rash appears.
- Pertussis: 5 days of appropriate antibiotic treatment (21 days from onset of cough, if untreated).
- Mumps: 5 days after onset of parotid gland swelling.
- Measles: 4 days after onset of rash.
- Hepatitis A virus infection: 1 week after onset of illness or jaundice or as directed by the health department (if the child's symptoms are mild).
- COVID-19 during the pandemic: according to CDC recommendations. (COVID-19 may currently be transitioning to endemic [ie, a normal, expected, seasonal, or background virus], which may affect whether testing and excluding are necessary in the future.)

In addition to the conditions listed previously, see the box titled "Three Key Criteria for Exclusion of Children Who Are Ill" earlier in this chapter. For more details and other diseases, see the Signs and Symptoms Chart in Chapter 5.

Procedures for a Child Who Requires Exclusion

While the child waits to be picked up from the ECE program or school, the educator should

- Move the child to a familiar and comfortable place where the child will be observed and cared for by someone who knows the child well. Moving the child who is ill will not expose people who have not already been exposed to the child's illness. It is best to keep the ill child in a comfortable corner of the child's usual care room, with as much separation from other children as can easily be arranged. If the child is coughing and sneezing, a separation of at least 3 feet will allow the heavy respiratory droplets to fall to the floor. Although the smaller aerosolized droplets may travel farther, the children in the group have already been exposed to these and little will be gained by moving the child to a space where new individuals may be exposed. During a pandemic, follow the CDC or local health department recommendations

- If child to staff ratio cannot be met by providing care for the ill child, it may be possible for supplemental staff to come help care for the other children until a family member or emergency contact person can pick up the child. Putting the ill child in the care of an unfamiliar EC educator and/or in a different space from where the child usually receives care may make it difficult to provide supportive care for the child and may expose previously unexposed individuals to infectious disease.
- Facilities that routinely provide care for ill children in a facility space designated for such care must follow special procedures for equipping and staffing this service, as defined in *Caring for Our Children*, Standard 3.6.2.2 (https://nrckids.org/CFOC).
- Continue to observe the child for new or worsening symptoms.
- Ask the parent/legal guardian to pick up the child as soon as possible as specified in written illness exclusion policies for the program.
- Program staff will share with the adult the ill child's symptoms and the staff's observations. Explain what is required for the child to return.
- The Symptom Record Form in Chapter 8 can be used to document information collected from all staff members involved that day in the child's care about the child's symptoms. The form will make it easier for the family to share valuable information with the child's health professional if the child's condition requires health professional advice.
- If the child seems well to the family and no longer meets criteria for exclusion, there is no need to ask for further information from the pediatric health professional when the child returns to care. Children who have been excluded from care do not necessarily need to have an in-person or virtual visit with a pediatric health professional. During a pandemic, follow the CDC or local health department recommendations.
- Ask the family member to share with the child's educator any advice received from the child's health professional during an office visit, by phone, or by any electronic transmission of information. Follow the advice of the child's health professional. If more information is needed to describe special care required by the returning child, the EC educator should obtain the parent/legal guardian's consent to contact the child's health professional to let the health professional know what information the program staff are seeking. This sharing of information with educators and administrative staff requires written parent consent. Note that if the family needs the health professional's advice, they may receive it electronically without needing an office visit. (See Sample Health Information Consent Form in Chapter 8.)
- Follow the advice provided by the child's health professional or by local public health officials about whether there is a need to inform others in the facility about a possible exposure to an infectious disease. The identity of the child should not be shared, but key elements of the risk to others may make early recognition and treatment of the disease in others possible. Prompt notification reduces the risk of spread of misinformation. Consider notifying families and staff members using the Sample Letter to Families About Exposure to Communicable Disease in Chapter 8, accompanied by the Quick Reference Sheet from Chapter 6 for that condition.
- Document actions in the child's file with date, time, symptoms, and actions taken (and by whom); sign and date the document.
- Sanitize toys and other items the child may have handled or put in their mouth and continue to practice good hand-hygiene techniques. (See the Glossary for the definition of *sanitize* and Chapter 2 for a discussion of the procedures to use.)

Reportable/Notifiable Conditions

The CDC designates infectious diseases that require notification of public health authorities in the United States at the national level. Additional conditions may be designated as needing to be reported to local and state public health authorities. (See https://ndc.services.cdc.gov/search-results-year.) Contact the local health department if there is a question about a condition on the list of reportable communicable diseases. If there are conflicting opinions from different health professionals about the management of a child with a reportable communicable disease, the health department has the legal authority to make a final determination.

Although laboratories and health professionals are expected to report these notifiable diseases, their reporting may not alert health authorities that the child attends an ECE program or is enrolled in school and may have exposed others. Delayed notification may preclude prompt responses to prevent illness among those exposed to the child in the ECE or school setting. If in doubt about whether to report, contact the local health department.

Generally, a designated staff member should contact the local health department and discuss what to do with a CCHC under the following circumstances:

- When a child or staff member has a reportable disease

- If a reportable illness occurs among staff members, children, or families involved with the program
- For assistance in managing a suspected outbreak (**Note:** Generally, an outbreak is considered to be 2 or more unrelated [ie, not siblings or members of the same household] children with the same diagnosis or symptoms in the same group within 1 week. Clusters of mild respiratory illness and ear infections are common and generally do not need to be reported.)

Designated staff members (eg, the program's Child Care Health Advocate) should work with a CCHC to develop policies and procedures for alerting staff members and families about their responsibility to report illnesses to the program and for the program to report diseases to the local health authorities. A Sample Letter to Families About Exposure to Communicable Disease is in Chapter 8.

Preparing for Managing Illness

Staff members should
- Prepare families for inevitable illnesses ahead of time, including having backup child care.
- At the time of enrollment and as necessary thereafter, review with families the inclusion/exclusion criteria in the facility's written policies (eg, before

influenza season). Make clear to family members that designated program staff members (not families) make the final decision about whether children who are ill may stay. Such decisions will be based on inclusion/exclusion criteria and staff ability to care for the child who is ill without compromising the care of other children in the program.
- Develop, with a CCHC, protocols and procedures for handling children's illnesses, including care plans and an inclusion/exclusion policy.
- Rely on the family's description of the child's behavior to determine whether the child is well enough to return, unless the child's status is unclear from the family's report. Only ask for a pediatric health professional's note to readmit a child if the health professional's advice is needed to determine whether the child is a health risk to others or the health professional's guidance is needed about any special care the child requires. See the Signs and Symptoms Chart in Chapter 5 for specific recommendations about visits to pediatric health professionals.
- Encourage families to develop a plan for times when their child may need to stay home and to make sure their emergency contact information at the center remains up to date.

Signs
and
Symptoms
Chart

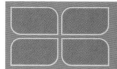

Signs and Symptoms Chart

The following chart lists, in alphabetical order, some of the most common signs and symptoms children in early childhood education (ECE) and school settings may develop when they have an infectious disease. Pediatric health professionals can use this chart to discuss with educators what signs and symptoms of illness require a health care visit. Educators can use this information to be aware of what might cause various signs and symptoms, when it is appropriate to notify the program's Child Care Health Consultant (if the program has one), when to notify the parent/legal guardian, and what criteria to use to determine when children should be excluded from and can return to an ECE program or school. Families should always be notified if a child is exhibiting signs or symptoms listed in the chart.

Note that the chart indicates when visits to a pediatric health professional are necessary. Not all children who are excluded from an ECE program or school require a visit to a pediatric health professional prior to return to care. However, if the educator is concerned about the nature of the child's specific illness

or needs instructions about how to care for the child, the child's parent/guardian can contact the child's health professional to ask for more information. The health professional may require further evaluation of the child to respond to this request. With parent/legal guardian consent, the child's health professional can give additional instructions to educators. Any form of communication is acceptable, including electronic or by phone. The Symptom Record Form (included in Chapter 8) can be used to gather and facilitate the transfer of symptoms and other useful information. The director, educator, or other staff member receiving the communication from the pediatric health professional should document in the child's record what is discussed with the health professional and any instructions the health professional gives. Children with special health care needs should have an individualized medical and emergency plan developed with a pediatric health professional that may list additional concerning symptoms or have extra instructions to meet their health care needs.

Signs and Symptoms Chart

Routine Exclusion Criteria Applicable to All Signs and Symptoms

- Child is unable to participate in program activities.
- Care would compromise staff's ability to care for other children.
- Child meets other exclusion criteria (see Chapter 4, "Call Emergency Medical Services [EMS] [911] Immediately If" and "Get Medical Attention Within 1 Hour" boxes and Conditions Requiring Temporary Exclusion section).

Sign or Symptom	Common Causes	Concerns or Symptoms	Notify Program's Health Consultant, If Program Has One	Notify Parent/Legal Guardian	Temporarily Exclude?	If Excluded, Readmit When
Cold Symptoms	*Viruses* • Adenovirus • Coronavirus (including SARS-CoV-2, the virus that causes COVID-19) • Enterovirus • Influenza virus • Parainfluenza virus • Respiratory syncytial virus (RSV) • Rhinovirus *Bacteria* • Mycoplasma • Pertussis	• Coughing • Hoarse voice, barky cough • Runny or stuffy nose • Scratchy throat • Sneezing • Fever • Watery and pink eyes	Not necessary unless epidemics occur (ie, RSV or vaccine-preventable disease like measles or varicella [chickenpox])	Yes	**No, unless** • Fever accompanied by behavior change. • Child looks or acts very ill. • Child has difficulty breathing. • Child has blood-red or purple rash not associated with injury. • Child meets routine exclusion criteria (see Conditions Requiring Temporary Exclusion in Chapter 4). • During the COVID-19 pandemic, refer to the Centers for Disease Control and Prevention (CDC) recommendations: https://www.cdc.gov/coronavirus/2019-ncov/community/schools-childcare/index.html.	Exclusion criteria are resolved.
Cough	• Common cold • COVID-19 • Lower respiratory infection (eg, pneumonia, bronchiolitis) • Croup • Asthma • Sinus infection • Bronchitis • Pertussis • Noninfectious causes like allergies	• Dry or wet cough. • Runny nose (clear, white, or yellow-green). • Sore throat. • Throat irritation. • Hoarse voice, barking cough. • Coughing fits. • Irritation in any part of the respiratory tract, from nose and mouth to lung tissue, can cause coughing.	Not necessary unless the cough is due to a vaccine-preventable disease, such as pertussis, which should be reported to the local public health department.	Yes	**No, unless** • Severe cough. • Rapid or difficult breathing. • Wheezing and not already evaluated and symptoms controlled by treatment. • Cyanosis (ie, blue color of skin or mucous membranes). • Pertussis is diagnosed and not yet treated. • Fever with behavior change. • Child meets routine exclusion criteria (see Conditions Requiring Temporary Exclusion in Chapter 4). • During the COVID-19 pandemic, refer to the CDC recommendations: https://www.cdc.gov/coronavirus/2019-ncov/community/schools-childcare/index.html.	Exclusion criteria are resolved.

▶continued

Sign or Symptom	Common Causes	Concerns or Symptoms	Notify Program's Health Consultant, If Program Has One	Notify Parent/ Legal Guardian	Temporarily Exclude?	If Excluded, Readmit When
Diaper Rash	• Irritation by rubbing of diaper material against skin wet with urine or stool • Infection with yeast or bacteria	• Redness • Scaling • Red bumps • Sores • Cracking of skin in diaper region	Not necessary	Yes	**No, unless** • Oozing sores that leak body fluids outside the diaper. • Child meets routine exclusion criteria (see Conditions Requiring Temporary Exclusion in Chapter 4).	Exclusion criteria are resolved.
Diarrhea	• Usually viral, less commonly bacterial or parasitic • COVID-19 • Noninfectious causes such as dietary (drinking too much juice), medications, inflammatory bowel disease, or cystic fibrosis	• Frequent loose or watery stools compared with child's normal pattern (Note that exclusively breastfed infants normally have frequent unformed and somewhat watery stools or may have several days with no stools.) • Abdominal cramps • Fever • Generally not feeling well • Vomiting occasionally present	**Yes, if** 1 or more cases of bloody diarrhea or 2 or more children or educators in same group experience diarrhea within a week	Yes	**Yes, if** • Directed by the local health department as part of outbreak management. • Stool is not contained in the diaper for diapered children. • Diarrhea is causing "accidents" for toilet-trained children. • Stool frequency exceeds 2 stools above normal for that child during the time the child is in the program because this may cause too much work for early childhood educators and make it difficult to maintain good sanitation. • Blood/mucus in stool. • Black stools. • No urine output in 8 hours. • Jaundice (ie, yellow skin or eyes). • Fever with behavior change. • Looks or acts very ill. • Child meets routine exclusion criteria (see Conditions Requiring Temporary Exclusion in Chapter 4). • During the COVID-19 pandemic, refer to the CDC recommendations: https://www.cdc.gov/coronavirus/2019-ncov/community/schools-childcare/index.html.	• Cleared to return by pediatric health professional for all cases of bloody diarrhea and diarrhea caused by Shiga toxin–producing *Escherichia coli*, *Shigella*, or *Salmonella* serotype Typhi until negative stool culture requirement has been met. • Diapered children have their stool contained by the diaper (even if the stools remain loose) and toilet-trained children do not have toileting accidents. • Stool frequency is no more than 2 stools above normal for that child during the time the child is in the program, or what has become normal for that child when the child seems otherwise well. • Exclusion criteria are resolved.

Signs and Symptoms Chart (*continued*)

Sign or Symptom	Common Causes	Concerns or Symptoms	Notify Program's Health Consultant, If Program Has One	Notify Parent/ Legal Guardian	Temporarily Exclude?	If Excluded, Readmit When
Difficult or Noisy Breathing	• Common cold • COVID-19 • Croup • Epiglottitis • Bronchiolitis • Asthma • Pneumonia • Object stuck in airway • Exposed to a known trigger of asthma symptoms (eg, animal dander, pollen)	• Common cold: stuffy/runny nose, sore throat, cough, or mild fever. • Croup: barking cough, hoarseness, fever, possible chest discomfort (symptoms worse at night), or very noisy breathing, especially when breathing in. • Epiglottitis: gasping noisily for breath with mouth wide open, chin pulled down, high fever, or bluish (cyanotic) nails and skin; drooling, unwilling to lie down. • Bronchiolitis and asthma: child is working hard to breathe; rapid breathing; space between ribs looks like it is sucked in with each breath (retractions); wheezing; whistling sound with breathing; cold/cough; irritable and unwell. Takes longer to breathe out than to breathe in. • Pneumonia: deep cough, fever, rapid breathing, or space between ribs looks like it is sucked in with each breath (retractions). • Object stuck in airway: symptoms similar to croup (listed previously). • Exposed to a known trigger of asthma symptoms and the child is experiencing breathing that sounds or looks different from normal for that child.	Not necessary except for epiglottitis	Yes	**Yes, if** • Fever with behavior change. • Child looks or acts very ill. • Child has difficulty breathing. • Rapid breathing. • Wheezing if not already evaluated and symptoms controlled by treatment. • Cyanosis (ie, blue color of skin or mucous membranes). • Cough interferes with activities. • Noisy, high-pitched breath sounds can be heard when the child is at rest (stridor). • Child has blood-red or purple rash not associated with injury. • Child meets routine exclusion criteria (see Conditions Requiring Temporary Exclusion in Chapter 4). • During the COVID-19 pandemic, refer to the CDC recommendations: https://www.cdc.gov/coronavirus/2019-ncov/community/schools-childcare/index.html. *Note:* Emergency care may be needed for some of the conditions herein (see Situations That Require Medical Attention Right Away in Chapter 4).	Exclusion criteria are resolved.

Sign or Symptom	Common Causes	Concerns or Symptoms	Notify Program's Health Consultant, If Program Has One	Notify Parent/ Legal Guardian	Temporarily Exclude?	If Excluded, Readmit When
Earache	• Viruses (common cold) followed by bacteria	• Fever • Pain or irritability • Difficulty hearing • "Blocked ears" • Drainage • Ear tugging or pulling in young children	Not necessary	Yes	**No, unless** child meets routine exclusion criteria (See Conditions Requiring Temporary Exclusion in Chapter 4.)	Exclusion criteria are resolved.
Eye Irritation, Pinkeye	• Bacterial infection of the membrane covering 1 or both eyes and eyelids (bacterial conjunctivitis) • Viral infection of the membrane covering 1 or both eyes and eyelids (viral conjunctivitis) • Allergic irritation of the membrane covering 1 or both eyes and eyelids (allergic conjunctivitis) • Chemical irritation of the membrane covering the eye and eyelid (irritant conjunctivitis) (eg, swimming in heavily chlorinated water, air pollution, smoke exposure)	• Bacterial infection: pink color of the "whites" of eyes and thick yellow/green discharge. Eyelid may be irritated, swollen, or crusted. • Viral infection: pinkish/red color of the whites of the eye; irritated, swollen eyelids; watery discharge with or without some crusting around the eyelids; may have associated cold symptoms. • Allergic and chemical irritation: red, painful, tearing, itchy, puffy eyelids; runny nose, sneezing; watery/stringy discharge with or without some crusting around the eyelids.	**Yes, if** 2 or more children have red eyes with watery discharge	Yes	*For bacterial conjunctivitis* **No.** Exclusion is not required for this condition. Pediatric health professionals may vary on whether to treat this condition with antibiotic medication. The role of antibiotics in treatment and preventing spread is unclear. Most children with pinkeye get better after 5 or 6 days without antibiotics. *For red eyes with intense pain* Refer to pediatric health professional. *For other eye problems* **No, unless** child meets other exclusion criteria (See Conditions Requiring Temporary Exclusion in Chapter 4.) *Note:* One type of viral conjunctivitis spreads rapidly and requires exclusion. If 2 or more children in the group have watery red eyes without any known chemical irritant exposure, exclusion may be required, and health authorities should be notified to determine if the situation involves the uncommon epidemic conjunctivitis caused by a specific type of adenovirus. Herpes simplex conjunctivitis (red eyes with blistering/vesicles on eyelid) occurs rarely and would also require exclusion if there is eye watering.	• *For bacterial conjunctivitis, once parent has discussed with pediatric health professional.* Antibiotics may or may not be prescribed. • Exclusion criteria are resolved.

▶ continued

Signs and Symptoms Chart (*continued*)

Sign or Symptom	Common Causes	Concerns or Symptoms	Notify Program's Health Consultant, If Program Has One	Notify Parent/Legal Guardian	Temporarily Exclude?	If Excluded, Readmit When
Fever	• Any viral, bacterial, or parasitic infection • Vigorous exercise • Reaction to medication or vaccine • Other noninfectious illnesses (eg, rheumatoid arthritis, malignancy)	Flushing, tired, irritable, decreased activity *Notes* • Fever alone is not harmful. When a child has an infection, raising the body temperature is part of the body's normal defense against germs. Children can have higher than normal temperatures if they are outside doing vigorous exercise. • Rapid elevation of body temperature sometimes triggers a febrile seizure in young children; this usually is outgrown by age 6 years. The first time a febrile seizure happens, the child requires medical evaluation. These seizures are frightening but are usually brief (less than 15 minutes) and do not cause the child any long-term harm. Parents should inform their child's health professional every time the child has a seizure, even if the child is known to have febrile seizures. **Warning:** *Do not give aspirin. It has been linked to an increased risk of Reye syndrome (a rare and serious disease affecting the brain and liver).*	Not necessary	Yes	**No, unless** • Behavior change or other signs of illness in addition to fever or child meets other routine exclusion criteria (see Conditions Requiring Temporary Exclusion in Chapter 4). • Child meets routine exclusion criteria (see Conditions Requiring Temporary Exclusion in Chapter 4). • During the COVID-19 pandemic, refer to the CDC recommendations: https://www.cdc.gov/coronavirus/2019-ncov/community/schools-childcare/index.html. *Note:* A temperature considered meaningfully elevated above normal, although not necessarily an indication of a significant health problem for infants and children older than 2 months, is above 101 °F (38.3 °C) from any site (axillary, temporal/forehead, oral, or rectal). *Get medical attention* when infants younger than 4 months have unexplained fever. In any infant younger than 2 months, a temperature above 100.4 °F (38.0 °C) is considered meaningfully elevated and requires that the infant get medical attention promptly, within 1 to 2 hours if possible. The fever is not harmful; however, the illness causing it may be serious in this age group.	Exclusion criteria are resolved.

Sign or Symptom	Common Causes	Concerns or Symptoms	Notify Program's Health Consultant, If Program Has One	Notify Parent/ Legal Guardian	Temporarily Exclude?	If Excluded, Readmit When
Headache, Stiff or Painful Neck	• Any bacterial/viral infection • Other noninfectious causes	• Tired and irritable • Can occur with or without other symptoms	Not necessary	**Yes**	**No, unless** child meets routine exclusion criteria (See Conditions Requiring Temporary Exclusion in Chapter 4.) *Note:* Notify pediatric health professional in the case of sudden, severe headache with fever, vomiting, or stiff neck that might signal meningitis. A stiff neck would be concerning if the back of the neck is painful or the child can't look at their belly button (putting chin to chest)—different from soreness in the side of the neck.	Exclusion criteria are resolved.
Itching	• Ringworm • Chickenpox • Pinworm • Head lice • Scabies • Allergic (hives) or irritant reaction (eg, poison ivy) • Dry skin or eczema • Impetigo	• Ringworm: itchy ring-shaped patches on skin or bald patches on scalp. • Chickenpox: blister-like spots surrounded by red halos on scalp, face, and body; fever; irritable. • Pinworm: anal itching. • Head lice: small insects or white egg sheaths that look like grains of sand (nits) in hair. • Scabies: severely itchy red bumps on warm areas of body, especially between fingers or toes. • Allergic or irritant reaction: raised (hives), circular, mobile rash; reddening of the skin; blisters occur with local reactions (poison ivy, contact reaction). • Dry skin or eczema: dry areas on body. More often worse on cheeks, in front of elbows, and behind knees. In infants, may be dry areas on face and anywhere on body but not usually in diaper area. If swollen, red, or oozing, think about infection.	**Yes, for** infestations such as lice and scabies; if more than 1 child in group has impetigo or ringworm; for chickenpox	**Yes**	*For chickenpox* **Yes, until lesions are fully crusted** *For ringworm, impetigo, scabies, and head lice* At the end of the day, the child should see a pediatric health professional and, if any of these conditions are confirmed, the child should start treatment before returning. If treatment is started before the next day, no exclusion is necessary. However, the child may be excluded until treatment has started. *For pinworm, allergic or irritant reactions like hives, and eczema* **No, unless** • Appears infected as a weeping or crusty sore. • There is a concern for food allergy when hives are accompanied by breathing difficulties (eg, wheezing, noisy breathing), severe irritability, explosive diarrhea, or vomiting within 15 to 30 minutes of food exposure.	• Exclusion criteria are resolved. • On medication or treated as recommended by a pediatric health professional if treatment is indicated for the condition.

▲ continued

Signs and Symptoms Chart (continued)

Sign or Symptom	Common Causes	Concerns or Symptoms	Notify Program's Health Consultant, If Program Has One	Notify Parent/Legal Guardian	Temporarily Exclude?	If Excluded, Readmit When
Itching (continued)		• Impetigo: areas of crusted yellow, oozing sores. Often around mouth or nasal openings or areas of broken skin (insect bites, scrapes).			*Note:* Although exclusion for these conditions is not necessary, families should seek advice from the child's health professional for how to care for these health problems. *For any other itching* **No, unless** the child meets routine exclusion criteria (See Conditions Requiring Temporary Exclusion in Chapter 4.)	
Mouth Sores	• Oral thrush (yeast infection) • Herpes or coxsackievirus infection • Canker sores	• Oral thrush: white patches on tongue, on gums, and along inner cheeks • Herpes or coxsackievirus infection: pain on swallowing; fever; painful, white/red spots in mouth; swollen lymph nodes (neck glands); fever blister, cold sore; reddened, swollen, painful lips • Canker sores: painful ulcers inside cheeks or on gums	Not necessary	Yes	**No, unless** • Drooling steadily related to mouth sores. • Fever with behavior change. • Child meets routine exclusion criteria (see Conditions Requiring Temporary Exclusion in Chapter 4).	Exclusion criteria are resolved.
Rash	Many causes • Viral: roseola infantum, fifth disease, chickenpox, herpesvirus, molluscum contagiosum, warts, cold sores, shingles (herpes zoster), and others • Skin infections and infestations: ringworm (fungus), scabies (parasite), impetigo, abscesses, and cellulitis (bacteria) • Scarlet fever (strep infection) • Severe bacterial infections: meningococcus, pneumococcus, *Staphylococcus* (methicillin-susceptible *S aureus*; methicillin-resistant *S aureus*), *Streptococcus*	• Skin may show similar findings with many different causes. Determining cause of rash requires a competent pediatric health professional evaluation that takes into account information other than just how rash looks. *However, if the child appears well other than the rash, a pediatric health professional visit is not necessary.* • Viral: usually signs of general illness such as runny nose, cough, and fever (except not for warts or molluscum). Some viral rashes have a distinctive appearance. • Minor skin infections and infestations: see Itching. • More serious skin infections: redness, pain, fever, pus.	For outbreaks, such as multiple children with impetigo within a group	Yes	**No, unless** • Rash with behavior change or fever. • Has oozing/open wound that can't be covered. • Has bruising not associated with injury. • Has joint pain and rash. • Rapidly spreading rash consisting of pinpoint round spots with reddish-purple color. • Tender, red area of skin, especially if it is increasing in size or tenderness. • Child meets routine exclusion criteria (see Conditions Requiring Temporary Exclusion in Chapter 4).	• On antibiotic medication for required period (if indicated). • Infestations (lice and scabies) and ringworm can be treated at the end of the day with immediate return the following day. • Exclusion criteria are resolved.

▶ continued

Sign or Symptom	Common Causes	Concerns or Symptoms	Notify Program's Health Consultant, If Program Has One	Notify Parent/ Legal Guardian	Temporarily Exclude?	If Excluded, Readmit When
Rash (*continued*)	• Noninfectious causes: allergy (hives), eczema, contact (irritant) dermatitis, medication related, poison ivy, vasculitis	• Severe bacterial infections: rare. These children usually have fever with a rapidly spreading blood-red rash and may be very ill. • Allergy may be associated with a raised, itchy, pink rash with bumps that can be as small as a pinpoint or large welts known as hives. See also Itching for what might be seen for allergy or contact (irritant) dermatitis or eczema. • Vasculitis rash can be itchy, with small or large red or purple spots that resemble bruises, sometimes with red puffy hands or feet.			• Diagnosed with a vaccine-preventable condition, such as chickenpox.	
Sore Throat (pharyngitis)	• Viral: common cold viruses that cause upper respiratory infections, including SARS-CoV-2, the virus that causes COVID-19 • Strep throat	• Viral: verbal children will complain of sore throat; younger children may be irritable with decreased appetite and increased drooling (refusal to swallow). Often see symptoms associated with upper respiratory illness, such as runny nose, cough, and congestion. • Strep throat: red tissue with white patches on sides of throat, at back of tongue (tonsil area), and at back wall of throat. Unlike viral pharyngitis, strep throat infections are *not* typically accompanied by cough or runny nose and usually occur in children older than 3 years. • Tonsils may be large, even touching each other. Swollen lymph nodes (sometimes called "swollen glands") occur as body fights off the infection.	Not necessary	Yes	**No, unless** • Inability to swallow. • Excessive drooling with breathing difficulty. • Fever with behavior change. • Child meets routine exclusion criteria (see Conditions Requiring Temporary Exclusion in Chapter 4). • During the COVID-19 pandemic, refer to the CDC recommendations: https://www.cdc.gov/coronavirus/2019-ncov/community/schools-childcare/index.html. *Note:* Most children with red back of throat or tonsils, pus on tonsils, or swollen lymph nodes have viral infections. If strep is present, 12 hours of antibiotics is required before return to care. Tests for strep infection are not usually necessary for children younger than 3 years because children younger than 3 years do not typically develop rheumatic heart disease—the primary reason for treatment of strep throat.	• Able to swallow. • If strep, on medication at least 12 hours. • Exclusion criteria are resolved.

Signs and Symptoms Chart (*continued*)

Sign or Symptom	Common Causes	Concerns or Symptoms	Notify Program's Health Consultant, If Program Has One	Notify Parent/ Legal Guardian	Temporarily Exclude?	If Excluded, Readmit When
Stomachache	• Viral gastroenteritis or strep throat • COVID-19 • Problems with internal organs of the abdomen such as stomach, intestine, colon, liver, spleen, or bladder • Nonspecific, behavioral, and dietary causes • If combined with hives, may be associated with a severe allergic reaction	• Viral gastroenteritis or strep throat: vomiting and diarrhea or cramping are signs of a viral infection of the stomach or intestine. Strep throat may cause stomachache with sore throat, headache, and possible fever (see Sore Throat). • Problems with internal organs of the abdomen: persistent severe pain in abdomen. • Nonspecific stomachache: vague complaints without vomiting/ diarrhea or much change in activity.	If multiple cases in same group within 1 week	Yes	**No, unless** • Severe pain causing child to double over or scream. • Abdominal pain after injury. • Bloody/black stools. • No urine output for 8 hours. • Diarrhea (see Diarrhea). • Vomiting (see Vomiting). • Yellow skin/eyes. • Fever with stomachache and/or behavior change. • Looks or acts very ill. • Child meets routine exclusion criteria (see Conditions Requiring Temporary Exclusion in Chapter 4). • During the COVID-19 pandemic, refer to the CDC recommendations: https://www.cdc.gov/coronavirus/2019-ncov/community/schools-childcare/index.html.	• Pain resolves. • Exclusion criteria are resolved.
Swollen Glands (properly called swollen lymph nodes)	• Viruses: normal body defense response to viral infection in the area where lymph nodes are located (ie, in the neck for any upper respiratory infection). • Bacteria: lymph nodes may be enlarging, one-sided, and painful.	• Normal lymph node response: swelling at front, sides, and back of the neck and ear; in the armpit or groin; or anywhere else near an area of an infection. Usually, these nodes are less than 1" across. • Bacterial infection of lymph nodes: swollen, warm lumps under the skin with overlying pink skin, tender to the touch, usually located near an area of the body that has been infected. Usually, these nodes are larger than 1" across.	Not necessary	Yes	**No, unless** • Difficulty breathing or swallowing. • Red, tender, warm glands. • Fever with behavior change. • Child meets routine exclusion criteria (see Conditions Requiring Temporary Exclusion in Chapter 4).	• Child is on antibiotics (if indicated). • Exclusion criteria are resolved.
Urinating Frequently, Unusually Having Urine Accidents	• Urinary infection • Irritation of urogenital tissues by chemicals such as bubble bath	Wet underclothing, uncomfortable while sitting, pulling at underclothing	Not necessary	Yes	No	Exclusion criteria are resolved.

Sign or Symptom	Common Causes	Concerns or Symptoms	Notify Program's Health Consultant, If Program Has One	Notify Parent/ Legal Guardian	Temporarily Exclude?	If Excluded, Readmit When
Vomiting	• Viral infection of the stomach or intestine (gastroenteritis), including COVID-19 • Coughing strongly • Other viral illness with fever • Noninfectious causes: food allergy (vomiting, sometimes with hives), trauma, ingestion of toxic substance, dietary and medication related, headache	Diarrhea, vomiting, or cramping for viral gastroenteritis	For outbreak	Yes	**Yes, if** • Vomited more than 2 times in 24 hours • Vomiting and fever • Vomiting with hives • Vomit that appears green/bloody • No urine output in 8 hours • Recent history of head injury • Looks or acts very ill • Child meets routine exclusion criteria (See Conditions Requiring Temporary Exclusion in Chapter 4.) • During the COVID-19 pandemic, refer to the CDC recommendations: https://www.cdc.gov/coronavirus/2019-ncov/community/schools-childcare/index.html.	• Vomiting ends. • Exclusion criteria are resolved.

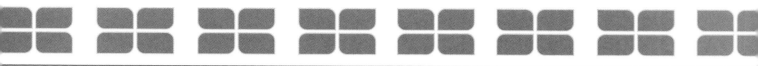

CHAPTER 6

Quick
Reference
Sheets

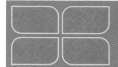

Quick Reference Sheets

This chapter contains a series of Quick Reference Sheets about some of the infections and infestations that commonly occur in children in early childhood education (ECE) and school settings. The Quick Reference Sheets are arranged in alphabetical order according to what the conditions and diseases are commonly called, not necessarily their scientific names (eg, chickenpox instead of varicella zoster).

Each sheet contains information about common signs and symptoms, incubation and contagious periods, spread, infection control, the role of the parent or educator, exclusion criteria, and return-to-care criteria. Copy these Quick Reference Sheets to facilitate communication among parents, educators, and pediatric health professionals. No permission is necessary to make single copies for noncommercial, educational purposes.

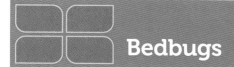

Bedbugs

What are bedbugs?

These are small insects that feed on human blood by biting through the skin. Bedbugs are most active between 2:00 and 5:00 am. They can travel 10 to 15 feet to feed and go without feeding for up to 6 months. Their bites may look like a small rash and are itchy. Bedbugs are not known to transmit or spread any disease. Bedbugs are not commonly found in early childhood education (ECE) and school settings because the conditions that promote the most activity occur at night when people are sleeping. But they can "hitchhike" on clothing and backpacks from a child's home into the educational setting.

What are the signs or symptoms?

- Bites typically occur on exposed skin, such as the face, neck, arms, and hands. These are itchy bites, which often occur in a row, on areas of skin that are exposed during the night.
- Bites often have a red dot where the bite occurred in the middle of a raised red bump.
- Look for specks of blood, rusty spots from crushed bugs, or dung spots the size of a pen point on bedsheets and mattresses or behind loose wallpaper.
- Look for reddish/brown live bugs, about ⅛ of an inch, in crevices or seams of bedding.

What are the incubation and contagious periods?

- Bedbugs do not reproduce on humans like scabies or lice. They bite humans at night and then hide in cracks or crevices on mattresses, cushions, or bed frames during the day.
- Children or staff members may bring bedbugs to school in book bags and outer garments and clothes.

How are they spread?

- Bedbugs are not spread from one person to another. They are not an indication that people or their homes are dirty. They may hide in belongings or clothing that allows them to spread to others in ECE and school settings.
- These insects crawl at the speed of a ladybug.

How do you control them?

- Avoid overreacting. One bedbug is not an infestation. It is not necessary to send the child home. Do not throw anything away. Nap mats and mattresses can be cleaned.
- Bedbugs in ECE and school settings are almost always "hitchhikers" brought from home and usually do not represent a problem at the program.
- Educate staff members and families about bedbugs.
- Reduce clutter and limit items that travel back and forth between homes and the facility.
- Clean up any bedbug debris with detergent and water.
- Seal cracks and crevices to eliminate hiding places for bedbugs and other pests. Caulk and paint wooden baseboards or molding around ceilings.
- Separate the backpack and coat of one child from those of another child to avoid cross contamination.
- Provide enough space between coat hooks so each child's belongings do not touch those of another child.
- Empty and clean cubbies, lockers, and child storage areas at least once every season.
- Inspect the nap area regularly (preferably by a trained pest control operator). Use a flashlight to examine nap mats, mattresses (especially seams), bedding, cribs, and other furniture in the area.
- In the unlikely event bedbugs are identified in the facility, contact a professional exterminator. Extermination involves vacuuming and one of the following approaches: application of the least toxic (preferably "bio-based") products, heating the living area to 122 °F (50 °C) for about 90 minutes, freezing infested articles, or (if necessary) use of synthetic chemical insecticides. Use integrated pest management, which involves a combination of nonchemical strategies, such as maintenance and sanitation, followed by pesticides, if other methods are not effective, but avoiding sprays of toxic chemicals that pollute the air, water, and land.
- Laundering bedding and clothing (hot water and hot drying cycle for 30–60 minutes), vacuuming cracks and crevices (in furniture, equipment, walls, and floors), and freezing smaller articles that may have been used as hiding places for bedbugs may reduce infestation until extermination can be performed. Dispose of the vacuum cleaner filter and bags in a tightly sealed plastic bag.
- Use encasements/covers around the mattress, box spring, and pillows to trap bedbugs. These encasements/covers are readily available by searching the internet for "mattress or pillow encasement." They are marketed for bedbug or allergy control.

What are the roles of the educator and the family?

- Usually, the educator will not know which children with insect bites have been bitten by bedbugs because they are hard to distinguish from other insect bites.
- Children with bedbug bites are not infested and so do not require treatment to prevent spread to others.
- Fingernails should be kept short to avoid damaging and infecting the skin due to itching. Observe for signs of skin infection, such as boils, abscesses, or cellulitis (see Boil/Abscess/Cellulitis Quick Reference Sheet).
- Affected children may receive steroid skin creams or oral antihistamines to relieve the itch.

Exclude from educational setting?

No.

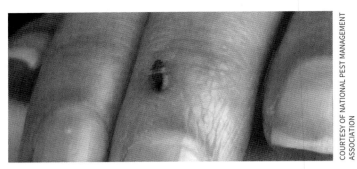

Bedbug

COURTESY OF NATIONAL PEST MANAGEMENT ASSOCIATION

Comments

- Unlike lice or scabies, bedbugs do not infest or require treatment of that person. Bedbugs infest the living area and require extermination. Bedbugs are most active at night and are attracted to heat and exhaled carbon dioxide.
- Good resources for identifying and controlling bedbugs are the US Environmental Protection Agency (www.epa.gov/bedbugs, https://www.epa.gov/ipm/bed-bugs-and-schools) and the New York City Department of Health and Mental Hygiene (www.nyc.gov/bedbugs).

American Academy of Pediatrics

DEDICATED TO THE HEALTH OF ALL CHILDREN®

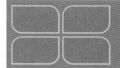

Bites (Human and Animal)

Human Bites

Biting is very common among young children but usually does not lead to serious infectious disease issues. If the skin is broken, bacteria introduced into the wound can cause a tissue infection that needs to be treated by a health professional. Blood-borne diseases could be a concern if the biter breaks the skin and blood is drawn into the biter's mouth or if the biter has bleeding gums or mouth sores, which transfers germs to the bitten person. Hepatitis B virus, HIV, and hepatitis C virus are examples of blood-borne disease-causing germs. However, the risk of transmission of these viruses is very low in early childhood education (ECE) and school settings. For HIV, there have not been any episodes of transmission in an ECE or school setting.

What are the roles of the educator and the family?

- Provide first aid to the child who was bitten by washing any broken skin and applying a cold compress to any bruise.
- Notify the parent/guardian of the biter and of the bitten child, if possible without identifying the biter to the family of the child who was bitten or the child who was bitten to the family of the biter.
- Recommend a pediatric health professional visit if the skin is broken because, in some cases, preventive antibiotics may be indicated.
- Initially focus on the injured child, rather than on the child who did the biting. Later, try to determine why the biting happened. Biting may occur when a child is excited, frustrated, or angry. See if future biting situations can be prevented by identifying what may cause these behaviors and avoiding them, distracting the child before biting occurs, or offering alternative activities. Suggest the child use words to express frustration or anger. Offer a harmless, vigorous physical activity the child can do when frustrated or angry. If the biting behavior of a child is repetitive despite 3 or 4 weeks of using these suggested measures, consider seeking additional professional help to develop an effective management plan. Consult the program's mental health consultant and your Child Care Health Consultant (if your program has one) or the child's health professional. Use the following resources:
  - Play Nicely, a free video for parents and EC educators about how to handle aggressive behavior in young children (www.playnicely.org).
  - Head Start Early Childhood Learning & Knowledge Center fact sheet about addressing biting (https://eclkc.ohs.acf.hhs.gov/mental-health/article/biting-fact-sheet-families)
  - Early Childhood Education Linkage System (ECELS)–Healthy Child Care Pennsylvania of the Pennsylvania Chapter of the American Academy of Pediatrics (https://ecels-healthychildcarepa.org). Search for "biting" and "challenging behavior" to locate resources. The ECELS materials may be used at no cost. Pennsylvania EC educators may pay a fee to have ECELS staff review their responses to the self-learning module assessment questions and obtain state-authorized training credits for using the self-learning module.

Exclude from educational setting?

No, unless the bite caused broken skin or prolonged bleeding, which may require treatment by a pediatric health professional, or the child who was bitten or the child who bit the other child is unable to participate and staff members determine they cannot care for the child without compromising their ability to care for the health and safety of the other children in the group.

Readmit to educational setting?

Yes, when all the following criteria are met:

When the child is able to participate and staff members determine they can care for the child without compromising their ability to care for the health and safety of the other children in the group

Animal Bites/Rabies

Animal bites are common. Dog bites account for 85% to 90% of bite wounds, perhaps because dogs are very common pets and have a great deal of contact with humans. Many adults allow interactions between children and dogs. Children can behave unpredictably, and dogs have normal protective instincts. The combination can result in injuries for children. The rate of infection after dog bites is 5% to 20%. After cat bites, the rate of infection is as high as 80%. (See Infections Caused by Interactions of Humans With Pets and Wild Animals in Chapter 8 for a discussion of diseases spread by cats, including "cute" kittens.)

An animal bite that breaks or punctures the skin needs immediate wound care to reduce the risk of infection. The wound should be washed out with water and then promptly evaluated by a health professional for the following reasons:

- First, there is a chance of developing a bacterial infection. The longer the animal's mouth germs stay in the wound, the greater the potential of infection that will need antibiotics. Some wounds require preventive antibiotics. The health professional needs to decide whether the wound should be left open or closed with materials such as special tape or stitches. All animal bites need to be watched closely for signs of infection until they are fully healed.
- Second, the situation in which the animal bite occurred should be evaluated for the possibility of transmission of rabies. Although any mammal bite can transmit rabies, bites of some wild animals (eg, bats, raccoons, skunks, foxes, coyotes, bobcats) and some stray and unvaccinated pet dogs and cats are of greatest concern for transmitting the rabies virus. Wild animals should not be kept or allowed to visit ECE or school facilities. Children should not have direct contact with wild animals in any setting. Rodents (mice, squirrels, and gerbils) and rabbits can, but rarely do, carry rabies (woodchucks are an exception). Rabies has occurred in animals in petting zoos, pet stores, animal shelters, and county fairs.

Rabies is a very serious viral infection that infects the nervous system. The virus spreads from a rabies-infected animal's saliva into the bite site. Rabies is usually transmitted by the bite of wild animals. However, the virus can be spread by unimmunized pets and, in rare cases, immunized pets that have been infected with the rabies virus. The possibility that an animal is infected with rabies is greatest when the animal is unimmunized and the bite was unprovoked. If a pet or wild animal bites and breaks the skin, the situation requires urgent medical attention. Because the rabies virus spreads from the animal's saliva and enters the bite site, the bite wound should be immediately and thoroughly cleaned as soon as possible. The bitten person should be referred for immediate evaluation by a health professional. If possible, the animal should be observed by a veterinarian for signs of rabies.

Report all suspected exposure to rabies promptly to public health authorities and be sure health professionals are involved in deciding about appropriate treatment right away. Signs or symptoms of rabies in humans include anxiety, difficulty swallowing, seizures, and paralysis. Once signs or symptoms develop, rabies is nearly always a fatal disease.

How do you control rabies?

- By immunizing dogs and cats with rabies vaccination

- By avoiding contact with wild or stray animals, particularly those acting peculiarly or aggressively
- By not allowing children to touch dead animals

What are the roles of the educator and the family?

- Provide first aid by washing any broken skin and applying a cold compress to any bruise.
- Teach children to avoid contact with stray, wild, or dead animals.
- Make sure any animal in a child's environment is healthy and a suitable pet for children, fully immunized, and on a flea-, tick-, and worm-control program (when appropriate). If a pet is on-site at the ECE facility, a certificate from a veterinarian indicating the pet meets this list of conditions and how long the certificate is valid should be on file.
- All contact between animals and children should be supervised by an educator.
- Contact a health professional if
  - A child or an adult is bitten by a pet or an unknown or wild animal.
  - There is redness, swelling, drainage, or pain at the site of the bite.
  - The skin is broken.
  - A bat is found in a room with sleeping children or if children have touched a bat. Bat bites are not easily detected.
- If you can do so safely, capture or confine the animal for an evaluation. If you cannot make the animal available for evaluation, note the size, appearance, and any distinguishing characteristics of the animal (eg, if it was wearing a collar; if so, if it had tags).
- If there is a chance a person has been exposed to rabies, arrange for urgent medical attention.

Exclude from educational setting?

No, unless the child is unable to participate and staff members determine they cannot care for the child without compromising their ability to care for the health and safety of the other children in the group.

Readmit to educational setting?

Yes, when all the following criteria are met:

When the child is able to participate and staff members determine they can care for the child without compromising their ability to care for the health and safety of the other children in the group

American Academy of Pediatrics

DEDICATED TO THE HEALTH OF ALL CHILDREN®

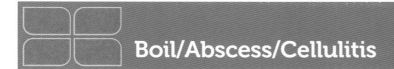

Boil/Abscess/Cellulitis

What are boils, abscesses, and cellulitis?

These are bacterial infections of the skin that usually begin from a scratch or bug bite and may progress to a red nodule that fills with pus. *Boils* are superficial infections with a thin layer of skin over fluid. *Abscesses* are generally larger and deeper with redness and painful swelling over an area filled with pus. *Cellulitis* is an infection within the skin and the area just beneath it; the skin is red and tender to touch. The area of cellulitis can spread quickly.

What are the signs or symptoms?

Abscesses and boils tend to be softer in the middle over the fluid or pus than at the edges. They may drain when the skin over the infected area opens and lets the fluid or pus out. Signs of cellulitis include areas of redness and skin tenderness. The skin over these infections is usually warmer than the surrounding normal areas of skin because of the body's reaction to the infection.

What are the incubation and contagious periods?

The incubation period is unknown. Common skin bacteria (staphylococcus and streptococcus) are usually the cause of boils/abscesses/cellulitis. These bacteria are present on the skin of most children and usually do not cause a problem. However, skin bacteria may cause infection when there is a break in the skin or the bacterial infection overpowers normal defenses against infection. Having a methicillin-resistant *Staphylococcus aureus* (MRSA) skin infection is no more serious than other staphylococcal skin infections (see also *Staphylococcus aureus* [Methicillin-Resistant (MRSA) and Methicillin-Sensitive (MSSA)] Quick Reference Sheet). Regardless of the bacteria, these skin infections are contagious when the infected area is open and draining. People who carry the bacteria in their noses and throats and on their skin may pass the bacteria on to others. However, for a skin infection to occur, the bacteria must get through a break in the skin.

How is it spread?

Person-to-person contact with pus and skin bacteria and, to a lesser extent, contaminated environmental surfaces and objects

How do you control it?

- Use good hand-hygiene technique at all the times listed in Chapter 2.
- Any skin condition that may cause skin breaks, such as eczema, is a risk factor for having a skin infection and passing this on to others. Educators with eczema on their hands should practice good eczema control. They should ask their health professional how to prevent dry or cracked skin while continuing to perform required frequent hand hygiene. Also, they should ask whether they need to wear gloves during activities that involve touching the skin of the children. For children who have eczema, use a care plan that involves the child's family and pediatric health professional to control this skin condition.
- Cover lesions if they are draining.
- Culturing children who do not have infections to determine if they harbor MRSA in their noses or throats or on their skin is not indicated.
- Infected children may need antibiotic treatment for tissue infections. Small abscesses may be surgically drained without antibiotics. If antibiotics are prescribed, they should be given according to the pediatric health professional's instructions on the prescription label.
- If more than one child in the program experiences skin infections that require surgical drainage or antibiotics, contact the Child Care Health Consultant or local health department.

What are the roles of the educator and the family?

- Use good hand hygiene technique at all the times listed in Chapter 2.
- Also practice good hand hygiene after changing bandages or dressings. Practice Standard Precautions.

Exclude from educational setting?

No, unless
- The child is unable to participate and staff members determine they cannot care for the child without compromising their ability to care for the health and safety of the other children in the group.
- The child meets other exclusion criteria (see Conditions Requiring Temporary Exclusion in Chapter 4).

• A draining lesion cannot be covered, or the covering cannot be maintained because the drainage comes through the covering to contaminate other surfaces.

Readmit to educational setting?

Yes, when all the following criteria are met:

When exclusion criteria are resolved, the child is able to participate, and staff members determine they can care for the child without compromising their ability to care for the health and safety of the other children in the group

Comments

• Having a MRSA infection, or harboring MRSA bacteria (carrier), is not a reason for exclusion.
• Occasionally, multiple people within a family or ECE setting may become recurrently infected with boils/abscesses. This may be due to *S aureus* (MRSA or other types).
• Using nasal antibiotic ointment and special cleansers (chlorhexidine or bleach in bathwater) may reduce repeated staphylococcal infections within families. However, reexposure can occur in the community because staphylococcus commonly lives on the skin and in the noses of noninfected (colonized) individuals. This treatment should only be done under the guidance of a health professional.

American Academy of Pediatrics

DEDICATED TO THE HEALTH OF ALL CHILDREN®

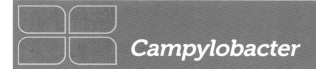

Campylobacter

What is *Campylobacter*?

A type of bacteria that can cause infection of the intestines

What are the signs or symptoms?

- Diarrhea (often bloody)
- Fever
- Vomiting
- Abdominal cramping
- Malaise

What are the incubation and contagious periods?

- Incubation period: 2 to 5 days but can be longer.
- Contagious period: Excretion of *Campylobacter* is shortened by antibiotic treatment. Without treatment, excretion of bacteria typically continues for 2 to 3 weeks (and up to 7 weeks in some cases) and relapse of symptoms may occur.

How is it spread?

- Contact with stool from infected birds, farm animals (eg, chickens, turkeys), or pets (eg, dogs, cats, hamsters, birds—especially young animals).
- Contaminated water.
- Unpasteurized milk.
- Contaminated food (eg, raw or undercooked poultry).
- Person-to-person via the fecal-oral route occurs occasionally, particularly from very young children (most likely during the diarrhea phase). This generally involves an infected child contaminating their own fingers and then touching an object that another child touches. The child who touched the contaminated surface then puts their fingers into their own mouth or another person's mouth.

How do you control it?

- Use good hand-hygiene technique at all the times listed in Chapter 2, especially after toilet use or handling soiled diapers, and particularly before and after contact with raw poultry or dog or cat feces and anything to do with food preparation or eating.
- Ensure proper surface disinfection that includes cleaning and rinsing of surfaces that may have become contaminated with stool (feces) with detergent and water and application of a US Environmental Protection Agency–registered disinfectant according to the instructions on the product label.

- Ensure proper cooking and storage of food.
- Exclude infected staff members who handle food.
- Cook poultry thoroughly.
- Use antibiotics as prescribed.
- Exclude for specific types of symptoms (see the section Exclude from educational setting?).

What are the roles of the educator and the family?

- A child or staff member with *Campylobacter* may have bloody diarrhea, which should trigger a medical evaluation.
- There are multiple causes of bloody diarrhea. Until the cause of the diarrhea is identified, apply the recommendations for a child or staff member with diarrhea from any cause (see Diarrhea Quick Reference Sheet).
  – Report the condition to the staff member designated by the early childhood education program or school for decision-making and action related to care of ill children or staff members. That person, in turn, alerts possibly exposed family and staff members to watch for symptoms and notifies the Child Care Health Consultant.
  – Ensure staff members follow the control measures listed in the section How do you control it?
  – Report outbreaks of diarrhea (more than 2 children and/or staff members in the group) to the Child Care Health Consultant, who may report to the local health department.
- If you know a child or staff member in the program has *Campylobacter*
  – Follow the advice of the child's or staff member's health professional.
  – Report the infection to the local health department, as the health professional who makes the diagnosis may not report that the infected child is a participant in an early childhood education program or school. This could lead to loss of precious time for controlling the spread of the disease.
  – Reeducate staff members about strict and frequent handwashing, diapering, toileting, food handling, and cleaning and disinfection procedures.
  – In an outbreak, follow the directions of the local health department.
    - Avoid milk that is not pasteurized and water that is not chlorinated.
    - Do not allow a staff member with diarrhea to be involved with food handling or feeding of children.

Exclude from educational setting?

Yes, if

- The local health department determines exclusion is needed to control an outbreak.
- Stool is not contained in the diaper for diapered children.
- Diarrhea is causing "accidents" for toilet-trained children.
- Stool frequency exceeds 2 stools above normal for that child during the time the child is in the program because this may cause too much work for educators and make it difficult for them to maintain sanitary conditions.
- There is blood or mucus in stool.
- The child has a dry mouth, no tears, or no urine output in 8 hours (suggesting the child's diarrhea may be causing dehydration).
- The child is unable to participate and staff members determine they cannot care for the child without compromising their ability to care for the health and safety of the other children in the group.
- The child meets other exclusion criteria (see Conditions Requiring Temporary Exclusion in Chapter 4).

Readmit to educational setting?

Yes, when all the following criteria are met:

- Once diapered children have their stool contained by the diaper (even if the stools remain loose) and when toilet-trained children do not have toileting accidents
- Once stool frequency is no more than 2 stools above normal for that child during the time the child is in the program, even if the stools remain loose
- When the child is able to participate and staff members determine they can care for the child without compromising their ability to care for the health and safety of the other children in the group

Note: It is not necessary to demonstrate negative *Campylobacter* stool culture test results to be readmitted to the educational setting.

Comment

Outbreaks are possible, but uncommon, in educational settings.

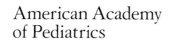

American Academy of Pediatrics

DEDICATED TO THE HEALTH OF ALL CHILDREN®

Single copies of this Quick Reference Sheet may be made for noncommercial, educational purposes. The information contained in this publication should not be used as a substitute for the medical care and advice of a pediatric health professional. There may be variations in treatment that a pediatric health professional may recommend based on individual facts and circumstances.

The American Academy of Pediatrics is an organization of 67,000 primary care pediatricians, pediatric medical subspecialists, and pediatric surgical specialists dedicated to the health, safety, and well-being of all infants, children, adolescents, and young adults.

American Academy of Pediatrics website—www.HealthyChildren.org   © 2023 American Academy of Pediatrics. All rights reserved.

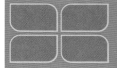

Chickenpox (Varicella-Zoster Infections)

What is chickenpox?

An illness with rash and fever caused by the varicella-zoster virus

What are the signs or symptoms?

* Rash (ie, small red spots and bumps developing into very small fluid-filled sacs on the skin [vesicles] over 3–4 days and then forming scabs or "crusts").
* Discrete groupings ("crops") of vesicles will come out over several days. Someone who has chickenpox for more than a day will have some red bumps, vesicles, and scabbed-over vesicles all at the same time.
* Rash may appear inside mouth, ears, genital areas, and scalp.
* The rash is usually quite itchy.
* Fever, runny nose, cough.

What are the incubation and contagious periods?

* Incubation period: Usually 14 to 16 days; occasionally as short as 10 days and as long as 21 days after contact.
* Contagious period: Chickenpox is highly contagious to people who have not previously been vaccinated or had the disease. The most contagious period is while the rash is spreading; a child may also be contagious 1 to 2 days before the rash appears. An infected person no longer spreads the virus when all the vesicles have scabs or crusts and no new skin vesicles are forming.
* Although uncommon, a previously immunized person can have a mild form of chickenpox, which is contagious.

How is it spread?

* Contact with the skin vesicles of someone with chicken pox or an uncovered shingles rash (see Shingles [Herpes Zoster] Quick Reference Sheet).
* Airborne route: Inhalation of virus that becomes airborne after fluid escapes from inside the vesicles or breathing small particles containing virus floating in the air. The particles come from the vesicles or a child's respiratory secretions as droplets after a cough or sneeze. These germ-containing particles dry out quickly in the air or fall onto surfaces. After drying out and attaching to dust particles, they can become suspended in the air again. The particles travel along air currents and can infect people in the same or another room. Even brief exposure or

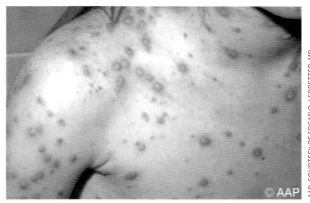

Child with chickenpox rash

AAP, COURTESY OF EDGAR O. LEDBETTER, MD

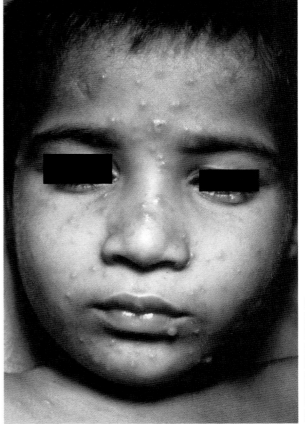

Varicella lesions on the face of a 4-year-old

AAP, COURTESY OF PAUL WEHRLE, MD

shared airflow poses a high risk of infection for people who have not had the disease before, have not been protected by the chickenpox vaccine, or have a problem with their immune system.

How do you control it?

- Chickenpox is a vaccine-preventable infection. Immunize according to the current recommendations—when a child is 12 to 15 months of age and with a second dose at 4 to 6 years of age.
- Vaccinate older children, teens, and adults who are susceptible (ie, those who have not received 2 doses of vaccine or who have not had the natural infection—the occurrence of a natural infection will need to be determined by a health professional).
- Exclude infected children and educators until entire rash is crusted over.
- Use good surface-sanitation technique and good hand-hygiene technique at all the times listed in Chapter 2.
- Ventilate room air with fresh outdoor air.
- Children with chickenpox who are mildly ill and able to come to a program that cares for ill children require a room with separate ventilation with exhaust to and air exchange with the outside.

What are the roles of the educator and the family?

- Report the infection to the staff member designated by the early childhood education (ECE) program or school for decision-making and action related to care of ill children. That person, in turn, alerts possibly exposed family and staff members and the parents of unvaccinated children to watch for symptoms and notifies the Child Care Health Consultant.
- Report the infection to the local health department. The health professional who makes the diagnosis may not report that the infected child is a participant in an ECE program or school, and this could lead to a delay in controlling the spread.
- Specifically notify all adults (staff and volunteers) and families of children who have not had chickenpox or 2 doses of the chickenpox vaccine to contact their health professionals. Within 24 hours of exposure, be sure to advise those who might be pregnant or have a problem with their immune system to check with their health professionals about what to do. Pregnant women who have previously had chickenpox infection or vaccination should not have a pregnancy-related problem if exposed to chickenpox. However, pregnant women should be encouraged to confirm their protection with their own health professionals. Adults and children need 2 doses of chickenpox vaccine for full protection.

- Use good hand-hygiene technique at all the times listed in Chapter 2 and after any contact with soiled articles or skin vesicles.
- Do not give aspirin to ill children, as it may increase their risk of contracting Reye syndrome, a serious complication associated with the use of aspirin in someone infected with chickenpox and other viral illnesses (eg, influenza).

Exclude from educational setting?

Yes. Chickenpox is a highly communicable illness for which routine exclusion of infected children is warranted. See the Comments section for information about shingles, vaccine-related chickenpox, and chickenpox in previously vaccinated children.

Readmit to educational setting?

Yes, when all the following criteria are met:
- When all vesicles have scabs (usually 6 days after start of rash) or, in immunized children who have a mild infection with no crusts, once no new red bumps have appeared for at least 24 hours
- When the child is able to participate and staff members determine they can care for the child without compromising their ability to care for the health and safety of the other children in the group

Comments

- Initial chickenpox infections in adults can be extremely serious and may result in death.
- The chickenpox virus stays for a lifetime in an inactive form in the body's nerve cells. Shingles (herpes zoster) occurs when someone has fully recovered from chickenpox and, later, the inactive virus in their body's nerve cells becomes active (see Shingles [Herpes Zoster] Quick Reference Sheet).
- Rash from varicella vaccination can occur in 3% to 5% of children 5 to 26 days after vaccination. This condition is mild and causes a few red bumps at or near the injection site or very widely scattered bumps over the entire body. Bumps near the injection site may be covered with a nonporous bandage and clothing, and the child may continue to participate. In a child with a more widespread rash, the child might have been exposed to natural chickenpox and become infected before the vaccine had time to work. A pediatric health professional should decide when a child with a widespread rash can continue to participate in an ECE program or school.

- Rarely, children get chickenpox a second time. These cases usually are very mild with less fever and fewer bumps and blisters than the first time. However, these children are still contagious and should not come to an educational setting until the vesicles scab over.
- It is possible for children to get chickenpox despite being vaccinated. The first dose of this vaccine is about 85% effective at preventing mild chickenpox and 97% effective at preventing severe chickenpox. Two doses of vaccine are recommended and are much more effective than 1 in preventing infection. Chickenpox in previously immunized children is usually mild with less fever and fewer bumps and vesicles than in unimmunized children. These children are contagious and should stay home until the vesicles scab over and no new lesions have appeared in 24 hours.

American Academy of Pediatrics

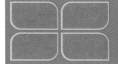

Clostridioides difficile (Formerly Known as *Clostridium difficile*; Also Called "C diff")

What is *Clostridioides difficile*?

- Spore- and toxin-forming bacteria that cause diarrhea
- Often associated with recent antibiotic use

What are the signs or symptoms?

- Usually the illness is mild and causes
  - Non-bloody diarrhea
  - Mild abdominal pain
  - Low-grade fever
- Rarely, more severe illness occurs, especially in immunocompromised children, and causes
  - High fever
  - Abdominal cramps
  - Very ill appearance
  - Very bloated abdomen
  - Occasional blood in the stool
- In children younger than 5 years (especially infants), *Clostridioides difficile* bacteria or protein toxin may be detected in the stool, yet the child has no symptoms. It is unclear why so many children harbor the bacteria but do not become ill.

What are the incubation and contagious periods?

- Incubation period: Unknown. Illness can occur 5 days to 10 weeks after antibiotic therapy.
- Contagious period: Unknown because infants can harbor the bacteria and not cause illness in themselves or others.

How is it spread?

- Fecal-oral route: Contact with feces of children who are infected. This generally involves an infected child contaminating their own fingers and then touching an object that another child touches. The child who touched the contaminated surface then puts their fingers into their own mouth or another person's mouth.
- *C difficile* spores are also present in soil and the environment.

How do you control it?

- Use good hand-hygiene technique at all the times listed in Chapter 2, especially after toilet use or handling soiled diapers and before anything to do with food preparation or eating. Alcohol-based sanitizers are not effective in killing *C difficile* spores. Soap and water will wash away the spores.
- Ensure proper surface disinfection that includes cleaning and rinsing of surfaces that may have become contaminated with stool (feces) with detergent and water and application of a US Environmental Protection Agency–registered disinfectant according to the instructions on the product label.
- Exclude infected staff members who handle food.
- Exclusion for specific types of symptoms (see the section Exclude from educational setting?).

What are the roles of the educator and the family?

- A child or staff member with *C difficile* may have bloody diarrhea, which should trigger a medical evaluation.
- There are multiple causes of bloody diarrhea. The following recommendations apply for a child or staff member with diarrhea from any cause (see Diarrhea Quick Reference Sheet):
  - Report the condition to the staff member designated by the early childhood education program or school for decision-making and action related to care of ill children or staff members. That person, in turn, alerts possibly exposed family and staff members to watch for symptoms and notifies the Child Care Health Consultant.
  - Ensure staff members follow the control measures listed in the section How do you control it?
  - Report outbreaks of diarrhea (more than 2 children and/or staff members in the group) to the Child Care Health Consultant, who may report to the local health department.
- If you know a child or staff member in the program has *C difficile*
  - Follow the advice of the child's or staff member's health professional.
  - Report the infection to the local health department, as the health professional who makes the diagnosis may not report that the infected child is a participant in an early childhood education program or school, and this could lead to delay in controlling the spread of the disease.
  - Reeducate staff members to ensure strict and frequent handwashing, diapering, toileting, food handling, and cleaning and disinfection procedures.
  - In an outbreak, follow the direction of the local health department.

Note: *C difficile* spores will not be killed by alcohol-based hand sanitizers. Soap and water is more effective. Using gloves is also an effective means of preventing spread, although they are not required.

Exclude from educational setting?

Yes, if

- The local health department determines exclusion is needed to control an outbreak.
- Stool is not contained in the diaper for diapered children.
- Diarrhea is causing "accidents" for toilet-trained children.
- Stool frequency exceeds 2 stools above normal for that child during the time the child is in the program because this may cause too much work for educators and make it difficult for them to maintain sanitary conditions.
- There is blood or mucus in stool.
- The ill child's stool is all black.
- The child has a dry mouth, no tears, or no urine output in 8 hours (suggesting the child's diarrhea may be causing dehydration).
- The child is unable to participate and staff members determine they cannot care for the child without compromising their ability to care for the health and safety of the other children in the group.
- The child meets other exclusion criteria (see Conditions Requiring Temporary Exclusion in Chapter 4).

Readmit to educational setting?

Yes, when all the following criteria are met:

- Once diapered children have their stool contained by the diaper (even if the stools remain loose) and when toilet-trained children do not have toileting accidents
- Once stool frequency is no more than 2 stools above normal for that child during the time the child is in the program, even if the stools remain loose
- When the child is able to participate and staff members determine they can care for the child without compromising their ability to care for the health and safety of the other children in the group

Note: It is not necessary to demonstrate negative *C difficile* stool test results to be readmitted to the educational setting. *C difficile* is caused by antibiotic use; however, it is treated with a different antibiotic than the one that caused the infection.

American Academy of Pediatrics

DEDICATED TO THE HEALTH OF ALL CHILDREN®

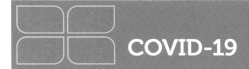

COVID-19

What is COVID-19?

A contagious disease caused by a respiratory virus called SARS-CoV-2

What are the signs or symptoms?

Some children who are infected with COVID-19 have no symptoms. If symptoms are present, they are usually mild.

- Fever or chills
- Cough
- Shortness of breath or difficulty breathing
- Fatigue
- Muscle or body aches
- Headache
- New loss of taste or smell
- Sore throat
- Nasal congestion or runny nose
- Nausea or vomiting
- Diarrhea

What are the incubation and contagious periods?

- Incubation period: 2 to 14 days, with a mean of 2 to 4 days
- Contagious period: From 2 days before signs or symptoms appear until 10 days after the onset of symptoms. Vaccination may shorten the contagious period.

How is it spread?

- Respiratory (droplet) route: Contact with large droplets that form when a child talks, coughs, sneezes, or sings. These droplets can land on or be rubbed into the eyes, nose, or mouth. The droplets do not stay in the air; they usually travel no more than 3 feet and fall onto the ground. This is the most common mode of spread of SARS-CoV-2.
- Airborne route: Breathing small particles containing virus floating in the air. These particles first come from a child's respiratory secretions as droplets after a cough or sneeze. These germ-containing particles dry out quickly in the air or fall onto surfaces and then dry out and attach to dust particles, which become suspended again in the air. These particles travel along air currents and can infect people more than 3 feet apart in the same or in another room. This is a mode of spread of SARS-CoV-2, although room-to-room transmission has not been proven

in early childhood education (ECE) programs or schools.
- Contact route: Thought to be the least common route of spread of SARS-CoV-2, the virus is spread when children carrying the virus contaminate surfaces or objects with their respiratory or oral secretions. Other children can then become infected after touching these contaminated surfaces or objects and then putting their fingers in their own mouth, eyes, or nose.

How do you control it?

- Follow the latest Centers for Disease Control and Prevention (CDC) recommendations, "Operational Guidance for K-12 Schools and Early Care and Education Programs to Support Safe In-Person Learning," available at https://www.cdc.gov/coronavirus/2019-ncov/community/schools-childcare/k-12-childcare-guidance.html.
- Routinely check that children complete the COVID-19 vaccine series according to the most recent immunization recommendations at www.cdc.gov/vaccines.
- Use good hand-hygiene technique at all the times listed in Chapter 2.
- Prevent contact with respiratory secretions. Teach children and educators to practice respiratory etiquette (covering mouth when coughing or sneezing by using facial tissue or upper sleeve or elbow). Teach everyone to remove any mucus or debris on skin or other surfaces and perform hand hygiene right after using facial tissues or having contact with mucus.
- Dispose of facial tissues that contain nasal secretions after each use.
- Perform hand hygiene after contact with any soiled items.
- Mask children 2 years and older if indicated by high local case counts or health department or state/tribal regulations or in the setting of an outbreak.
- Reduce crowding as much as possible.
- Increase ventilation by opening windows. Working with a ventilation consultant can optimize ventilation systems because healthy indoor air can help reduce the risk of spreading viral infections. More information about working with a ventilation consultant is available from the Head Start Early Childhood Learning & Knowledge Center at https://eclkc.ohs.acf.hhs.gov/publication/tips-working-ventilation-consultant.

- Increase outdoor time for class, play, or eating, staff and weather permitting.
- Create a cohort (prevent mixing of people into different rooms) of children and staff members by rooms as much as possible.

What are the roles of the educator and the family?

- Ensure all adults that come in contact with children at home and in the ECE program and school are fully immunized against COVID-19, especially all educators, because prior to immunizations being available, spread most commonly occurred from an infected adult to a child.
- Follow the latest COVID-19 guidance from the CDC and your state and local health department.

Exclude from educational setting?

Yes, if

- The child is unable to participate and staff members determine they cannot care for the child without compromising their ability to care for the health and safety of the other children in the group.
- The child meets other exclusion criteria (see Conditions Requiring Temporary Exclusion in Chapter 4)—specifically, the child has fever and behavior change or fever with other signs or symptoms of respiratory illness like cough, sore throat, sneeze, or runny nose.
- Your state or local health department recommends exclusion for managing high case counts or in the setting of an outbreak.
- Recommended by the CDC ("Operational Guidance for K-12 Schools and Early Care and Education Programs to Support Safe In-Person Learning," available at https://www.cdc.gov/coronavirus/2019-ncov/community/schools-childcare/k-12-childcare-guidance.html).

Readmit to educational setting?

Yes, when all the following criteria are met:

When exclusion criteria are resolved, fever has been absent for 24 hours without fever-reducing medicines, the child is able to participate, and staff members determine they can care for the child without compromising their ability to care for the health and safety of the other children in the group

Comments

- Note that SARS-CoV-2 mutates frequently, changing the predominant symptoms, contagious period, and effectiveness of immunizations. Please check the website for this book (www.aap.org/midupdates), the CDC (https://www.cdc.gov/coronavirus/2019-ncov/community/schools-childcare/index.html), and *Caring for Our Children* (https://nrckids.org/CFOC) for the latest updates.
- In general, research shows that COVID-19 does not spread rapidly or widely in ECE programs or schools compared with homes. This is in contrast to influenza and respiratory syncytial virus infections, for which ECE programs and schools are the primary drivers of the spread of infection into the community.
- Child-to-child, child-to-adult, adult-to-adult, and adult-to-child spread have all been documented in ECE programs and schools.
- COVID-19 can be a serious disease that causes complications, like myocarditis (inflammation of the heart tissue) and multisystem inflammatory syndrome of childhood (a condition in which multiple body parts become inflamed). Children with COVID-19 in the United States may need to be hospitalized and can die.
- Follow the latest immunization recommendations (https://www.cdc.gov/vaccines/hcp/acip-recs/index.html) and ensure that all eligible people (children and staff) are immunized against COVID-19.
- The role of testing to diagnose children with COVID-like symptoms and to determine when children can return to care continues to evolve based on available science. See the latest recommendations by the CDC, "Operational Guidance for K-12 Schools and Early Care and Education Programs to Support Safe In-Person Learning," at https://www.cdc.gov/coronavirus/2019-ncov/community/schools-childcare/k-12-childcare-guidance.html.
- Masking has been shown to reduce COVID-19 transmission in school-aged children. National survey studies of child care professionals suggest that masking of children 2 years and older has been associated with fewer ECE program closures (https://pubmed.ncbi.nlm.nih.gov/35084484). Masking has a role in reducing transmission when community transmission is high.

American Academy of Pediatrics

DEDICATED TO THE HEALTH OF ALL CHILDREN®

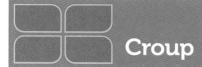

Croup

What is croup?

A respiratory illness primarily affecting infants and children 6 months to 3 years of age caused by multiple different viruses and characterized by a hoarse voice and barky cough. The symptoms of croup are caused by the primary area of infection, which is the larynx, commonly known as the voice box, and the trachea, commonly known as the windpipe. Parainfluenza viruses are the most common cause of croup; however, many other viruses (ie, respiratory syncytial virus, measles, influenza, rhinoviruses, COVID-19, and enteroviruses) may sometimes cause croup.

What are the signs or symptoms?

- Barky cough (like a seal).
- Hoarse or whispery voice.
- Noisy breathing on inspiration (breathing in) called *stridor.*
- Runny nose.
- Fever may be present.
- Occasionally, children with croup may develop respiratory distress, which can be a medical emergency. This distress may include labored and noisy breathing, sucking in of the skin above and between the ribs, flaring of the nostrils, exaggerated motion of the abdomen with breathing, and anxiousness. Children with these symptoms require urgent medical attention, need to be treated in the emergency department, and may need to be hospitalized.

What are the incubation and contagious periods?

- Incubation period: 2 to 6 days for most parainfluenza viruses but may vary for other viruses.
- Contagious period: As with most respiratory viruses, viruses that cause croup can be spread for 1 week or longer.

How is it spread?

- Respiratory (droplet) route: Contact with large droplets that form when a child talks, coughs, or sneezes. These droplets can land on or be rubbed into the eyes, nose, or mouth. The droplets do not stay in the air; they usually travel no more than 3 feet and fall onto the ground.
- Contact with the respiratory secretions from or objects contaminated by children who carry respiratory viruses.

How do you control it?

- Use good hand-hygiene technique at all the times listed in Chapter 2.
- Prevent contact with respiratory secretions. Teach children and educators to cover their noses and mouths when sneezing or coughing with a disposable facial tissue, if possible, or with an upper sleeve or elbow if no facial tissue is available in time. Teach everyone to remove any mucus or debris on skin or other surfaces and perform hand hygiene right after using facial tissues or having contact with mucus to prevent the spread of disease by contaminated hands. Change or cover clothing with mucus on it.
- Dispose of facial tissues that contain nasal secretions after each use.
- Ensure immunizations are up to date for all children. This may reduce croup caused by measles or influenza.

What are the roles of the educator and the family?

- Observe the child for signs of respiratory distress such as labored and noisy breathing, sucking in of the skin above and between the ribs, flaring of the nostrils, exaggerated motion of the abdomen with breathing, and anxiousness. Try to keep the child calm because being upset and crying can worsen the cough and work of breathing. Cold, moist air can decrease swelling and noisy breathing, so if the temperature outside is cold, dress the child warmly and then go outside. If these symptoms persist longer than 10 minutes, call emergency medical services (EMS) (911).
- Report the infection to the staff member designated by the early childhood education program or school for decision-making and action related to care of ill children. That person, in turn, alerts possibly exposed family and staff members to watch for symptoms of respiratory virus infection. The viruses that can cause croup may cause other respiratory symptoms.
- Practice control measures at home and educational settings.

Exclude from educational setting?

No, unless

- Child exhibits respiratory distress as described previously. (Call EMS [911].)
- The child is unable to participate and staff members determine they cannot care for the child without compromising their ability to care for the health and safety of the other children in the group.
- The child meets other exclusion criteria (see Conditions Requiring Temporary Exclusion in Chapter 4).

Readmit to educational setting?

Yes, when all the following criteria are met:

When exclusion criteria are resolved, the child is able to participate, and staff members determine they can care for the child without compromising their ability to care for the health and safety of the other children in the group

Comment

A child who develops high-pitched breath sounds (stridor) caused by a narrowed airway or respiratory distress may be treated with steroids. As long as the symptoms of stridor or respiratory distress have resolved, the child may return to care.

American Academy
of Pediatrics

DEDICATED TO THE HEALTH OF ALL CHILDREN®

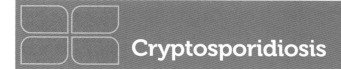

Cryptosporidiosis

What is cryptosporidiosis?

An intestinal infection caused by a parasite (*Cryptosporidium hominis* or *Cryptosporidium parvum*)

What are the signs or symptoms?

- Acute watery diarrhea.
- Fever.
- Vomiting.
- Abdominal cramps.
- Fatigue.
- Lack of appetite.
- Many individuals are infected and infectious without signs or symptoms.
- Illness may last 1 to 20 days (average of 10 days) in normal children; can last much longer in immuno-compromised children.

What are the incubation and contagious periods?

- Incubation period: 7 days is average but can vary from 3 to 14 days.
- Contagious period: Passage of the parasite in the stool can occur for 2 weeks after symptoms have resolved.

How is it spread?

- Fecal-oral route: Contact with feces of children who are infected. This generally involves an infected child contaminating their own fingers and then playing in communal water (during water play) or touching an object that another child touches. The child who has contact with the communal water or touched the contaminated surface then puts their fingers into their own mouth or another person's mouth. About 2% to 4% of children without symptoms in ECE settings pass *Cryptosporidium* oocysts (eggs; the infectious form of the parasite) in their stools.
- Most commonly spread through contaminated swimming or wading water or other water used for recreation by more than one person. Young children commonly let some fecal material escape into the water while they are playing. The largest outbreaks of waterborne disease occur in the summer months and involve children who are younger than 5 years. Contaminated municipal water supplies can cause outbreaks too.

- The parasite is resistant to chlorine, which is commonly used to prevent infections from water used for swimming. For this reason, *Cryptosporidium* is the leading cause of treated recreational water–associated outbreaks of diarrhea. *Cryptosporidium* oocysts that spread diarrheal disease can remain infectious for more than 10 days in chlorine concentrations typically required for swimming pools.
- Outbreaks can occur in early childhood education (ECE) settings and are thought to be spread person-to-person at high rates, as well as from contaminated water sources.
- The parasite can be transmitted from animals in petting zoos and contaminated feces on farms and in the wild.

How do you control it?

- Use good hand-hygiene technique at all the times listed in Chapter 2, especially after toilet use or handling soiled diapers and before anything to do with food preparation or eating.
- Ensure proper surface disinfection that includes cleaning and rinsing of surfaces that may have become contaminated with stool (feces) with detergent and water and application of a US Environmental Protection Agency–registered disinfectant according to the instructions on the product label.
- Ensure proper cooking and storage of food.
- Exclude infected staff members who handle food.
- Exclusion for specific types of symptoms (see the section Exclude from educational setting?).
- Children with *Cryptosporidium* diarrhea should not participate in water play activities for 2 weeks after diarrhea has resolved.
- Use a combination of water disinfection and proper pool maintenance. For children younger than 8 years, consider restricting communal water play to water contact above the waist (eg, water table). or limiting play in a body of water that involves getting wet below the waist to one person before the water is replaced by fresh water (eg, a portable wading pool). Advise swimmers and waders to use the toilet before using recreational water to reduce the likelihood they will release feces into the water. Encourage recreational water users to shower before and after use and avoid swallowing the water. Some recreational pools have a routine call at 2-hour intervals for children younger than 8 years to leave the pool for a toilet break.

What are the roles of the educator and the family?

- Usually, educators will not know a child has crypto-sporidiosis because the condition is not distinguishable from other common forms of watery diarrhea. So, the following recommendations apply for a child with diarrhea from any cause (see Diarrhea Quick Reference Sheet):
  - Report the condition to the staff member designated by the ECE program or school for decision-making and action related to care of ill children or staff members. That person, in turn, alerts possibly exposed family and staff members to watch for symptoms and notifies the Child Care Health Consultant.
  - Ensure staff members follow the control measures listed in the section How do you control it?
  - Report outbreaks of diarrhea (more than 2 children and/or staff members in the group) to the Child Care Health Consultant, who may report to the local health department.
- If a child has a known cryptosporidiosis infection
  - Follow the advice of the child's or staff member's health professional.
  - Report the infection to the local health department, as the health professional who makes the diagnosis may not report that the infected child is a participant in an ECE program or school, and this could lead to loss of precious time for controlling the spread of the disease. In an outbreak, follow the directions of the local health department.
  - Reeducate staff members about strict and frequent handwashing, diapering, toileting, food handling, and cleaning and disinfection procedures.
  - In an outbreak, follow the directions of the local health department.

Exclude from educational setting?

Yes, if

- The local health department determines exclusion is needed to control an outbreak.
- The child is unable to participate and staff members determine they cannot care for the child without compromising their ability to care for the health and safety of the other children in the group.
- Stool is not contained in the diaper for diapered children.
- Diarrhea is causing "accidents" for toilet-trained children.
- Stool frequency exceeds 2 stools above normal for that child during the time the child is in the program because this may cause too much work for educators and make it difficult for them to maintain sanitary conditions.
- There is blood or mucus in stool.
- The child has a dry mouth, no tears, or no urine output in 8 hours (suggesting the child's diarrhea may be causing dehydration).

Note: For educators and children without symptoms (ie, recently recovered or exposed), testing stool cultures, treatment, and exclusion are not necessary.

Readmit to educational setting?

Yes, when all the following criteria are met:

- Once diapered children have their stool contained by the diaper (even if the stools remain loose) and when toilet-trained children do not have toileting accidents
- Once stool frequency is no more than 2 stools above normal for that child during the time the child is in the program, even if the stools remain loose
- When the child is able to participate and staff members determine they can care for the child without compromising their ability to care for the health and safety of the other children in the group

Note: It is not necessary to demonstrate negative *Cryptosporidium* stool test results to be readmitted to the educational setting.

American Academy of Pediatrics

DEDICATED TO THE HEALTH OF ALL CHILDREN®

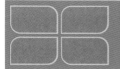

Cytomegalovirus (CMV) Infection

What is cytomegalovirus infection?

A very common viral infection in children

What are the signs or symptoms?

- Generally, no symptoms occur in young children.
- Older children and adults may have a generalized illness with fever. Sometimes the liver or spleen may become enlarged.
- Cytomegalovirus (CMV) infection of a pregnant mother's fetus can be very harmful.

What are the incubation and contagious periods?

Probably several weeks to months. Once a person is infected, the virus is shed intermittently in the saliva and urine for the rest of that person's life. Up to 70% and usually 30% to 40% of normal children aged 1 to 3 years in early childhood education (ECE) settings excrete CMV in their saliva and urine, respectively. Nearly everyone is infected with CMV during their lifetime.

How is it spread?

- Person-to-person contact with blood, saliva, urine, human (breast) milk, and other secretions from infected people
- Mother to baby before, during, and after birth
- Blood transfusions from an infected person
- During kissing and sexual activities

How do you control it?

- Attention to proper hand-hygiene technique at all the times listed in Chapter 2. This is especially important for women of childbearing age who work with young children or whose young children are enrolled in ECE settings. Avoid exchange of saliva directly or via objects (eg, moistening a pacifier with the mouth), and wash hands and objects carefully after contact with urine.
- Do not kiss children on the lips or allow them to put their fingers or hands in another person's mouth.
- Do not share cups or eating utensils.

What are the roles of the educator and the family?

- Use good hand-hygiene technique at all the times listed in Chapter 2.
- Review Standard Precautions, particularly hand hygiene, especially for women of childbearing age who work with or have their own children younger than 3 years who participate in educational settings.
- Women of childbearing age who have any contact with groups of children or have their own children younger than 3 years who participate in ECE settings should discuss their risk of CMV exposure with their health professionals. Although most women are already immune to some strains of CMV, the potential consequences to the fetus exposed to a strain of CMV to which the mother is not immune can be very serious. Risk-reduction measures include conscientious handwashing. Staff members who care for children may consider taking care of older children or working in an administrative role during pregnancy. Programs should inform these women about the risk to their fetus if they become pregnant, urge them to discuss this risk with their health professional, and have them sign a document indicating their understanding of this risk. (See Letter to Staff About Occupational Health Risks and Staff Health Assessment Form in Chapter 8.)

Exclude from educational setting?

No, unless
- The child is unable to participate and staff members determine they cannot care for the child without compromising their ability to care for the health and safety of the other children in the group.
- The child meets other exclusion criteria (see Conditions Requiring Temporary Exclusion in Chapter 4).

Readmit to educational setting?

Yes, when all the following criteria are met:

When exclusion criteria are resolved, the child is able to participate, and staff members determine they can care for the child without compromising their ability to care for the health and safety of the other children in the group

Comments

- Cytomegalovirus is the most common viral infection that babies are born with, affecting 0.5% to 1.0% of all births. Most infected newborns do not have any illness or disability. However, 10% to 20% of infected newborns have sensorineural hearing loss, developmental disabilities, cerebral palsy, or vision disturbances.
- The risk of CMV exposure is greatest in settings in which children who are younger than 3 years are cared for. It must be assumed that exposure to the virus among children and caregivers will occur. Hand hygiene substantially reduces but does not eliminate the spread of infection because young children have frequent runny noses, drool on and mouth objects, touch many surfaces, and need diapering or toileting assistance.
- Because this virus is so common in ECE settings, exclusion of a CMV-infected child to reduce disease transmission has no benefit. Testing young children for excretion of the virus or performing CMV antibody tests for young children because they are in an ECE setting is not appropriate because infection with the virus is so prevalent.
- Cytomegalovirus exposure risk during pregnancy: Although most adults have their first CMV infection during childhood and are immune to the strains of CMV that have infected them, a pregnant woman who works with infants and toddlers or who is a mother with a child in an ECE program is at increased risk of having a CMV infection during her pregnancy and infecting her fetus. This could be her first CMV infection or an infection with a different strain of CMV than she previously experienced.

To alert health professionals responsible for the health assessment of staff members of childbearing age about the need of their patient to be counseled about CMV risk, ECE program directors/administrators should be sure CMV risk assessment and counseling are items on the staff health assessment form. In addition, it may be helpful for directors/administrators to attach this Quick Reference Sheet and the Fifth Disease (Human Parvovirus B19) Quick Reference Sheet to the note in the box below to help health professionals review with their patient the increased risk of exposure to the fetus if the woman is infected during her pregnancy. Health professionals are not necessarily aware of the increased exposure to these viruses for women who work with young children in ECE programs.

Dear Health Professional:

Your patient works in a setting where she has contact with young children in groups. Human parvovirus B19 and cytomegalovirus (CMV) occur commonly and are often asymptomatic among young children. Exposure of a woman who lacks immunity to human parvovirus B19 and/or CMV during pregnancy poses some risk to her fetus. Please discuss with your patient her childbearing intentions and whether she might want to consider the following risk-reduction measures when she might become pregnant:

- Conscientious handwashing after any contact with saliva, urine, or blood
- Care of children who are older than 3 years
- Working in a role other than direct care of young children

About Serologic Testing

Because different strains of CMV circulate among young children, especially those in early childhood education programs, a serologic test for CMV informs about risk but does not completely guarantee immunity from exposure to novel strains. However, a serologic test for human parvovirus B19 is a reliable indicator of immunity.

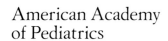

American Academy of Pediatrics

DEDICATED TO THE HEALTH OF ALL CHILDREN®

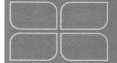

Dental Caries (Early Childhood Caries, Tooth Decay, or Cavities)

What is early childhood caries?

Early childhood caries (tooth decay, which leads to cavities) is the most common chronic infectious disease of childhood. Tooth decay is an infectious disease process that damages tooth structure and eventually makes holes (cavities) in the teeth. The consequence of early childhood tooth decay is more than unattractive teeth. Early childhood caries can cause severe pain, speech difficulty, and poor nutrition and interfere with sleep. It can start serious infections elsewhere in the body, such as the brain, lungs or heart. Treatment for tooth decay can require expensive dental services. These services in young children often require general anesthesia and treatment in an operating room. Dental caries is nearly entirely preventable.

The caries process begins when plaque builds up on teeth, usually because of poor toothbrushing habits and inappropriate nutrition. Plaque is a sticky substance produced by bacteria that live near the gumline of the teeth. Children become infected sometime early in life with the bacteria that can cause caries. Adults and other children can transfer bacteria to an infant or child's mouth. The bacteria in plaque break down sugars in the food and beverages given to children. As the bacteria break down the sugars, they produce acids that can damage the hard surface of teeth, called *enamel*. After consuming a sugary food or drink, it can take up to 40 minutes for the saliva to neutralize the acid environment in the mouth to return to safe levels.

What are the signs or symptoms?

Caries begins as a change in color of the tooth, indicating acid is starting to break down the hard enamel surface. Usually, the first changes are white spots at the gumline on the upper front teeth. Without special equipment, these spots are hard to see at first, even for a physician or dentist. If a child with early signs of tooth decay is not treated, the damage will continue. Next, the tooth starts to look yellow, brown, or black in the area where decay of the tooth is happening. If the process is not stopped, the whole tooth can be eaten away by the acid. The tooth and gum area may become painful. The child may be left with only a broken-off stub of tooth in the gum. A serious infection of the root of the tooth, gum, and jawbone can occur, with the risk of further complications. Because the enamel in primary teeth is thinner than the enamel in permanent teeth, this whole process can take place in just a few months.

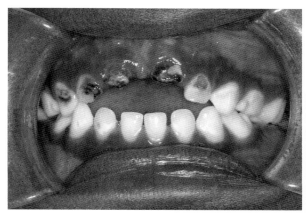

ROCIO B. QUINONEZ, DMD, MS, MPH

Child with dental caries

How is it spread?

The bacteria that cause caries are transmitted by seemingly innocent acts of sharing objects that enter the mouth. For example, the bacteria can be spread by sharing a cup, moistening a pacifier or cleaning it off in a person's mouth before giving it to a baby, pretasting food, sharing spoons and toothbrushes that involves transfer of saliva, and, less commonly, kissing on the mouth.

How do you control it?

To prevent early childhood caries, focus on 5 measures.

1. Start toothbrushing with fluoridated toothpaste once the first teeth erupt.
2. Harden the enamel with appropriate intake of and exposure to fluoride.
3. Limit total juice consumption (diluted or undiluted) per 24 hours as follows: Infants younger than 1 year: avoid giving any juice, unless medically indicated; children 1 to 3 years of age, no more than 4 ounces; children 4 to 6 years of age, no more than 6 ounces; children 7 to 18 years of age, no more than 8 ounces. Other sugary beverages should be avoided in all age-groups. Have the child drink water after eating and after drinking juice to minimize the exposure of the teeth to acid.
4. Any juice consumed should be limited to what the child drinks in a single sitting. Do not let the child carry around a beverage during the day or sleep with it during naps or nighttime. Juice should not be sipped from any cup, including a sippy cup, or sucked on from a bottle over a prolonged period.
5. Teach children to drink from a cup as soon as they are ready to learn how to do it, usually by 1 year of age.

What are the roles of the educator and the family?

- Take care of your own teeth. Early childhood educators should brush their teeth 2 times a day, preferably after the first meal of the day and before bed. Be a good role model for children.
- Practice good oral health for the children.
  - Brush children's teeth at least 2 times a day, preferably after a meal and before bed.
  - Teach and practice toothbrushing in early childhood education settings. If brushing with toothpaste occurs at home twice a day, toothpaste may not be required at the program. However, because many families do not accomplish twice-daily toothbrushing at home, do not assume it is occurring.
  - Infants without teeth do not need any gum care. There is no strong evidence that wiping gums with a cloth is of any benefit.
  - After a child's first tooth comes in, twice-daily toothbrushing can begin.
    - ❖ Children younger than 3 years should use a smear of toothpaste the equivalent of a grain of rice.
    - ❖ At 3 years of age, children should start to use a pea-sized amount of fluoridated toothpaste.
  - Encourage all children to spit after brushing. Many will not be able to do this consistently until about 8 years of age. It is safe for them to swallow this amount of fluoride toothpaste without spitting it out.
  - Children will need supervision and assistance with toothbrushing until 8 years of age. Educators should have clean hands when assisting a child with toothbrushing. The most important areas to clean are at the gumline and in all the spots that can trap food. That is why the inter-tooth surfaces need to be flossed to remove food from these spaces.
- The first dental visit should occur within 6 months after the first tooth comes through the gum. This is an ideal time for planning when and how to do toothbrushing and for the first application of fluoride varnish. Checking the child's teeth should also be part of routine preventive health care provided by the child's health professional. Children with special health care needs should be seen by a dentist as soon as the first tooth comes in and every 3 to 6 months thereafter to keep their teeth in good condition.
- Practices that may help reduce the risk of caries
  - Do not taste an infant's heated cereal (or other foods) for safe temperature and then use the same spoon to feed the infant.
  - Put any child-mouthed toy out of reach and clean it before another child has a chance to mouth it.
  - Encourage staff and families to be sure adults and children have oral health examinations every 6 months to reduce the concentration of caries-causing bacteria on their teeth—and, possibly, the ability of caries-causing bacteria to do damage to their teeth.
  - Limit snacking, meals, milk, and beverages other than water to planned times that are spread at least 2 to 3 hours apart rather than allowing grazing on food and sugar-containing fluids (eg, milk, juice) throughout the day. Infants younger than 1 year should not be offered juice.
  - Avoid sweet or sticky foods as snacks. When sticky foods are part of the menu, try to follow up with something crunchy, like an apple or some celery.
  - Avoid letting children repeatedly sip from a bottle, sippy cup, or another container any drinks, except water. Bottle propping or allowing children to drink from a bottle while napping causes prolonged contact of sugars on the teeth and promotes caries. Drinking water is always a good idea after eating, as it may rinse off some food or drink substance from the surface of teeth.

Exclude from educational setting?

No.

Comment

The American Academy of Pediatrics recommends that all infants receive oral health risk assessments by their pediatric health professional beginning at 6 months of age. They should also be referred to a dentist if they do not have one established, especially those at high risk for dental caries (eg, history of caries, limited-income status, lack of fluoride in the water). There is strong evidence that fluoride reduces caries. Children are very seldom able to spit out the toothpaste after brushing and usually swallow it. The use of a smear of toothpaste (an amount equivalent to a grain of rice) for brushing in early childhood is not harmful even if swallowed. There is evidence that fluoride in excess of the recommendations above at an early age may cause white staining or pitting of the teeth (fluorosis). Most children with fluorosis have a mild cosmetic problem but experience no other harm. Application of fluoride varnish by pediatric health professionals or dentists to children's teeth every 3 to 6 months is now recommended for all children. Fluoride varnish does not cause fluorosis.

American Academy of Pediatrics

DEDICATED TO THE HEALTH OF ALL CHILDREN®

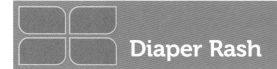

Diaper Rash

What is diaper rash?

Red and irritated skin in the diaper area. There are many causes. The most common are fungal, irritant contact, and seborrheic dermatitis.

- Fungal diaper rash is caused by a yeast called *Candida albicans*. It can happen naturally or commonly during or after a course of antibiotics.
- Irritant contact dermatitis is caused by skin rubbing against a wet, soiled diaper.
- Seborrheic dermatitis does not have a clear cause but may also be due to a fungus called *Malassezia*.

What are the signs or symptoms?

- Redness in the diaper area.
- Fungal
  - Rash is worse in the skinfolds (creases) within the diaper area.
  - Redness often bordered by red pimples ("satellite lesions").
  - Rash may have a shiny appearance.
  - Sores or cracking or oozing skin present in severe cases.
- Irritant contact
  - The rash spares the creases and emphasizes areas in contact with the diaper (inner thighs, genital areas, and buttocks).
  - Absence of satellite lesions.
- Seborrheic
  - Red, greasy scales in diaper area. May also be located on scalp, face, ears, and neck.

What are the incubation and contagious periods?

- Incubation period for fungal diaper rash: Unknown.
- Contagious period: The yeast that infects the diaper area is widespread in the environment, normally lives on the skin, and is found in the mouth and stool. *Candida* diaper rash may occur with or following antibiotic use. Repetitive or severe *Candida* diaper rash could signal immune problems.

How is it spread?

- Yeast.
  - *C albicans* is present in the intestinal tract and mucous membranes of healthy people.
  - A warm environment (eg, diaper area) fosters growth and spread.
- None of these causes of diaper rash are spread from one child to another.

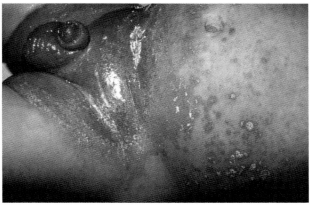

Candida rash with typical spread of affected skin to thighs and abdomen in a male infant

COURTESY OF CDC

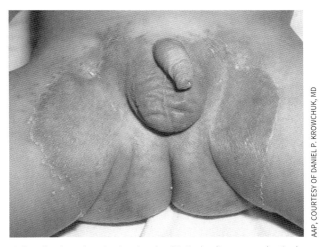

Pink and red patches that involve the skin in the diaper area that is characteristic of candidal diaper dermatitis. Scaling skin and spreading to the thighs and abdomen is present.

AAP, COURTESY OF DANIEL P. KROWCHUK, MD

How do you control it?

- Use good hand-hygiene technique at all the times listed in Chapter 2.
- Candidal (yeast) diaper rash: Treat with an antifungal cream so the quantity of yeast in any area is reduced to levels the body can control.
- Contact/irritant diaper dermatitis: Keep the skin dry and reduce irritation through friction from rubbing of a diaper or other clothing. Avoid soaps or wipes that contain fragrance. Frequent diaper changes, air exposure, or avoiding rubbing of material against the involved skin may help.
- Seborrhea: Treatment with antifungal cream or shampoo may help.

What are the roles of the educator and the family?

- Report the infection to the staff member designated by the early childhood education program or school for decision-making and action related to care of ill children. That person, in turn, alerts the parents/guardians so they can seek treatment for the child.
- Administer prescribed medication as instructed by the child's health professional.

Exclude from educational setting?

No.

American Academy of Pediatrics

DEDICATED TO THE HEALTH OF ALL CHILDREN®

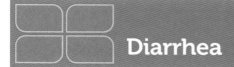

Diarrhea

What is diarrhea?

Diarrhea is an illness in which someone develops more watery or more frequent stools than is typical for that person. Diarrhea can be caused by changes in diet, such as drinking an excessive amount of fruit juice or eating more than the usual amounts of certain foods, and the use of some medications. Diarrhea can also be the result of a problem with the intestines, such as inability to absorb nutrients or allergy to foods. Infections with some viruses, bacteria, parasites, and toxins produced by certain bacteria can cause diarrhea.

- Viruses: rotaviruses, enteric adenoviruses, astroviruses, *Sapovirus*, enteroviruses, and noroviruses
- Bacteria: *Shigella, Salmonella, Campylobacter*, Shiga toxin–producing *Escherichia coli, Clostridioides difficile*
- Parasites: *Giardia duodenalis, Cryptosporidium*

What are the signs or symptoms?

- Frequent loose or watery stools
- Abdominal cramps and tenderness
- Fever
- Not feeling well
- Blood in stool

Note: Individuals can be infected and infectious with minimal or no signs or symptoms.

What are the incubation and contagious periods?

See the Quick Reference Sheet for each specific disease.

How is it spread?

- Fecal-oral route: Contact with feces of children who are infected. This generally involves an infected child contaminating their own fingers and then touching an object that another child touches. The child who touched the contaminated surface then puts their fingers into their own mouth or another person's mouth.
- Water or food contaminated by human or animal feces (eg, swimming pools).
- Contact with raw or undercooked poultry or beef.
- Contact with animals in the child's environment (eg, puppies, reptiles, poultry), during trips to sites with animals (eg, farms, pet stores, petting zoos), or in the wild.

What are some types of diarrhea?

- Viruses cause most diarrheal illness in early childhood education (ECE) settings. Rotavirus was the most common virus associated with severe diarrhea in young children. Rotavirus vaccine was included in the routine immunizations of infants in 2006. Now, diarrhea caused by this virus is much less common. Rotavirus tends to cause illness in winter. Enteroviruses are more common in the summer than other times of the year. Noroviruses, now the most common viral cause of diarrhea in children, occur year-round. Noroviruses often cause outbreaks of diarrhea and vomiting. Other viral infections may include diarrhea as one symptom (see the Quick Reference Sheet for each specific disease for more information).
- Diarrheal infections from bacteria are less common. They may cause bloody diarrhea. A health professional should always evaluate anyone with bloody diarrhea. The evaluation should include 1 or more tests, usually including stool cultures to identify the type of bacteria involved.
- Diarrhea from intestinal diseases unrelated to infections, foods, juices, or medicines is not infectious and usually is not severe enough to cause dehydration.

How do you control it?

- Ensure immunization of infants for rotavirus, following the most recent immunization schedule.
- Use good hand-hygiene technique at all the times listed in Chapter 2, especially after toilet use or handling soiled diapers and before anything to do with food preparation or eating.
- Ensure proper surface disinfection that includes cleaning and rinsing of surfaces that may have become contaminated with stool (feces) with detergent and water and application of a US Environmental Protection Agency–registered disinfectant according to the instructions on the product label.
- Ensure proper cooking and storage of food.
- Exclude infected staff members who handle food.
- Exclude for specific types of symptoms (see the section Exclude from educational setting?).

What are the roles of the educator and the family?

- Report the condition to the staff member designated by the ECE program or school for decision-making and action related to care of ill children and staff members. That person, in turn, alerts possibly exposed family and staff members to watch for symptoms.
- Ensure staff members follow the control measures listed in the section How do you control it?
- Report outbreaks of diarrhea (more than 2 children and/or staff members in the group) to the Child Care Health Consultant, who, in turn, may report the problem to the local health department.
- Require a medical evaluation for any child or staff member with diarrhea and blood or mucus in the stool.

Exclude from educational setting?

Yes, if

- The local health department determines exclusion is needed to control an outbreak.
- Stool is not contained in the diaper for diapered children.
- Diarrhea is causing "accidents" for toilet-trained children.
- Stool frequency exceeds 2 stools above normal for that child during the time the child is in the program because this may cause too much work for EC educators and make it difficult for them to maintain sanitary conditions.
- There is blood or mucus in the ill child's stool.
- The ill child's stool is all black.
- The child has a dry mouth, no tears, or no urine output in 8 hours (suggesting the child's diarrhea may be causing dehydration).
- The child is unable to participate and staff members determine they cannot care for the child without compromising their ability to care for the health and safety of the other children in the group.
- The child meets other exclusion criteria (see Conditions Requiring Temporary Exclusion in Chapter 4).

Readmit to educational setting?

Yes, when all the following criteria are met:

- For blood or mucus in the stool: A health professional must clear the child or staff member for readmission.
- For a diarrhea outbreak: Readmit following the requirements of the local health department authorities. State laws may govern exclusion for these conditions and should be followed by the health professional who is clearing the child or staff member for readmission. The following organisms may require negative stool testing before the child can return:
  - *Shigella:* At least 1 negative stool culture result (rules vary by state) obtained after antibiotic treatment is complete (if prescribed).
  - Shiga toxin–producing *E coli:* 2 negative stool culture results obtained at least 48 hours after antibiotic treatment is complete (if antibiotic is prescribed). Studies have not shown a benefit of antibiotics for this condition.
  - *Salmonella* Typhi and Paratyphi: Typically, 3 negative stool culture results obtained at least 48 hours after antibiotic treatment is complete but check state or local health department guidelines.
- Once the frequency of bowel movements is no more than 2 stools above normal for that child during the time the child is in the program, allow return to the ECE program of diapered children who have their stool contained by the diaper (even if the stools remain loose) and of toilet-trained children who are not having toileting accidents. A child who has had diarrhea may establish a new normal pattern that may include more frequent stools for a period after the child has recovered from diarrhea and seems otherwise well.
- When the child is able to participate and staff members determine they can care for the child without compromising their ability to care for the health and safety of the other children in the group.

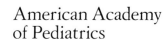

American Academy of Pediatrics

DEDICATED TO THE HEALTH OF ALL CHILDREN®

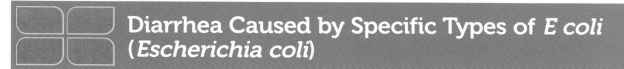

Diarrhea Caused by Specific Types of *E coli* (*Escherichia coli*)

What is *Escherichia coli* (*E coli*) diarrhea?

Although many types of *Escherichia coli* (*E coli*) bacteria live normally in the intestinal tract, at least 5 types are known to cause diarrhea. Shiga toxin–producing *E coli* has caused numerous outbreaks in early childhood education (ECE) settings. Infections with Shiga toxin–producing *E coli* may be associated with other severe problems, such as bleeding from irritation of the bowel, kidney damage, and blood cell damage, also known as hemolytic uremic syndrome. Other diarrhea-producing types are enteropathogenic *E coli*, enteroinvasive *E coli*, and enteroaggregative *E coli*. In children and adults who travel to resource-limited countries, enterotoxigenic *E coli* is the most serious and the most likely to be diagnosed. Currently, there are not readily available and reliable diagnostic tests for the others.

What are the signs or symptoms?

- Loose stools, which may be watery and bloody
- Abdominal pain
- May have fever

What are the incubation and contagious periods?

- Incubation period: Average 3 to 4 days for Shiga toxin–producing *E coli* but ranges from 10 hours to 8 days for all types.
- Contagious period: For Shiga toxin–producing *E coli*, at least 2 weeks and, in some cases, much longer.

How is it spread?

- Ingesting the bacteria through food or water contaminated with human or animal (eg, cattle, sheep, deer) feces, undercooked ground beef, unpasteurized milk, or other products contaminated with cattle feces. Contamination has occurred in improperly treated apple cider, raw vegetables, yogurt, and drinking water in recreation areas.
- Fecal-oral route: Contact with feces of children who are infected. This generally involves an infected child contaminating their own fingers and then touching an object that another child touches. The child who touched the contaminated surface then puts their fingers into their own mouth or another person's mouth.
- Exposure to animal feces by direct contact with animals, as in petting zoos, farms, or other contact between animals and people.
- Outbreaks in water parks have been reported.

How do you control it?

- Use good hand-hygiene technique at all the times listed in Chapter 2, especially after toilet use or handling soiled diapers and before anything to do with food preparation or eating.
- Ensure proper surface disinfection that includes cleaning and rinsing of surfaces that may have become contaminated with stool (feces) with detergent and water and application of a US Environmental Protection Agency–registered disinfectant according to the instructions on the product label.
- Ensure proper washing of raw vegetables (eg, grape and cherry tomatoes).
- Ensure proper cooking and storage of food. Cook all ground beef thoroughly so there is no pink meat. Use only pasteurized milk and juice products.
- Exclude infected staff members who handle food.
- Prevent contamination with human and animal feces.
- Make sure someone has notified local public health authorities that the infected child or adult attends or works at an ECE facility if Shiga toxin–producing *E coli* is identified by a health professional. It is a major public health issue. Local public health authorities should be notified immediately and will be involved. They may close the facility to new enrollees.
- Prevent enrolled children from being transferred for care to other groups or facilities where they may expose other susceptible children.
- Pay close attention to reducing communal exposure to water, such as water tables where the play occurs in a fashion that enhances the risk of transfer of germs from one child to another. Water tables with free-flowing fresh water or separate water bins for each child reduce this risk.
- Exclusion for specific types of symptoms (see the section Exclude from educational setting?).

What are the roles of the educator and the family?

- A child or staff member with Shiga toxin–producing *E coli* may have bloody diarrhea, which should trigger a medical evaluation.
- There are multiple causes of bloody diarrhea. The following recommendations apply for a child or staff member with diarrhea from any cause (see Diarrhea Quick Reference Sheet):
  - Report the condition to the staff member designated by the ECE program or school for decision-making and action related to care of ill children and staff members. That person, in turn, alerts possibly exposed family and staff members to watch for symptoms and notifies the Child Care Health Consultant.
  - Ensure staff members follow the control measures listed in the section How do you control it?
  - Report outbreaks of diarrhea (more than 2 children or staff members in the group) to the Child Care Health Consultant, who may contact the local health department.
- If you know a child or staff member has Shiga toxin–producing *E coli* in the program
  - Follow the advice of the child's or staff member's health professional.
  - Report the infection to the local health department, as the health professional who makes the diagnosis may not report that the infected person is a participant in an ECE program or school, and this could lead to loss of precious time for controlling the spread of the disease.
  - Reeducate staff members to ensure strict and frequent handwashing, diapering, toileting, food handling, and cleaning and disinfection procedures.
  - Follow the direction of the local health department. A potential outbreak with Shiga toxin–producing *E coli* is a public health emergency.

Exclude from educational setting?

Yes, if Shiga toxin–producing *E coli* is identified and for any type of *E coli* diarrhea if

- The local health department determines exclusion is needed to control an outbreak.
- Stool frequency exceeds 2 stools above normal for that child during the time the child is in the program because this may cause too much work for EC educators and make it difficult for them to maintain sanitary conditions.

- There is blood or mucus in stool.
- The ill child or adult has stool that is all black.
- The child has a dry mouth, no tears, or no urine output in 8 hours (suggesting the child's diarrhea may be causing dehydration).
- The child is unable to participate and staff members determine they cannot care for the child without compromising their ability to care for the health and safety of the other children in the group.

Readmit to educational setting?

Yes, when all the following criteria are met:

- Test results from 2 stool cultures are negative for Shiga toxin–producing *E coli*. These stool tests should be performed more than 48 hours after antibiotics have been discontinued, if they were started. Public health professionals will need to review the situation and approve the child's readiness to return.
- Once diapered children have their stool contained by the diaper (even if the stools remain loose) and when toilet-trained children do not have toileting accidents.
- Once stool frequency is no more than 2 stools above normal for that child during the time the child is in the program, even if the stools remain loose.
- When the child is able to participate and staff members determine they can care for the child without compromising their ability to care for the health and safety of the other children in the group.

Comments

- Outbreaks of Shiga toxin–producing *E coli* diarrhea have been associated with the death of young children. Management requires informing parents/guardians carefully about the problem, identifying the source of contamination, and containing the spread of disease with the recommended control measures.
- Antibiotics are not recommended for diarrhea caused by Shiga toxin–producing *E coli*.
- Many ECE programs and schools include visits to petting zoos or visits by animals into the classroom as a routine activity. There is a risk of exposure of young children to animal feces in such activities, which can result in diarrheal illness. Emphasizing good hand hygiene for all children after animal encounters or contact is recommended.

American Academy of Pediatrics

DEDICATED TO THE HEALTH OF ALL CHILDREN®

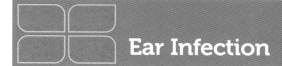

Ear Infection

What is an ear infection?

There are 2 common types of ear infections: otitis media (middle ear infection) and otitis externa (swimmer's ear). Most ear infections of young children occur in the middle ear.

- Otitis media: The middle ear is the space behind the eardrum where tiny bones attached to the eardrum transmit sound across the air space of the middle ear to the inner ear. Otitis media occurs when mucus containing bacteria collects in the middle ear space, usually during or shortly after a viral upper respiratory infection (ie, a cold). Ear infections can be very painful. In older children, most ear infections resolve by themselves in a few days. However, in children younger than 24 months, ear infections can last longer. These younger children may benefit from antibiotics. Sometimes, pressure from the infection breaks the eardrum, and pus drains from the ear. There are several factors that increase the risk of middle ear infections.

  - Young age: Young children have an inexperienced immune system, get frequent viral respiratory infections, and have ineffective drainage of fluid and mucus from the middle ear because of a blocked eustachian tube. The eustachian tube drains the middle ear to the back of the throat near the back of the nose. In young children, the eustachian tube is small and more horizontal in their throats and is more easily blocked by mucus in the nose and throat.
  - Children in educational settings: Children who are exposed to large groups of other children have more frequent colds, increasing the odds of an ear infection.
  - Smoke exposure: Exposure to tobacco smoke increases the risk of middle ear infections.

- Otitis externa (swimmer's ear): Moisture and bacteria from water in a pool, lake, or stream promotes infection of the lining of the ear canal, producing painful swelling. Pus may collect in the ear canal.

What are the signs or symptoms?

- Pain inside the ear.
- Pain when moving the earlobe (mostly with infection of the ear canal).
- Fussing, irritability, crying, poor feeding, or ear pain.
- Fever may be present.
- Ear drainage.

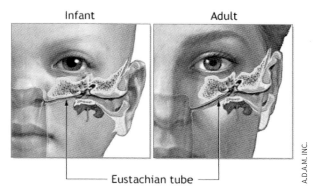

Infant   Adult

Eustachian tube

A.D.A.M. INC.

Cross section of the ear. Children have a more horizontal eustachian tube, which predisposes them to getting and keeping fluids in the middle ear.

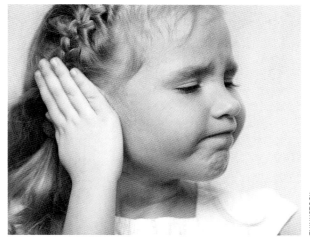

THINKSTOCK

Child with ear infection

What are the incubation and contagious periods?

- Incubation period: For middle ear infection, the incubation period is related to the type of virus or bacteria that is causing fluid buildup in the middle ear. For swimmer's ear, signs or symptoms usually appear within a day or so after swimming or getting water in the ear canal.
- Contagious period: Ear infections are not contagious.

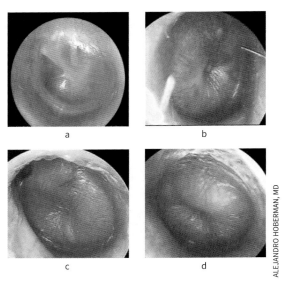

a, Normal tympanic membrane (TM); b, TM with mild bulging; c, TM with moderate bulging; d, TM with severe bulging

How is it spread?

Middle ear infections are a complication of a respiratory infection. The virus or bacteria that led to the middle ear infection may be contagious but no more worrisome than other germs that cause the common cold. Swimmer's ear is a bacterial infection of the skin in the ear canal. Drainage from ear infections can contain bacteria and should be treated as wound drainage.

How do you control it?

- For a middle ear infection
  - Prevention
    - ❖ Promote breastfeeding, which reduces the number of ear infections.
    - ❖ Promote immunizations, which help reduce the number of ear infections caused by specific bacteria (eg, *Streptococcus pneumoniae*).
    - ❖ Avoid exposure to cigarette smoke.
  - Get treatment instructions from a pediatric health professional. Sometimes, ear drops that numb the eardrum or an oral pain-reducing medication (ie, acetaminophen or ibuprofen) is all that is needed. Sometimes, the health professional will prescribe antibiotics. In children younger than 24 months using antibiotics improve symptoms faster.
- For ear canal infections (swimmer's ear)
  - Prevent infection by rinsing out ear canals with warm, clean water or a solution of 1:1 vinegar and rubbing alcohol after swimming. Sometimes,

pediatric health professionals will recommend a special ear wash after swimming if the child has a lot of trouble with ear canal infections.
  - Dry the ears by allowing the water to drain out onto a towel.
  - Get treatment instructions from a pediatric health professional.
- For a child with ear drainage
  - Have the child evaluated by a pediatric health professional. Drainage from the ear is a common occurrence if a child has ear tubes. Ear drainage does not require exclusion.

What are the roles of the educator and the family?

Observe the child's signs or symptoms and arrange for family members to contact the child's health professional for management instructions.

Exclude from educational setting?

No, unless

- The child is unable to participate and staff members determine they cannot care for the child without compromising their ability to care for the health and safety of the other children in the group.
- The child meets other exclusion criteria (see Conditions Requiring Temporary Exclusion in Chapter 4).

Readmit to educational setting?

Yes, when all the following criteria are met:

When exclusion criteria are resolved, the child is able to participate, and staff members determine they can care for the child without compromising their ability to care for the health and safety of the other children in the group

Comment

Some children in early childhood education programs get many ear infections each year. These children may receive surgically placed ear tubes to ventilate the middle ear and drain any fluid buildup from the middle ear into the ear canal. Parents/guardians should understand that the ear infections are a result of the child's age, smaller ear structures, and exposure to groups of other children and to cigarette smoke. Changing early childhood education facilities is unlikely to reduce ear infections.

American Academy of Pediatrics

DEDICATED TO THE HEALTH OF ALL CHILDREN®

Single copies of this Quick Reference Sheet may be made for noncommercial, educational purposes. The information contained in this publication should not be used as a substitute for the medical care and advice of a pediatric health professional. There may be variations in treatment that a pediatric health professional may recommend based on individual facts and circumstances.

The American Academy of Pediatrics is an organization of 67,000 primary care pediatricians, pediatric medical subspecialists, and pediatric surgical specialists dedicated to the health, safety, and well-being of all infants, children, adolescents, and young adults.

American Academy of Pediatrics website—www.HealthyChildren.org   © 2023 American Academy of Pediatrics. All rights reserved.

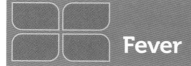

Fever

What is fever?

Fever is an elevation of the normal body temperature. Fever is most commonly caused by the body's response to a viral or bacterial infection, but it can have causes other than infection, such as juvenile idiopathic arthritis, a reaction to a vaccine or medication, or cancer.

What is considered a fever?

For infants and children older than 2 months, a body temperature above 101 °F (38.3 °C) from any site (axillary, oral, temporal/forehead, or rectal) is considered meaningfully elevated above normal. For infants younger than 2 months, a body temperature above 100.4 °F (38.0 °C) is considered meaningfully elevated above normal. These temperature elevations are not necessarily an indication of a significant health problem.

Children's temperatures may be elevated for a variety of reasons, most of which do not indicate serious illness.

Does fever mean a child is contagious?

- Children with fever are not always contagious. Noncontagious causes of fever include urinary tract infections, ear infections, and causes unrelated to infections.
- The most common cause of fever is a viral upper respiratory infection (the common cold). Although the common cold is contagious, it is not particularly harmful to others. Some children have a fever and never develop other symptoms, and the fever resolves by itself. Many infections cause a child to be contagious for several days before a fever develops. Some infections cause a child to remain contagious long after the fever has resolved. Finally, many children spread germs without ever developing a fever or other symptoms.

Is fever harmful to the child?

- No. Most (virtually all) fevers that occur because of infectious diseases are not harmful. The very high body temperatures in heatstroke are harmful. Children should never be left unattended in a car because the temperature can rise quickly and cause heatstroke (hot, dry, red skin with lethargy) and even death in a young child. Exercising in excessively hot weather or in overheated indoor rooms can also be harmful.

- Children with fever are usually less active.
- Children with fever need to drink more to avoid dehydration. Dehydration may occur because fever depletes body fluids, which should be replaced with increased fluid intake.
- Some young children with fever may have a brief seizure called a *febrile seizure*. Most brief seizures associated with fever last less than 15 minutes, occur in children younger than 6 years, and are not harmful. They are frightening to witness but do not result in any kind of brain damage. However, a child who has experienced a seizure with fever for the first time should be referred to a pediatric health professional for evaluation. Referral to a pediatric health professional is not needed only if the child's seizure fits the pattern of a previously identified febrile seizure disorder for that child and the program has been taught by a health professional how to manage a febrile seizure for that child.
- Fever is one way the body may respond to an infection. When fever develops, all the infection-fighting mechanisms tend to speed up and can help the body fight the infection. Children may have high elevations in body temperature and appear relatively well. Therefore, fever is not a good indication of severity of illness.
- Behavior is a much more reliable indicator of the significance of illness than the presence and height of fever. However, high elevations in body temperatures can sometimes affect behavior. Children who appear to be moderately ill with a fever should be referred for a medical evaluation.

What are the roles of the educator and the family?

- Measure a temperature only if a child is acting ill (ie, has a behavior change).
- If a child who is acting ill has a fever, notify the staff member designated by the early childhood education program or school for decision-making and action related to care of ill children. That person, in turn, should alert the parents/guardians to pick up the child.
- Treating the fever is not necessary unless the child is uncomfortable. Evidence suggests fever helps the body fight infection. Acetaminophen (eg, Tylenol) or ibuprofen (eg, Advil, Motrin) may be considered for the child's comfort if the child feels ill. Generally, there is no rush to reduce a child's temperature. Aspirin should never be administered to children with fever because of the potential risk of Reye

syndrome. Reye syndrome is a serious complication associated with the use of aspirin in someone infected with a viral illness.

- Any child receiving a medication should have a note from the child's health professional. The medication bottle should have the child's name and clear dosing instructions on it. If a child has a fever and behavior change and the requirement for a note and clearly labeled medication is met, the program can administer fever-reducing medication while waiting for parents/legal guardians to come pick up the child.
- There is no need to cool the child to try to bring down an elevated body temperature. A known exception is if the child's elevated temperature is not a fever but the result of exposure to extreme heat, often associated with vigorous exercise or an excessively hot environment (heat exhaustion or heatstroke); such instances are medical emergencies that require immediate first aid and health professional care.
- Infants younger than 4 months with an unexplained fever should be evaluated by a pediatric health professional. Any infant younger than 2 months with a temperature above 100.4 °F (38.0 °C) should get medical attention immediately—within an hour if possible. The fever is not harmful; however, the illness causing it may be serious in infants younger than 2 months.

Exclude from educational setting?

Only if

- Fever is noted in an infant younger than 2 months (60 days).
- Unexplained fever occurs in an infant who is younger than 4 months.
- Fever is associated with behavior change or other signs of illness or other conditions that require exclusion (see Conditions Requiring Temporary Exclusion in Chapter 4). The signs of illness are anything (other than the fever) that indicates the child's condition is different from what is usual when the child is healthy. Exclusion for fever and signs of illness transfers the responsibility from the early childhood education or school facility to the family to monitor the child.
- The child is unable to participate and staff members determine they cannot care for the child without compromising their ability to care for the health and safety of the other children in the group.
- The child has not completed the recommended vaccine series, until it is clear the child does not have a vaccine-preventable illness.

Readmit to educational setting?

Yes, when all the following criteria are met:

When exclusion criteria are resolved, the child is able to participate, and staff members determine they can care for the child without compromising their ability to care for the health and safety of the other children in the group

Note: A pediatric health professional visit is not required after every exclusion for fever. Requiring exclusion for a specific amount of time for the child who had a fever to be fever-free is not necessary as long as the criteria for readmission listed previously are met.

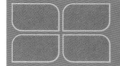

Fifth Disease (Human Parvovirus B19)

What is fifth disease?

Common viral infection with rash occurring 4 to 14 days (up to 21 days) after the start of the viral infection

What are the signs or symptoms?

- Fever.
- Headache.
- Tired, muscle aches.
- Uncommon symptoms are itchiness, cough, diarrhea or vomiting, runny nose, and joint aches.
- Red "slapped-cheek" rash appears 4 to 14 days (up to 21 days) after these signs or symptoms. This characteristic rash is followed shortly by a lacelike-appearing rash proceeding from trunk to arms, buttocks, and thighs.
- Rash may disappear and reappear after exposure to heat for weeks; once rash appears, the child is no longer contagious and usually does not feel ill.
- Individuals can be infected and infectious without ever having any signs or symptoms.
- Disease can be severe in people with sickle cell disease or certain blood disorders, as well as those with compromised immune systems.

What are the incubation and contagious periods?

- Incubation period: 4 to 14 days but can be as long as 21 days.
- Contagious period: Until the rash appears.
- Outbreaks occur in late winter and early spring.

How is it spread?

- Respiratory (droplet) route: Contact with large droplets that form when a child talks, coughs, or sneezes. These droplets can land on or be rubbed into the eyes, nose, or mouth. The droplets do not stay in the air; they usually travel no more than 3 feet and fall onto the ground.
- Exposure to blood or blood products (very rare).
- A baby can be infected before birth from infection of a pregnant mother (rare).

How do you control it?

- Use good hand-hygiene technique at all the times listed in Chapter 2.
- Sanitation of contaminated items.
- Disposal of tissues containing nose and throat secretions.

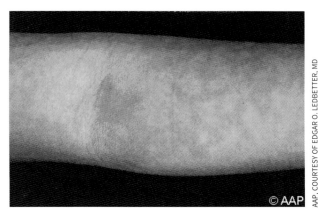

AAP, COURTESY OF EDGAR O. LEDBETTER, MD

Child's leg with lacelike-appearing rash

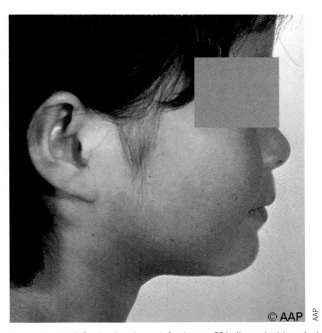

© AAP

AAP

Parvovirus B19 infection (erythema infectiosum, fifth disease) with typical facial erythema, commonly referred to as the "slapped-cheek sign"

What are the roles of the educator and the family?

- Report the infection to the staff member designated by the early childhood education (ECE) program or school for decision-making and action related to care of ill children. That person, in turn, alerts possibly exposed family and staff members to watch for symptoms. In particular, children with conditions of an underlying blood disorder, such as sickle cell disease, or a compromised immune system may become seriously ill if infected with human parvovirus B19 and so notifying parents of these children about an exposure to fifth disease is important.

- Susceptible pregnant educators and pregnant mothers of children in ECE programs or school should carefully practice hand hygiene to reduce their risk of human parvovirus B19 infection and infection from other viruses that could harm a fetus. Directors should have educators read and sign the Letter to Staff About Occupational Health Risks and ensure completion and review of the Staff Health Assessment Form (see Chapter 8).
- Prevent contact with respiratory secretions. Teach children and educators to cover their noses and mouths when sneezing or coughing with a disposable facial tissue, if possible, or with an upper sleeve or elbow if no facial tissue is available in time. Teach everyone to remove any mucus or debris on skin or other surfaces and perform hand hygiene right after using facial tissues or having contact with mucus to prevent the spread of disease by contaminated hands.
- Dispose of facial tissues that contain nasal secretions after each use.

Exclude from educational setting?

No, unless

- The child is unable to participate and staff members determine they cannot care for the child without compromising their ability to care for the health and safety of the other children in the group.
- The child meets other exclusion criteria (see Conditions Requiring Temporary Exclusion in Chapter 4).

Readmit to educational setting?

Yes, when all of the following criteria are met:

When exclusion criteria are resolved, the child is able to participate, and staff members determine they can care for the child without compromising their ability to care for the health and safety of the other children in the group

Comment

Pregnant family members and educators who expect to have contact with their own or other children who receive care in ECE settings should consult with their health professionals about the risk, although low, to the fetus if the pregnant mother is infected with parvovirus. These women should understand the risk to their fetus and ways to reduce that risk. At enrollment, the program should explain the importance of hand hygiene to reduce the risk of sharing infections for children, staff, and family members. Contact with their own young children who are enrolled in ECE programs increases the risk of exposure of women to parvovirus that may cause problems for their fetus, if they are pregnant.

To alert health professionals responsible for the health assessment of staff members of childbearing age to the need of their patient to be counseled about parvovirus risk, ECE program directors/administrators should be sure parvovirus risk assessment and counseling are items that are addressed on the staff health assessment form. In addition, it may be helpful for directors/administrators to attach this Quick Reference Sheet and the Cytomegalovirus (CMV) Infection Quick Reference Sheet to the note in the box below to alert health professionals to increased risk of exposure to the fetus if the woman is infected during her pregnancy. Health professionals are not necessarily aware of the increased exposure to these viruses for women who work with young children in ECE settings.

Dear Health Professional:

Your patient works in a setting where she has contact with young children in groups. Human parvovirus B19 and cytomegalovirus (CMV) occur commonly and are often asymptomatic among young children. Exposure of a woman who lacks immunity to human parvovirus B19 and CMV during pregnancy poses some risk to her fetus. Please discuss with your patient her childbearing intentions and whether she might want to consider the following risk-reduction measures when she might become pregnant:

- Conscientious handwashing after any contact with saliva, urine, or blood
- Care of children who are older than 3 years
- Working in a role other than direct care of young children

About Serologic Testing

Because different strains of CMV circulate among young children, especially those in early childhood education programs, a serologic test for CMV informs about risk but does not completely guarantee immunity from exposure to novel strains. However, a serologic test for human parvovirus B19 is a reliable indicator of immunity.

American Academy of Pediatrics

DEDICATED TO THE HEALTH OF ALL CHILDREN®

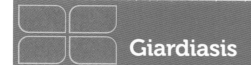

Giardiasis

What is giardiasis?

The most common intestinal infection caused by a parasite (*Giardia duodenalis*) in the United States. This parasite is often found in streams, springs, ponds, lakes, and other natural bodies of water.

What are the signs or symptoms?

- Acute watery diarrhea.
- Excessive gas (flatulence).
- Distended and painful abdomen.
- Decreased appetite.
- Weight loss.
- Many individuals are infected and infectious without signs or symptoms.
- Some individuals may have symptoms that last for weeks to months.

What are the incubation and contagious periods?

- Incubation period: 1 to 3 weeks.
- Contagious period: Highly variable but can be months. Most contagious during diarrhea phase.

How is it spread?

- Fecal-oral route: Contact with feces of children who are infected. This generally involves an infected child contaminating their own fingers and then touching an object that another child touches. The child who touched the contaminated surface then puts their fingers into their own mouth or another person's mouth.
- Ingestion of contaminated water (from people or animals) or food. Drinking water from an untreated source or playing or swimming in water contaminated with human or animal feces.
- Water tables and other water play have been associated with outbreaks of giardiasis in early childhood education (ECE) facilities.

How do you control it?

- Use good hand-hygiene technique at all the times listed in Chapter 2, especially after toilet use or handling soiled diapers and before anything to do with food preparation or eating.
- Ensure proper surface disinfection that includes cleaning and rinsing of surfaces that may have become contaminated with stool (feces) with detergent and water and application of a US Environmental Protection Agency–registered disinfectant according to the instructions on the product label.
- Ensure proper cooking and storage of food.
- Exclude infected staff members who handle food.
- Exclusion for specific types of symptoms (see the section Exclude from educational setting?).

Note: Treatment and exclusion of carriers (individuals who have the parasite but are not sick) is not effective for outbreak control.

What are the roles of the educator and the family?

- Usually, educators will not know a child has a *Giardia* infection because the condition is not distinguishable from other common forms of watery diarrhea. The following recommendations apply for a child with diarrhea from any cause (see Diarrhea Quick Reference Sheet):
  - Report the condition to the staff member designated by the ECE program or school for decision-making and action related to care of ill children and staff members. That person, in turn, alerts possibly exposed family and staff members to watch for symptoms and notifies the Child Care Health Consultant.
  - Ensure staff members follow the control measures listed in the section How do you control it?
  - Report outbreaks of diarrhea (more than 2 children and/or staff members in the group) to the Child Care Health Consultant, who may report to the local health department.
- If a child has a known *Giardia* infection
  - Follow the advice of the child's health professional.
  - Report the infection to the local health department, as the health professional who makes the diagnosis may not report that the infected child is a participant in an ECE program or school, and this could lead to delay in controlling the spread of the disease.
  - Reeducate staff members to ensure strict and frequent handwashing, diapering, toileting, food handling, and cleaning and disinfection procedures.
  - In an outbreak, follow the directions of the local health department.
- Administer medication as prescribed. Some infections are self-limited and treatment is not required.

Exclude from educational setting?

Yes, if

- The local health department determines exclusion is needed to control an outbreak.
- Stool is not contained in the diaper for diapered children.
- Diarrhea is causing "accidents" for toilet-trained children.
- Stool frequency exceeds 2 stools above normal for that child during the time the child is in the program because this may cause too much work for educators and make it difficult for them to maintain sanitary conditions.
- There is blood or mucus in stool.
- The ill child's stool is all black.
- The child has a dry mouth, no tears, or no urine output in 8 hours (suggesting the child's diarrhea may be causing dehydration).
- The child is unable to participate and staff members determine they cannot care for the child without compromising their ability to care for the health and safety of the other children in the group.

Readmit to educational setting?

Yes, when all the following criteria are met:

- Once diapered children have their stool contained by the diaper (even if the stools remain loose) and when toilet-trained children do not have toileting accidents
- Once stool frequency is no more than 2 stools above normal for that child during the time the child is in the program, even if the stools remain loose
- When the child is able to participate and staff members determine they can care for the child without compromising their ability to care for the health and safety of the other children in the group

Comments

- *Giardia* organisms are common in the stools of young children in ECE programs and schools.
- Outbreaks in educational settings may occur.
- For educators and children without symptoms (ie, recently recovered or exposed), testing stool cultures, treatment, and exclusion are not necessary.
- Negative *Giardia* stool test results are not required for readmission to an educational setting.

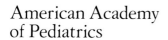

American Academy of Pediatrics

DEDICATED TO THE HEALTH OF ALL CHILDREN®

The American Academy of Pediatrics is an organization of 67,000 primary care pediatricians, pediatric medical subspecialists, and pediatric surgical specialists dedicated to the health, safety, and well-being of all infants, children, adolescents, and young adults.

American Academy of Pediatrics website—www.HealthyChildren.org

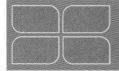

Haemophilus influenzae Type b (Hib)

What is *Haemophilus influenzae* type b?

- A type of bacteria that causes infections. Infections caused by *Haemophilus influenzae* type b (Hib) can be prevented by the Hib vaccine, which is one of the routine childhood immunizations.
- These bacteria can infect ears, eyes, and sinuses and cause serious infections, such as epiglottis (ie, infection of the flap that covers the windpipe) and infection of skin, lungs, blood, joints, and coverings of the brain (meningitis).
- Not to be confused with "the flu," a disease caused by influenza, a virus.
- There are *H influenzae* types other than type b that are less dangerous. Those bacteria commonly cause ear and sinus infections.

What are the signs or symptoms?

Depends on the site of infection. May include
- Fever
- Vomiting
- Irritability
- Stiff neck
- Rapid onset of difficulty breathing
- Cough
- Warm, red, swollen joints
- Swelling and discoloration of the skin, particularly of the cheek and around the eye

What are the incubation and contagious periods?

- Incubation period: Unknown
- Contagious period: Until antibiotic treatment has begun

How is it spread?

- Respiratory (droplet) route: Contact with large droplets that form when a child talks, coughs, or sneezes. These droplets can land on or be rubbed into the eyes, nose, or mouth. The droplets do not stay in the air; they usually travel no more than 3 feet and fall onto the ground.
- Contact with the respiratory secretions from or objects contaminated by children who carry these bacteria.

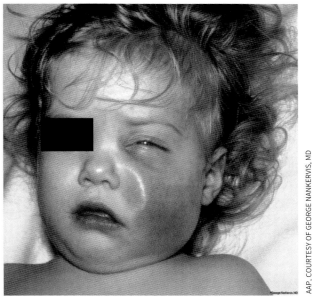

AAP, COURTESY OF GEORGE NANKERVIS, MD

A classic presentation of *Haemophilus influenzae* type b (Hib) facial cellulitis in a 10-month-old. This once-common infection has been nearly eliminated among children who have been immunized with the Hib vaccine.

How do you control it?

- *Haemophilus influenzae* type b infection is a vaccine-preventable disease. Children should receive the vaccine according to the most recent immunization recommendations.
- Preventive antibiotics (chemoprophylaxis) for exposed children and staff may be considered on the advice of the local health department if a child is seriously ill with meningitis or blood infection due to Hib. For this reason, alerting the local health department if a child has been diagnosed with Hib is very important. This is not commonly needed now that Hib immunization is widespread. Immunized people are protected if they encounter a sick individual with a Hib infection.

What are the roles of the educator and the family?

- Report the infection to the staff member designated by the early childhood education (ECE) program or school for decision-making and action related to care of ill children. That person, in turn, alerts possibly exposed family and staff members and the parents of unimmunized or incompletely immunized children to watch for symptoms. The designated staff person also notifies the Child Care Health Consultant.

- Report the infection to the local health department. If the health professional who makes the diagnosis does not inform the local health department that the infected child is a participant in an ECE program or school, this could lead to a delay in controlling the spread.
- Household members and children (especially those younger than 4 years) who are under-immunized or unimmunized and attending an ECE setting where 2 or more cases of Hib infection occur within 60 days may need to take an antibiotic to prevent the spread of this disease and should be offered the vaccine. Do not exclude children and staff members who have been exposed as long as they have no other reasons for exclusion.
- Ensure exposed children who develop a fever are seen by a pediatric health professional as soon as possible.
- Use good hand-hygiene technique at all the times listed in Chapter 2.
- Clean and sanitize surface areas and items that are contaminated by children's respiratory (nasal and cough) secretions.

Exclude from educational setting?

Yes.

Exclude all children with a diagnosis of Hib infection.

Readmit to educational setting?

Yes, when all the following criteria are met:

- After the child has been cleared by a pediatric health professional
- When the child is able to participate and staff members determine they can care for the child without compromising their ability to care for the health and safety of the other children in the group

American Academy of Pediatrics

DEDICATED TO THE HEALTH OF ALL CHILDREN®

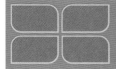

Hand-Foot-and-Mouth Disease

What is hand-foot-and-mouth disease?

A common set of symptoms associated with viral infections that are most frequently seen in the summer and fall. Despite its scary name, this illness is generally mild.

What are the signs or symptoms?

- Tiny blisters in the mouth and on the fingers, palms of hands, buttocks, and soles of feet that last a little longer than a week (one, few, or all of these body sites may be involved with the blisters).
- May see common cold signs or symptoms with fever, sore throat, runny nose, and cough. The most troublesome finding is blisters in the mouth, which make it difficult for the child to eat or drink. Other signs or symptoms, such as vomiting and diarrhea, can occur but are less frequent.
- Hand-foot-and-mouth disease may cause neurologic symptoms.

What are the incubation and contagious periods?

- Incubation period: 3 to 6 days.
- Contagious period: Virus may be shed for weeks to months in the stool after the infection starts; respiratory shedding of the virus is usually limited to 1 to 3 weeks.

How is it spread?

- Respiratory (droplet) route: Contact with large droplets that form when a child talks, coughs, or sneezes. These droplets can land on or be rubbed into the eyes, nose, or mouth. The droplets do not stay in the air; they usually travel no more than 3 feet and fall onto the ground.
- Contact with the respiratory secretions from or objects contaminated by children who carry these viruses.
- Fecal-oral route: Contact with feces of children who are infected. This generally involves an infected child contaminating their own fingers and then touching an object that another child touches. The child who touched the contaminated surface then puts their fingers into their own mouth or another person's mouth.

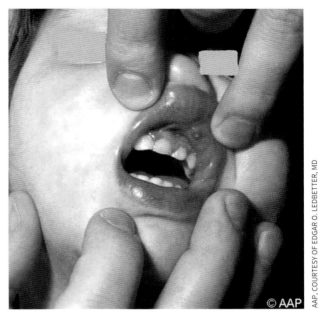

Child with blisters inside lips

AAP, COURTESY OF EDGAR O. LEDBETTER, MD

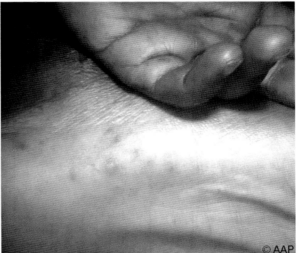

Child with blisters on hands and feet

AAP, COURTESY OF JERRI ANN JENISTA, MD

How do you control it?

- Prevent contact with respiratory secretions. Teach children and educators to cover their noses and mouths when sneezing or coughing with a disposable facial tissue, if possible, or with an upper arm sleeve or elbow if no facial tissue is available in time. Teach everyone to remove any mucus or debris on skin or other surfaces and perform hand hygiene right after using facial tissues or having contact with mucus to prevent the spread of disease by contaminated hands. Change or cover clothing with mucus on it.

- Dispose of facial tissues that contain nasal secretions after each use.
- Use good hand-hygiene technique at all the times listed in Chapter 2, especially after diaper changing.

What are the roles of the educator and the family?

- Report the infection to the staff member designated by the early childhood education program or school for decision-making and action related to care of ill children. That person, in turn, alerts possibly exposed family and staff members to watch for symptoms.
- Encourage the family to seek medical advice if the child is very uncomfortable with signs of illness from the infection, such as an inability to drink or eat, or if the child seems very ill.

Exclude from educational setting?

No, unless

- The child is unable to participate and staff members determine they cannot care for the child without compromising their ability to care for the health and safety of the other children in the group. Excessive drooling from mouth sores might be a problem that staff members will find difficult to manage for some children with this disease.
- The child meets other exclusion criteria (see Conditions Requiring Temporary Exclusion in Chapter 4).

Readmit to educational setting?

Yes, when all the following criteria are met:

When exclusion criteria are resolved, the child is able to participate, and educators determine they can care for the child without compromising their ability to care for the health and safety of the other children in the group

Notes: Exclusion will not reduce disease transmission because some children may shed the virus without becoming recognizably ill and other children who became ill may shed the virus for weeks in the stool.

In some cases, the local health department may require children with hand-foot-and-mouth disease to stay home to control an outbreak.

American Academy of Pediatrics

DEDICATED TO THE HEALTH OF ALL CHILDREN®

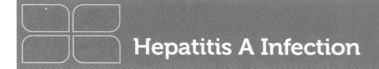

Hepatitis A Infection

What is hepatitis A infection?

- A viral infection causing liver inflammation.
- An acute, usually self-limited illness.
- Hepatitis A is spread by the fecal-oral route. Hepatitis B and C are blood-borne hepatitis viruses. (See Chapter 1 for more details.)

What are the signs or symptoms?

- Children younger than 6 years usually have few or no signs or symptoms. Symptoms are common in older children and adults.
- Fever.
- Jaundice (ie, yellowing of skin or whites of eyes).
- Abdominal discomfort.
- Fatigue.
- Dark-brown urine.
- Nausea, loss of appetite.
- Occasionally, diarrhea can occur.

What are the incubation and contagious periods?

- Incubation period: 15 to 50 days, with an average of 28 days.
- Contagious period: Most infectious in the 2 weeks before onset of signs or symptoms; the risk of transmission is minimal 1 week after onset of jaundice.

How is it spread?

Fecal-oral route: Contact with feces of children who are infected. This generally involves an infected child contaminating their own fingers and then touching a surface, an object, or food that another child touches. The child who touched the contaminated surface then puts their fingers into their own mouth or another person's mouth or on shared food.

How do you control it?

- Hepatitis A is a vaccine-preventable disease. The vaccine is recommended for all children 12 months and older. The immunization requires 2 doses, an initial dose and a second dose 6 to 18 months later.
- In an outbreak situation (a case of hepatitis A in a child or caregiver in an early childhood education [ECE] program or 2 or more cases of hepatitis A in household members of children in an ECE program), contacts should be vaccinated if not previously vaccinated or receive immune globulin shots. Local health authorities should be notified as soon as pos-

sible. They can help ensure all contacts have been notified and receive immune globulin or the hepatitis A vaccine. Giving hepatitis A vaccine immediately following exposure for those older than 12 months and younger than 40 years is equally effective as giving immune globulin. Furthermore, the vaccine will protect the person for a longer time against future hepatitis A infection than the immune globulin. When used, immune globulin should be given within 2 weeks of exposure.
- Staff members who work in ECE programs do not require the hepatitis A vaccine. However, the Centers for Disease Control and Prevention recommends hepatitis A vaccination for close personal contacts of children adopted from some countries where hepatitis A is common. The potential for exposure of educators to newly arrived international adoptees or children of newly immigrated families should be considered in deciding whether to get hepatitis A vaccine.
- Use good hand-hygiene technique at all the times listed in Chapter 2, especially after diaper changing.
- Early childhood education and school settings have been found to play a significant role in the community-wide spread of hepatitis A. Because young children usually have few or no signs or symptoms, spread within and outside an ECE setting may occur before the initial case is recognized.

What are the roles of the educator and the family?

- Report the infection to the staff member designated by the ECE program or school for decision-making and action related to care of ill children. That person, in turn, alerts possibly exposed family and staff members and the parents of unvaccinated children to watch for symptoms and notifies the Child Care Health Consultant.
- Report the infection to the local health department. If the health professional who makes the diagnosis does not inform the local health department that the infected child or staff member is a participant in an ECE program or school, this could lead to a delay in controlling the spread.
- Use good hand-hygiene technique at all the times listed in Chapter 2, with special attention after toileting or changing diapers.
- Teach children and remind adults to wash their hands after using the toilet and before any activity that potentially involves food or the mouth.

- Clean and disinfect surfaces in all areas. Hepatitis A virus can survive on surfaces for weeks.
- Contact a health professional and the local health department promptly to review the need for using vaccine or immune globulin for attendees and household members of attendees.
- Routinely check that children complete the hepatitis A vaccine series according to the most recent immunization recommendations.

Exclude from educational setting?

Yes.
- Children and adults, especially food handlers, with hepatitis A should be excluded for 1 week after onset of illness.
- Refer to a pediatric health professional.

Readmit to educational setting?

Yes, when all the following criteria are met:
- One week after onset of illness and after all contacts have received vaccine or immune globulin as recommended
- When the child is able to participate and staff members determine they can care for the child without compromising their ability to care for the health and safety of the other children in the group

Comments

- When an individual is infected and sick with hepatitis A treatment is limited to comfort measures.
- Hepatitis A outbreaks can occur in ECE settings. The first sign of an outbreak may be in adult caregivers (parents/guardians, staff members) because young children may not have symptoms.

American Academy of Pediatrics

DEDICATED TO THE HEALTH OF ALL CHILDREN®

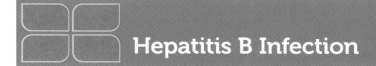

Hepatitis B Infection

What is hepatitis B?

- A viral infection causing liver inflammation.
- Hepatitis B can lead to serious illness, lifelong infection, liver failure, and liver cancer.
- Hepatitis B is a blood-borne infection. (See Chapter 1 for more details.)

What are the signs or symptoms?

- Flu-like (eg, muscle aches, nausea, vomiting).
- Jaundice (ie, yellowing of skin or whites of eyes, dark urine).
- Loss of appetite.
- Joint pains.
- Tiredness.
- Young children may show few or no signs or symptoms.
- Most people recover fully, but some carry the virus in their blood for a lifetime. Age at the time of infection is a major factor in whether hepatitis B will become a chronic infection.

What are the incubation and contagious periods?

- Incubation period: 45 to 160 days, with an average of 90 days
- Contagious period: As long as the virus is present in the blood of the infected person (can be for the lifetime of an infected person who is a chronic carrier)

How is it spread?

- Most commonly through
  - Blood or blood products.
  - Sexual contact.
  - Children born to infected mothers may become infected during birth.
- Uncommonly through
  - Saliva that contains blood
  - Contact with open sores or the fluid that comes from open sores (wound exudate)
  - Direct exposure to blood after injury, bites, or scratches that caused a skin break, introducing blood or body fluids from a carrier to another person
- Hepatitis B virus can remain contagious on surfaces for 7 days or more.

How do you control it?

- Hepatitis B is a vaccine-preventable disease. Babies should receive vaccine at or soon after birth, with additional doses of the vaccine according to the routine immunization schedule.
- Adults who are expected, as a condition of their employment, to come in contact with blood are required to be offered vaccine by their employers under US Occupational Safety and Health Administration (OSHA) regulations.
- Cover open wounds or sores.
- Do not permit sharing of toothbrushes or pacifiers.
- Standard Precautions should be followed when blood or blood-containing body fluids are handled. For blood and blood-containing substances, these are the same precautions described by OSHA as Universal Precautions.
  - Wear disposable gloves or, if using utility gloves, be sure the utility gloves are sanitized after use. Use barriers and techniques that minimize potential contact of mucous membranes or openings in the skin to blood.
  - Absorb as much of the spill as possible with disposable materials; put the contaminated materials in a plastic bag with a secure tie.
  - Clean contaminated surfaces with detergent and water, and then rinse with water. Floors, rugs, and carpeting should be cleaned by blotting to remove the fluid as quickly as possible and disinfected by spot-cleaning with a US Environmental Protection Agency (EPA)–registered detergent or disinfectant. Additional cleaning by shampooing or steam cleaning the contaminated surface may be necessary.
  - Disinfect the cleaned and rinsed surface using an EPA-registered disinfectant. Follow the manufacturer's instruction for preparation and use of the disinfectant. For guidance on disinfectants, refer to Chapter 8, Selecting an Appropriate Sanitizer or Disinfectant.
  - Clean, rinse, and disinfect reusable household rubber gloves. Dry and store them away from any surface or object related to food. Discard disposable gloves.
  - Dispose of all soiled items in plastic bags with secure ties.
- Perform hand hygiene after cleaning and disinfecting are done, even though gloves were worn.

What are the roles of the educator and the family?

- Report the infection to the local health department. If the health professional who makes the diagnosis does not inform the local health department that the infected child is a participant in an early childhood education program or school, it could delay controlling the spread.
- Routinely check that children complete the hepatitis vaccine series according to the most recent immunization schedule.
- Practice Standard Precautions for handling blood and other body fluids at all times, as carriers of this infection may not be identified to staff members. Check and follow the facility's plan for handling exposure to blood-borne pathogens as required by OSHA.
- Contact the program's Child Care Health Consultant or the local health department and the infected child's health professional for a treatment and group management plan.

Exclude from educational setting?

Yes, if a child with known hepatitis B exhibits any of the following signs or symptoms:
- Weeping sores that cannot be covered.
- A bleeding problem.
- Biting or scratching behavior that would lead to bleeding by the child with hepatitis B.
- Generalized dermatitis that may produce wounds or weepy tissue fluids.
- The child is unable to participate and staff members determine they cannot care for the child without compromising their ability to care for the health and safety of the other children in the group.
- The child meets other exclusion criteria (see Conditions Requiring Temporary Exclusion in Chapter 4).

Readmit to educational setting?

Yes, when all the following criteria are met:
- When skin lesions are dry or covered
- When the child is able to participate and staff members determine they can care for the child without compromising their ability to care for the health and safety of the other children in the group

Comments

- The recommendation for universal immunization of newborns and children born and cared for in the United States has achieved high levels of immunity and protection against infection with hepatitis B, which has made the risk of infection in group care settings very small. Certain high-risk groups remain, such as injection drug users, those with more than one sex partner in the previous 6 months, and people from countries where universal immunization against hepatitis B is not practiced.
- Most children with hepatitis B infection should be admitted to an early childhood education program or school without restrictions. Admission of children with skin problems that bleed or ooze body fluids, bleeding problems, or aggressive behavior, including biting, should be handled on an individualized basis. If a child with known hepatitis B bites or is bitten by a child who is unimmunized or partially immunized against hepatitis B, the unimmunized/partially immunized child should be referred to a health professional or the local health department.
- Hepatitis C is also transmitted through blood and causes a disease similar to hepatitis B. It should be managed the same as hepatitis B.
- Hepatitis D is also transmitted through the blood but only occurs in those previously infected with hepatitis B. Hepatitis D can be a more severe disease. It is also managed just like hepatitis B.
- Currently, there are no hepatitis C or D vaccines available.

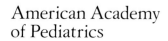

American Academy of Pediatrics

DEDICATED TO THE HEALTH OF ALL CHILDREN®

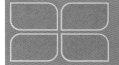

Herpes Simplex (Cold Sores)

What is herpes simplex?

- A viral infection that can cause a variety of signs and symptoms in different age-groups.
- In early childhood, herpes simplex most commonly causes blister-like sores in the mouth, around the lips, and on skin that is in contact with the mouth, such as a sucked thumb or finger.
- Virus is shed by people with or without signs or symptoms (often by adults).

What are the signs or symptoms?

- During the first or primary infection
  - Fever.
  - Irritability.
  - Tender, swollen lymph nodes.
  - Painful, small, fluid-filled blisters (called *vesicles*) in the mouth and on the gums and lips.
  - Vesicles weep clear fluid, bleed, and are slow to crust over.
- After the first infection, subsequent infections may occur with clusters of blisters on the lips, commonly called *cold sores* or *fever blisters*.
- Often, there are no signs or symptoms.

What are the incubation and contagious periods?

- Incubation period: 2 days to 2 weeks.
- Contagious period: During the first infection, people shed the virus for at least a week and, occasionally, for several weeks after signs or symptoms appear. After the first infection, the virus may be reactivated from time to time, producing cold sores on the lips. Compared to the first infection, people with recurrent cold sores shed smaller amounts of virus and only for 3 to 4 days after signs or symptoms appear. Virus shedding also occurs at lower levels in infected individuals who have no signs or symptoms.

How is it spread?

- Direct contact through kissing and contact with open sores.
- Contact with saliva (eg, from mouthed toys).
- Can be spread to other areas of the body by scratching or abrading skin after touching an open sore. This is especially problematic in a child with eczema.

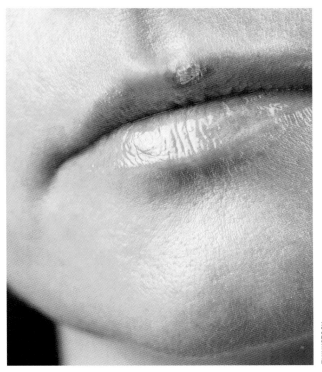

THINKSTOCK

Cold sore on lip

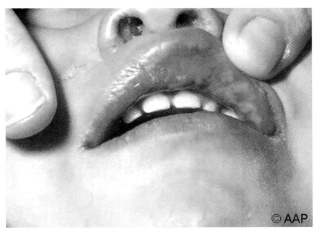

© AAP

AAP

Cold sores on inside of mouth

How do you control it?

- Use good hand-hygiene technique at all the times listed in Chapter 2.
- Avoid kissing or nuzzling children on the lips or hands.
- Do not share food or drinks between children or staff members.
- Do not touch sores.
- Avoid contact with saliva from mouthed toys or objects.
- Clean toys regularly. (See Chapter 2.)

What are the roles of the educator and the family?

- Report the infection to the staff member designated by the early childhood education program or school for decision-making and action related to care of ill children. That person, in turn, alerts possibly exposed family and staff members to watch for symptoms.
- Stress the importance of good hand hygiene and other measures aimed at controlling the transmission of infected secretions (eg, saliva, tissue fluid, fluid from a skin sore).
- Wash and sanitize mouthed toys, bottle nipples, and utensils that have come into contact with saliva or have been touched by children who are drooling and put fingers in their mouths.
- Try to avoid touching cold sores with hands, which is difficult but should be attempted. When sores have been touched, careful hand hygiene should follow immediately, using good hand-hygiene technique listed in Chapter 2.

Exclude from educational setting?

No, unless

- The child has ulcers and vesicles inside the mouth and does not have control of drooling.
- The child is unable to participate and staff members determine they cannot care for the child without compromising their ability to care for the health and safety of the other children in the group.
- The child meets other exclusion criteria (see Conditions Requiring Temporary Exclusion in Chapter 4).

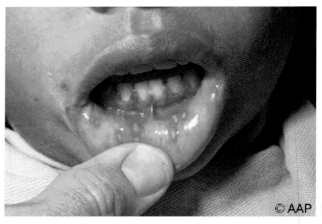

© AAP

Cold sores on inside of mouth

Readmit to educational setting?

Yes, when all the following criteria are met:

- When a child with ulcers or vesicles inside the mouth is no longer drooling or the ulcers or vesicles have resolved. A child with vesicles (blisters) on the body can return once these areas are covered with clothing or a bandage.
- When the child is able to participate and staff members determine they can care for the child without compromising their ability to care for the health and safety of the other children in the group.

Comments

- Children and educators with recurrent infection (ie, cold sores) do not need to be excluded as long as there is no drooling.
- A very serious eye infection can result when people with virus on their hands from cold sores transmit it to their eyes. Good hygiene, especially hand hygiene, cannot be overemphasized.
- Herpes simplex type 1 is the usual cause of mouth sores, while herpes simplex type 2 is the usual cause of genital sores. At times, type 1 causes infection in the genital area and type 2 causes infection in the mouth.

American Academy of Pediatrics

DEDICATED TO THE HEALTH OF ALL CHILDREN®

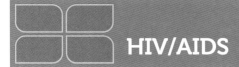

HIV/AIDS

What is HIV/AIDS?

Human immunodeficiency virus (HIV) infection affects the body in a variety of ways. In the most severe infection, the virus progressively destroys the body's immune system, causing a condition called acquired immunodeficiency syndrome (AIDS). With early testing and appropriate treatment, children in the United States rarely develop the severe signs and symptoms of HIV infection.

What are the signs or symptoms?

Children with HIV infection may show few signs or symptoms. Children with HIV infection may have

- Unexplained fevers
- Failure to grow and develop well
- Enlarged lymph nodes
- Swelling of salivary glands
- Enlargement of the liver and spleen
- Frequent infections, including pneumonia, diarrhea, and thrush (ie, a yeast infection on the surfaces of the mouth)
- Inflammation of the heart, salivary glands, liver, and kidneys
- Central nervous system disease
- Specific types of tumors

What are the incubation and contagious periods?

- Incubation period: If the infection is acquired before or during birth from infected mothers, children typically develop signs or symptoms between 12 and 18 months of age, although many remain symptom free for more than 5 years. With treatment, most children live into adulthood. However, approximately 15% to 20% of untreated children in the United States die before 4 years of age.
- Contagious period: Infected individuals can transmit the virus in their body fluids throughout their lifetime.

How is it spread?

- Contact of mucous membranes or openings in the skin with infected blood and body fluids that contain blood, semen, and cervical secretions; can also be spread from mother to baby through breastfeeding. If an infant has been mistakenly fed another infant's bottle of expressed human (breast) milk, the possible exposure to infectious disease should be treated just as if an unintentional exposure to other body fluids

had occurred. For a detailed discussion of what to do if the milk of one mother is fed to an infant of another mother, see *Caring for Our Children: National Health and Safety Performance Standards; Guidelines for Early Care and Education Programs*, Standard 4.3.1.4 (https://nrckids.org/CFOC).
- Contaminated needles or sharp instruments.
- Mother–baby transmission before or during birth.
- Sexual contact.
- HIV is not spread by the type of contact that occurs in early childhood education (ECE) and school settings, such as in typical classroom activities or with surfaces touched by infected people. It is not spread through non-bloody saliva, tears, stool, or urine.

How do you control it?

- Standard Precautions should be followed when blood or blood-containing body fluids are handled. For blood and blood-containing substances, these are the same precautions described by the US Occupational Safety and Health Administration (OSHA) as Universal Precautions.
  - Wear disposable gloves or, if using utility gloves, be sure the utility gloves are sanitized after use. Use barriers (eg, gloves) and cleanup techniques to minimize potential contact of mucous membranes or openings in the skin to blood.
  - Absorb as much of the spill as possible with disposable materials; put the contaminated materials in a plastic bag with a secure tie.
  - Clean contaminated surfaces with detergent and water, and then rinse with water. Floors, rugs, and carpeting should be cleaned by blotting to remove the fluid as quickly as possible and disinfected by spot-cleaning with a US Environmental Protection Agency (EPA)–registered detergent or disinfectant. Additional cleaning by shampooing or steam cleaning the contaminated surface may be necessary.
  - Disinfect the cleaned and rinsed surface using an EPA-registered disinfectant. Follow the manufacturer's instruction for preparation and use of the disinfectant. For guidance on disinfectants, refer to Chapter 8, Selecting an Appropriate Sanitizer or Disinfectant.
  - Clean, rinse, and disinfect reusable household rubber gloves. Dry and store them away from any surface or object related to food. Discard disposable gloves.
  - Dispose of all soiled items in plastic bags with secure ties.

- Perform hand hygiene after cleaning and disinfecting are done, even though gloves were worn.
- Children with HIV infection should not be excluded from ECE and school settings solely for the protection of other children or personnel. As long as affected children's health status enables participation, they should be admitted. Uncommonly, the risk of a child's transmission of blood-borne pathogens, through conditions such as generalized skin rash or bleeding problems, would merit assessment by the child's health professional and the ECE program director/administrator or school principal to see whether the child can participate.

What are the roles of the educator and the family?

- Parents/guardians of all children, including children with HIV, should be notified immediately if a case of a highly contagious disease, such as measles or chickenpox, occurs in an educational setting. Children with HIV infection may be at increased risk of severe complications from certain types of infections.
- Parents/guardians of a child with HIV are not required to reveal that their child is infected with HIV. They may choose to share the information confidentially so they can ask the program to observe their child more closely than other children for signs of illness that might require medical attention. If parents/guardians share HIV status of their children, this information is not to be disclosed to staff members without written permission of the parents/guardians. Only the child's parents/guardians and health professional have an absolute need to know the child is infected with HIV.
- Parents/guardians of children with HIV should consult with their children's health professional when their children have been exposed to a potentially harmful infectious disease.
- All staff members in ECE and school settings should receive annual education about Standard Precautions, which include OSHA requirements for Universal Precautions.

Exclude from educational setting?

No, unless

- The child has symptoms that require exclusion according to the child's individual care plan.

- The child is unable to participate and staff members determine they cannot care for the child without compromising their ability to care for the health and safety of the other children in the group.
- The child has weeping skin lesions that cannot be covered.
- The child has bleeding problems.
- Exposure to a highly contagious disease (eg, measles, chickenpox) occurs at the facility. Parents/guardians of children who have a compromised immune system can ask their child's primary health professional whether the child should receive preventive measures, including removal from the educational setting, to reduce the risk. Parents/guardians of all children in the facility should be notified immediately if their child has been exposed to chickenpox, tuberculosis, fifth disease (parvovirus B19), diarrheal disease, measles, or other infectious diseases through contact with other children in the facility.
- The child meets other exclusion criteria (see Conditions Requiring Temporary Exclusion in Chapter 4).

Readmit to educational setting?

Yes, when all the following criteria are met:

- A child who is known to have HIV and has been excluded because of risk of exposure to infections in an educational setting can return when the child's health professional determines it is safe for the child to return.
- When skin lesions are dry or covered.
- When the child is able to participate and staff members determine they can care for the child without compromising their ability to care for the health and safety of the other children in the group.

Comment

See *Caring for Our Children: National Health and Safety Performance Standards; Guidelines for Early Care and Education Programs*, 4th Edition, Standards 3.2.3.4, 3.6.1.1, 4.3.1.4, 7.6.3.1 through 7.6.3.4, 9.2.3.6, and 9.4.1.5 (https://nrckids.org/CFOC), or the Centers for Disease Control and Prevention HIV/AIDS website (https://www.cdc.gov/hiv/default.html) for more details on HIV/AIDS policies.

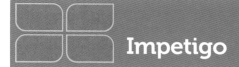

Impetigo

What is impetigo?

A common skin infection caused by streptococcal or staphylococcal bacteria

What are the signs or symptoms?

Small, red pimples or fluid-filled blisters (pustules) with crusted yellow scabs found most often on the face or on abraded areas anywhere on the body

What are the incubation and contagious periods?

- Incubation period: Variable. Bacteria that could cause impetigo commonly live harmlessly on the skin. Minor skin trauma may result in skin infections like impetigo.
- Contagious period: Until the skin sores are treated with antibiotics for at least 24 hours or the crusting lesions are no longer present.

How is it spread?

- Contact with the sores of an infected person or from contaminated surfaces.
- Germs enter an opening on skin (eg, cut, insect bite, burn, eczema) and cause oozing, leading to honey-colored crusted sores.
- Occurs year-round but most commonly in warm weather. Also occurs in cold weather when the skin around the nose and face is damaged by runny nasal secretions and nose wiping that irritates the skin.

How do you control it?

- Cover lesions, after which infected individuals should be treated with an appropriate antibiotic regimen (oral or topical) at the end of the day.
- Use good hand-hygiene technique at all the times listed in Chapter 2.
- Clean and sanitize surfaces.
- Clip fingernails to reduce further injury of tissues by scratching and subsequent spread through contaminated fingernails.
- In the event of an outbreak (more than one infected child in a group), consult with the local health department.
- The problem could involve staphylococcal bacteria (see *Staphylococcus aureus* [Methicillin-Resistant (MRSA) and Methicillin-Sensitive (MSSA)] Quick Reference Sheet).

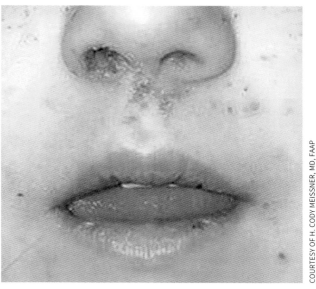

Impetigo. Crusted lesions inside and around nostrils start as red bumps.

COURTESY OF H. CODY MEISSNER, MD, FAAP

What are the roles of the educator and the family?

- Consult the child's health professional for a treatment plan.
- Use good hand-hygiene technique at all the times listed in Chapter 2.
- Clean infected area.
- Use medication recommended by the child's health professional.
- When possible, loosely cover infected area to allow airflow for healing and avoid contact with others in educational settings.
- Wear gloves. Perform hand hygiene after coming into contact with sores or when changing bandages in the educational setting and at home.
- Launder contaminated clothing articles daily.
- Notify the local health department if an outbreak occurs.

Exclude from educational setting?

Wash the affected area, cover the sores, and then, at the end of the day, the child should see a pediatric health professional. If impetigo is confirmed, the child should start treatment (oral or topical antibiotic) before returning. If treatment is started before the next day, no exclusion is necessary. However, the child may be excluded until treatment has started.

Readmit to educational setting?

Yes, when all the following criteria are met:

- As long as the lesions are covered, the child can return once appropriate treatment has started (oral or topical antibiotics). When possible, lesions should be kept covered until they are dry.
- When the child is able to participate and staff members determine they can care for the child without compromising their ability to care for the health and safety of the other children in the group.

Comments

- When impetigo is caused by group A *Streptococcus*, treatment and complication issues are similar to when this germ causes strep throat (see Strep Throat [Streptococcal Pharyngitis] and Scarlet Fever Quick Reference Sheet). However, acute rheumatic fever does not usually result from impetigo.
- Pediatric health professionals may use antibiotic ointment when there are only a few impetigo lesions and oral antibiotic(s) when there are many lesions.

American Academy of Pediatrics

DEDICATED TO THE HEALTH OF ALL CHILDREN®

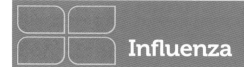

Influenza

What is influenza?

A contagious disease caused by a group of respiratory viruses called influenza viruses

What are the signs or symptoms?

- Sudden onset of fever
- Headache
- Chills
- Muscle aches and pains
- Sore throat
- Nasal congestion
- Cough
- Mild pinkeye (conjunctivitis)
- Decreased energy
- Abdominal pain
- Nausea and vomiting (These symptoms are always accompanied by respiratory symptoms like runny nose, cough, or sore throat and are not usually the only symptoms of influenza.)
- Croup (illness with barky cough and hoarseness), bronchiolitis (illness with wheezing and runny nose), or pneumonia

What are the incubation and contagious periods?

- Incubation period: 1 to 4 days, with a mean of 2 days
- Contagious period: From the day before signs or symptoms appear until at least 7 days after the onset of flu, although virus shedding can be longer in young children and those with compromised immune systems

How is it spread?

- Respiratory (droplet) route: Contact with large droplets that form when a child talks, coughs, or sneezes. These droplets can land on or be rubbed into the eyes, nose, or mouth. The droplets do not stay in the air; they usually travel no more than 3 feet and fall onto the ground.
- Contact with the respiratory secretions from or objects contaminated by children who carry influenza virus.

How do you control it?

- Annual immunization according to the most recent immunization schedule at www.cdc.gov/vaccines for all people 6 months and older, including all educators.
- Use good hand-hygiene technique at all the times listed in Chapter 2.
- Prevent contact with respiratory secretions. Teach children and educators to cover their noses and mouths when sneezing or coughing with a disposable facial tissue, if possible, or with an upper sleeve or elbow if no facial tissue is available in time. Teach everyone to remove any mucus or debris on skin or other surfaces and perform hand hygiene right after using facial tissues or having contact with mucus to prevent the spread of disease by contaminated hands. Change or cover clothing with mucus on it.
- Dispose of facial tissues that contain nasal secretions after each use.
- Perform hand hygiene after contact with any soiled items.
- Antiviral medications that treat influenza infection are most helpful if given early in the course of illness (first 48 hours).
- Reduce crowding as much as possible.

What are the roles of the educator and the family?

- Influenza is a serious disease that can cause complications, like pneumonia. Every year, children (and adults) die from influenza and its complications in the United States. Follow the recommendation to immunize all people 6 months and older.
- Avoid aspirin use for anyone with influenza. There is an increased risk of Reye syndrome, a serious complication associated with the use of aspirin in someone infected with influenza.

Exclude from educational setting?

Yes, if

- The child is unable to participate and staff members determine they cannot care for the child without compromising their ability to care for the health and safety of the other children in the group.
- The child meets other exclusion criteria (see Conditions Requiring Temporary Exclusion in Chapter 4) or, during flu season (when influenza is known to be prevalent in the community), the child has fever and behavior change or fever with other signs or symptoms of influenza illness, like cough, sore throat, sneeze, or runny nose.

Readmit to educational setting?

Yes, when all the following criteria are met:

When exclusion criteria are resolved, fever has been absent for 24 hours after any fever-reducing medicines have been given, the child is able to participate, and staff members determine they can care for the child without compromising their ability to care for the health and safety of the other children in the group

Comments

- Influenza immunization is very important in young children in early childhood education settings for the following reasons:
  - Influenza can be severe in young children and older adults. Hospitalization rates are similar in these 2 groups.
  - Death can occur in previously healthy children after influenza infection.
  - The risk of spread of influenza is very high among young children, and they bring the infection home to their families as well as spread it into the community.

- Health professionals can use a test to determine whether an ill person has influenza rather than other common viruses that cause respiratory symptoms. However, it is not practical to test all ill children to determine whether they have common cold viruses or influenza infection. Therefore, exclusion decisions are based on the symptoms and behavior of the child.
- During flu season, a child excluded with fever and respiratory symptoms (cough, runny nose, sneezing) should remain excluded until 24 hours of no fever without use of fever-reducing medications because children shed more of the influenza virus while they have a fever than when they are afebrile.
- Most children with flu-like symptoms (fever and respiratory symptoms) during flu season do not have influenza. They likely have infections from other viruses.
- Management strategies (control, exclusion, readmission) may be different and more stringent for pandemic influenza and under the guidance of the local public health authority. See Chapter 7 for a discussion of outbreaks, epidemics, and pandemics.

American Academy of Pediatrics

DEDICATED TO THE HEALTH OF ALL CHILDREN®

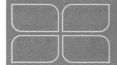

Lice (Pediculosis Capitis)

What are head lice?

- Small, tan/gray/white-colored insects (less than ⅛" long) that
  - Live on blood they draw from the scalp.
  - Live for days to weeks depending on temperature and humidity.
  - Crawl. They do not hop or fly.
  - Deposit tiny eggs (smaller than half a grain of rice), known as nits, on a hair shaft 3 to 4 mm (¼") from the scalp. They are attached to a hair shaft by female lice with a glue that holds them tightly in place. The eggs need the warmth from the scalp for hatching. The nits that are more than ¼" from the scalp have already hatched or have died. Removing nits requires fine-tooth combing that is tedious and difficult to do, especially when a person who is infested with head lice has long hair, hair extensions, or a hair style that involves extensive braiding.
  - Cannot live as adult insects for more than 48 hours away from the scalp.
  - Spread primarily by direct head-to-head contact, and less commonly by direct contact with clothing recently worn by someone who has head lice.
- Having an infestation with lice may cause irritation and scratching, which can lead to secondary skin infection.
- Families and educators often get very upset about lice. However, head lice do not carry disease. Head lice infestations occur in all socioeconomic groups and do not represent poor hygiene.
- Often, normal activities are disrupted because people become upset about these insect pests.

What are the signs or symptoms?

- Itching of skin where lice feed on the scalp or neck or complaints about itchiness by older children.
- Nits attached to hair, most easily seen behind ears and at or near the nape of the neck.
- Scratching behind ears and the nape of the neck.
- Open sores and crusting from secondary bacterial infection may cause swollen lymph nodes (glands).

What are the incubation and contagious periods?

- Incubation period: 7 to 12 days from laying to hatching of eggs. Lice can reproduce about 2 weeks after hatching if they are getting their blood meals from the scalp.

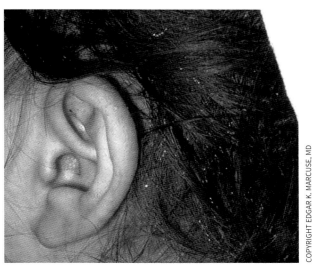

COPYRIGHT EDGAR K. MARCUSE, MD

Child with nits on hair behind ears and at nape of neck

- Contagious period: Until live lice are no longer present.

How are they spread?

- Primarily through direct head-to-head contact with infested hair. Shared objects (hats, headgear, and other objects) that contact the head are a possible but uncommon cause of spread of lice because the insects prefer to stay close to the blood supply on the scalp.
- Nits hatch best when they are kept warm by being on strands of hair that are within 3 to 4 mm (¼") of the scalp. However, research shows eggs can be laid on other surfaces and hatch more than 50% of the time.

How do you control them?

- By using medications (pediculicides) that kill lice and nits. Resistance of lice and nits to these chemicals has been reported, but the extent of resistance to the chemicals varies. Some chemicals may require 2 treatments. These chemicals are toxic to lice and may have some toxicity to humans, especially if used for age-groups for which the product is not recommended or without following the manufacturer's instructions. If a particular chemical fails to work, repeated use of that chemical is unlikely to be successful, and an alternative chemical that has been shown to be effective should be tried.

- Herbal and "natural" remedies, like ylang-ylang, tea tree, and lavender oils are not regulated by the US Food and Drug Administration, so their content, safety, and effectiveness cannot be assumed.
- Remedies using common household products (eg, salad oils, mayonnaise, petroleum jelly) have not been shown to be effective, and some (eg, kerosene) are dangerous.
- Some non–insecticide-based occlusive agents (dimethicone and isopropyl myristate) have shown promise.
- Mechanical removal of the lice and nits by combing them out of wet hair with a special fine-tooth comb may have some benefit compared with no treatment. It also may reduce confusion about whether the child has been successfully treated or is re-infested with lice. This treatment is tedious and very time-consuming, but it does damage and remove live lice. It requires washing the hair, applying conditioner, separating the hair into small sections to comb it thoroughly, and then repeating until no new nits are seen within ¼" from the scalp. It is unknown whether combing improves treatment success rates if the child is already receiving a chemical treatment at the same time.
- Household and close contacts should be examined and treated if they have infestations. Individuals who share the same bed with the infested child may also be treated, even if no live lice are found.
- Discourage activity that causes head-to-head contact. Avoid sharing clothing and headgear, like hats, bike helmets, or dress-up costumes.
- The following supplemental measures are options, not requirements, because spread is primarily from head to head:
  - Launder articles that were in contact with the infested individual, exposing them for 5 minutes to temperatures greater than 128.3 °F (53.5 °C) and then drying them in a dryer on the hot setting. Alternately, clothing and bedding can be dry-cleaned.
  - Toys, personal articles, bedding, other fabrics, and upholstered furniture that cannot be laundered with hot water and dried in a dryer or dry-cleaned can be kept away from people (eg, in a plastic bag) for 1 to 2 weeks if there is concern about lice having crawled from an infested child onto these articles.
  - Floors, carpets, mattresses, and furniture can be vacuumed (a safe alternative to spraying) to remove any strands of the infested person's hair that might have viable lice eggs. Chemical treatment of the environment is not necessary.

What are the roles of the educator and the family?

- Report the infestation to the staff member designated by the early childhood education program or school for decision-making and action related to care of ill children. That person, in turn, alerts possibly exposed family and staff members to watch for symptoms.
- Have parents/guardians consult with a health professional for a treatment plan.
- Check children observed scratching their heads for lice; if lice are found, check all contacts.
- Teach educators and families how to recognize lice and nits.

Exclude from educational setting?

- By the end of the day, families should consult the child's health professional to discuss whether treatment is indicated. If treatment is indicated and started before the next day, no exclusion is necessary. However, the child may be excluded until treatment has started.
- Some treatments must be repeated 7 to 10 days after the first treatment. Until the treatment course is completed, avoid any activity that involves the child in head-to-head contact with other children, such as group block building, art projects, games that involve head-to-head contact, or sharing of headgear in a dress-up corner, while using riding toys, or playing sports. Do not resume these activities until no new lice are seen and there are no nits within ¼" of the scalp for anyone in the group.

Readmit to educational setting?

Yes, when the child has received the treatment recommended by the child's health professional, even if nits are still present.

Comments

- The Centers for Disease Control and Prevention (CDC) recommends not using shampoo for several days after a lice-killing product has been applied to give the residual lice-killing product on the hair a chance to work on any live lice or viable nits. Also, the CDC suggests not using conditioner, oil, or any other occlusive product before applying the lice-killing product because these act as a barrier and may make the lice-killing medicine ineffective.
- No-nit policies that require children to be nit free are not recommended because they have not been shown to be effective in controlling outbreaks, may keep the child out of the program needlessly, and unduly burden the child's parents/guardians, who must implement this measure.

- Education of families and educators about the relatively benign consequences of head lice infestations should be attempted to reduce the level of disruption for the infested child and all others involved in the program. It may be necessary to arrange for a health professional to provide this education to overcome the widespread incorrect beliefs about this problem.
- Itching results from an allergic reaction to the lice saliva and, sometimes, from the treatment itself; itching often persists for weeks after the infestation has resolved.
- Schools and programs should work with a Child Care Health Consultant to create a lice protocol to ensure children are treated safely and effectively.

American Academy of Pediatrics

DEDICATED TO THE HEALTH OF ALL CHILDREN®

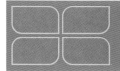

Lyme Disease (and Other Tick-borne Diseases)

What is Lyme disease?

An infection caused by a type of bacteria called a *spirochete* that is transmitted when particular types of ticks attach to a person's skin and feed on that person's blood. These ticks are very small—only a few millimeters (about the size of a freckle). The ticks that transit Lyme disease are found mainly in 3 areas of the United States: in the New England and eastern mid-Atlantic regions, in the upper Midwest, and on the West Coast. Also, they are seen in Europe, China, Japan, Canada, and in the countries that were part of the former Soviet Union. In the United States, the spirochete causing Lyme disease is called *Borrelia burgdorferi*.

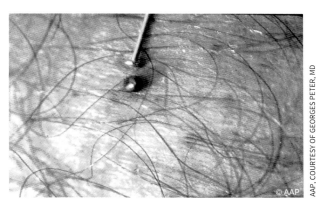

Child with a deer tick attached to skin (compared with the head of a sewing pin)

What are the signs or symptoms?

- Gradually expanding, large, circular or oval-shaped skin lesion (rash) with central clearing that appears after a tick bite. The individual lesion gets very large—usually 5 cm or greater in size. This lesion is present in children with early Lyme disease.
- Fever.
- Headache.
- Mild neck stiffness.
- Flu-like signs or symptoms.
- Inability to move some of the muscles in the face (facial palsy).
- Untreated Lyme disease usually resolves by itself, but a few infected people develop late Lyme disease with arthritis, neurologic problems, or meningitis.

What are the incubation and contagious periods?

- Incubation period: 1 to 32 days (usually around 11 days) from tick bite to appearance of rash.
- Contagious period: Lyme disease is not contagious except through blood transfusions or organ donation.

How is it spread?

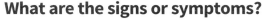

When infected ticks attach to and feed on humans long enough (minimum of 36 hours)

How do you control it?

- Avoid tick habitats (eg, tall grassy areas, bushes, wooded areas) if possible. Walk in the center of trails to limit brushing against trees, bushes, and high grasses.
- If children will be in tick-infested areas, dress them with hats, light-colored clothing, long sleeves, long pants tucked into socks, and closed shoes.
- Spray permethrin on clothing to prevent tick attachment. Apply the spray to the clothing when it is off the child in a well-ventilated area outdoors. Be sure to let the sprayed clothing dry before anyone wears it. Permethrin should not be applied directly to skin. Some clothing comes from the manufacturer permethrin treated. Permethrin-treated clothing offers better protection against ticks than diethyltoluamide (DEET) applied to the skin. DEET offers better protection than permethrin against mosquitoes.
- DEET may be applied to exposed skin according to Centers for Disease Control and Prevention (CDC) instructions (www.cdc.gov/westnile/faq/repellent.html) and the US Environmental Protection Agency (EPA) (www.epa.gov/insect-repellents/deet).
- DEET is safe when used according to the instructions on the product label. Be careful not to get it into the eyes or mouth because it can irritate these tissues. DEET is available in different concentrations. The concentration determines the length of time DEET will provide protection. Products with less than 10% active ingredient may only offer protection for 1 to 2 hours. Newer formulations of DEET that offer sustained-release or controlled-release (microencapsulated) formulations, even with lower active-ingredient concentrations, may provide longer protection times, up to 12 hours. Concentrations of

DEET above 50% do not offer much more protection time than those that contain 50% DEET. The CDC recommends using products containing 20% to 30% DEET on exposed skin to reduce biting by ticks that may spread disease.

- Products that combine DEET with sunscreen should not be used. Sunscreens need to be reapplied at least every 2 hours because they can be washed off by water play or sweating. Repeated application may increase the potential toxic effects of DEET.
  - Apply DEET sparingly on exposed skin; do not use under clothing. If repellent is applied to clothing, wash or dry-clean treated clothing before wearing again.
  - Do not use DEET on the hands of young children; avoid applying to areas around the eyes and mouth.
  - Do not use DEET over cuts, wounds, or irritated skin. Wash treated skin with soap and water after returning indoors; wash treated clothing.
  - Avoid spraying in enclosed areas; do not use DEET near food.
  - According to the EPA, there is no age restriction for DEET use. For infants and young children, use of products with the lowest effective DEET concentrations (ie, between 20% and 30%) seems most prudent. For infants and young children, DEET should be applied sparingly—preferably applied to clothing when possible. If DEET is used on the skin of infants and young children, it should be applied as a very small amount to exposed skin and only to skin children cannot put into their mouths.
  - Obtain written permission from the parent/guardian to use tick repellent and follow the instructions on the label. A pediatric health professional note is not required.
- Picaridin (also known as icaridin) is a repellent that will not damage certain fabrics and plastics that are stained by DEET. Picaridin products have a similar protection time to DEET of 2 to 12 hours.
- Lyme disease is treatable with antibiotics.

What are the roles of the educator and the family?

- Locate play areas away from heavily treed areas. Keep play areas mowed, leaves raked, and underbrush cleared. Put a barrier of dry wood chips or gravel between play areas and heavily treed areas to separate people from the bushes and tree leaves where ticks wait for a warm body to come by.

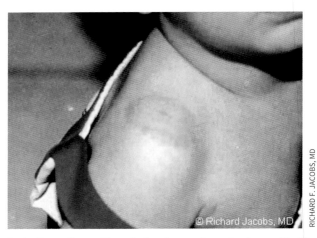

RICHARD F. JACOBS, MD

Rash of Lyme disease. The rash of erythema migrans in a 4-year-old with infection caused by *Borrelia burgdorferi*.

- Inspect children's skin and scalps after possible tick exposure. Tick checks should occur right after a possible exposure to an area that might have ticks. The sooner the ticks are removed, the better.
  - How to inspect for ticks: Look for these small insects on outer clothing. Then check the child's skin. If the outer clothing has ticks on it, the ticks can be killed by putting the clothing in a dryer on high heat for an hour. Ticks seek warm areas of the body to attach and get a blood meal. Inspect the scalp, the neck, behind the ears, and areas where clothing is closely held against the skin, like the sock and belt lines, armpits, and groin. Ticks are small before they feed but become as large as a kernel of corn when full of blood.
  - Removing ticks: Grasp the tick with tweezers close to the skin and use steady gentle traction without any twisting motion. Avoid crushing the tick or pulling too quickly so that none of the germ-containing insides or mouth parts are left behind. If fingers are used to remove ticks, protect the skin of the person removing the tick with facial tissue or cloth. After the tick is removed, thoroughly wash the bite area and the hands of anyone who might have touched the tick.
- Be sure to tell parents/guardians that the child has had a tick bite. Saving the tick for testing or identification is not recommended.

Exclude from educational setting?

No, unless

- The child is ill with a tick-borne disease, is unable to participate, and staff members determine they cannot care for the child without compromising their ability to care for the health and safety of the other children in the group.
- The child meets other exclusion criteria (see Conditions Requiring Temporary Exclusion in Chapter 4).

Readmit to educational setting?

Yes, when all the following criteria are met:

When exclusion criteria are resolved, the child is able to participate, and staff members determine they can care for the child without compromising their ability to care for the health and safety of the other children in the group

Other Tick-borne Diseases

Different types of ticks can transmit other diseases. They tend to be area specific and known to public health authorities in the local area. Tick-borne diseases may be caused by parasites, bacteria, or viruses the tick puts into a bite wound as it feeds. Control measures and exclusion and readmission criteria are the same for these tick-borne diseases as for Lyme disease. Infected individuals may not be aware of a recent tick bite.

Some of the following conditions are caused by bacteria and are treatable with antibiotics:

- Rocky Mountain spotted fever
  - Signs or symptoms: Severe headache, fever, muscle aches, nausea, vomiting, and a red, bumpy rash that begins on wrists and ankles and proceeds toward the center of the body. The illness may be severe or fatal in some cases.
  - Occurs more commonly than in the rest of the United States in these areas: along the Atlantic seaboard as far north as New Jersey and Pennsylvania and in the southeastern and south-central regions of the United States.
  - Incubation period: 2 to 14 days (average 1 week) after bite from dog tick or wood tick.

- Ehrlichiosis
  - Signs or symptoms: Similar to Rocky Mountain spotted fever, except the rash is less common. Less severe than Rocky Mountain spotted fever.
  - Occurs primarily in the southeastern and south-central regions of the United States, but occasionally may occur in other regions.
  - Incubation period: 5 to 14 days after bite from deer tick or lone star tick.

- Anaplasmosis
  - Signs or symptoms: Similar to Rocky Mountain spotted fever and ehrlichiosis, except rash is less common and disease is less severe
  - Occurs primarily in upper Midwest and northeastern United States, as well as northern California
  - Incubation period: 5 to 21 days after black-legged (deer) tick bite

- Tularemia
  - Signs or symptoms: Fever, chills, muscle aches, and headache. May involve painful bite site with swollen and draining lymph nodes; can also cause respiratory disease.
  - Occurs from tick or wild animal contact; handling dead animals, most commonly rabbits; ingestion of contaminated water or inadequately cooked meat; and other means (eg, it is considered by the CDC to be a bioterrorism agent).
  - Incubation period: Usually 3 to 5 days (range, 1–21 days) from exposure to the bacteria.

- Babesiosis (caused by a single-celled organism with a nucleus)
  - Signs or symptoms: Fever, chills or sweats, muscle or joint aches, and nausea or vomiting. Anemia may be severe, and disease can last for weeks or months.
  - Transmitted by the deer tick.
  - Incubation period: 1 to 5 weeks following tick bite.

American Academy of Pediatrics

DEDICATED TO THE HEALTH OF ALL CHILDREN®

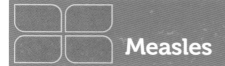

Measles

What is measles?

- A highly contagious and acute viral disease caused by the measles virus. Humans are the only natural host for the measles virus.
- Outbreaks occur when unimmunized people become infected and infect others who are not immunized. Measles was under control but has reemerged in states where vaccination rates have fallen.

What are the signs or symptoms?

- Fever, cough, runny nose, and red, watery eyes.
- Small, typically white spots in the cheek area inside the mouth (called Koplik spots).
- Appearance of rash at hairline spreading downward over body.
- May have diarrhea, pneumonia, or ear infection as a complication.
- Complications may be serious and result in a secondary bacterial pneumonia, brain inflammation, convulsions, deafness, intellectual disability, or death.

What are the incubation and contagious periods?

- Incubation period: 8 to 12 days (but up to 21 days in some cases) from exposure to onset of signs or symptoms
- Contagious period: From 1 to 2 days before the first signs or symptoms appear (4 days before the rash) until 4 days after the appearance of the rash

How is it spread?

- Airborne route: Breathing small particles containing virus floating in the air. These particles first come from a child's respiratory secretions as droplets after a cough or sneeze. These germ-containing particles dry out quickly in the air or fall onto surfaces and then dry out and attach to dust particles, which become suspended again in the air. These particles travel along air currents and can infect people in another room.
- Even brief exposure or shared airflow poses a high risk of infection for people who have not had the disease before, have not been protected by the measles vaccine, or have a problem with their immune system.

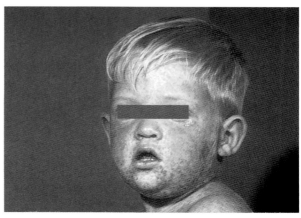

Face of a child with measles, characteristic of the third day of the rash

How do you control it?

- Measles is a vaccine-preventable infection. Immunize according to current schedule—when a child is 12 to 15 months of age and with a second dose at 4 to 6 years of age.
- Review immunization status of all children and staff members and identify those who are not protected by vaccine in the event there is a risk of exposure to someone with the disease that the vaccine prevents.
- Exclude infected children until 4 days after the rash starts when they are no longer contagious. Measles is a highly contagious infection. Because measles viruses are spread by the airborne route, infected children should not be cared for in any child care area and should be sent home as soon as possible. They should not be placed in a special room for children who are ill.
- Exclude exposed children and staff who have not been immunized (or who are incompletely immunized for their age) until they become immunized. If they are not immunized because of an accepted exemption from immunization, continue to exclude them until the local health department determines it is safe for them to return. (See the section Exclude from educational setting? for duration of exclusion of these individuals.)
- A single case of measles anywhere in the United States is considered to be a reportable outbreak.
- Use good hand-hygiene technique at all the times listed in Chapter 2 and routine infection control measures.

What are the roles of the educator and the family?

- Report the infection to the staff member designated by the early childhood education program or school for decision-making and action related to care of ill children. That person, in turn, alerts possibly exposed family and staff members and parents of unimmunized children to watch for symptoms and notifies the Child Care Health Consultant.
- Report the infection to the local health department. If the health professional who makes the diagnosis does not inform the local health department that the infected child is a participant in an early childhood education program or school, this could delay controlling the spread.
- Review and ensure all children have received measles, mumps, rubella (MMR) vaccine according to the current immunization schedule.
- Ensure staff members who have had fewer than 2 doses of vaccine are properly immunized unless they are documented to have had the disease or were born before 1957. Individuals born before 1957 are presumed immune because measles was so widespread before vaccine became available, although being in this group is not a guarantee of immunity. A laboratory test is available for testing immunity.
- During investigation of a suspected case, the educational facility should exclude exposed children with weakened immune systems or who have not received MMR vaccine routinely. In an outbreak, infants 6 to 11 months of age can be immunized and then re-immunized at 12 months of age. The 12-month immunization is still necessary because the child's immunity from the previous dose of vaccine may be blocked by the mother's measles antibodies that cross the placenta during pregnancy and are present in the child for a year.

Exclude from educational setting?

Yes.

- Measles is a highly communicable illness for which routine exclusion of infected children is warranted.
- Unimmunized children should be excluded. If unimmunized, exposed children are excluded for this reason, they may be readmitted on receiving measles immunization. If they remain unimmunized, they should be excluded for 21 days after the onset of rash in the last case of measles.
- Immune globulin may prevent or modify measles disease in an unimmunized susceptible person if given within 6 days of exposure, especially infants younger than 6 months, pregnant women, and those with immune deficiency.

Readmit to educational setting?

Yes, when all the following criteria are met:

- Four days after beginning of rash
- When the child is able to participate and staff members determine they can care for the child without compromising their ability to care for the health and safety of the other children in the group

Comment

The childhood and adolescent immunization program in the United States has resulted in a greater than 99% decrease in the reported incidence of measles since 1963. However, travelers from other countries where measles is more common may cause outbreaks among unimmunized people in the United States.

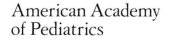
American Academy of Pediatrics

DEDICATED TO THE HEALTH OF ALL CHILDREN®

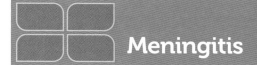

Meningitis

What is meningitis?

- An infectious disease causing swelling or inflammation of the tissue covering the spinal cord and brain.
- Three types of bacteria most commonly cause bacterial meningitis in young children after the newborn period.
  - *Neisseria meningitidis* (meningococcus)
  - *Streptococcus pneumoniae* (pneumococcus)
  - *Haemophilus influenzae* type b (Hib)
- With current immunizations, meningitis from these bacteria is rare.
- Most meningitis is caused by viruses. Although most cases of viral meningitis resolve without antimicrobial treatment or complications, they can be confused with bacterial meningitis in early stages.
- Viral meningitis typically occurs during summer and early fall in temperate climates.

What are the signs or symptoms?

- Fever (may be associated with a blood-red rash of meningococcus)
- Headache
- Nausea
- Loss of appetite
- Sometimes, a stiff neck (ie, pain or discomfort when trying to touch the chin to the chest; child is unwilling to bend head forward enough to look at her or his belly button)
- Irritability
- Photophobia (ie, eye discomfort when looking into bright lights)
- Confusion
- Drowsiness
- Seizures
- Coma

What are the incubation and contagious periods?

- Incubation period
  - For the most common cause of viral meningitis (enterovirus): 1 to 10 days, usually less than 4 days
  - For Hib: Unknown
  - For meningococcus and pneumococcus: 1 to 10 days
- Contagious period

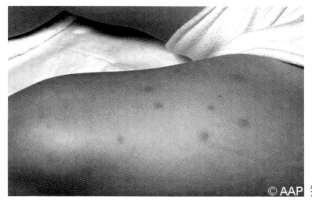

Skin lesions of early meningococcemia

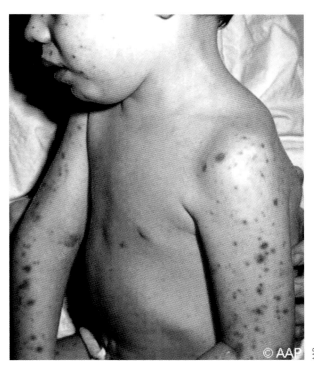

Meningococcemia showing striking involvement of the extremities

- For enterovirus viral meningitis: Shedding of the virus in feces can continue for several weeks, but shedding from the respiratory tract usually lasts a week or less.
- For Hib, meningococcus, and *S pneumoniae*: Until after 24 hours of antibiotics.

How is it spread?

- Contact with the respiratory secretions from or objects contaminated by children who carry these germs, such as sharing of food utensils and drinking vessels (meningococcus, Hib).
- Fecal-oral route (enterovirus): Contact with feces of children who are infected. This generally involves an infected child contaminating their own fingers and then touching an object that another child touches. The child who touched the contaminated surface then puts their fingers into their own mouth or another person's mouth.

How do you control it?

- Bacterial meningitis
  - Immunizations according to the latest schedule.
  - Preventive antibiotics may be indicated for close contacts.
  - Vaccinate unimmunized or under-immunized children as indicated by the local health department.
- Viral meningitis
  - Use good hand-hygiene technique at all the times listed in Chapter 2 and other routine infection control measures in Chapter 2.
  - Recommended immunizations prevent some viral meningitis in the United States from polio, measles, mumps, and chickenpox (varicella). However, these vaccine-preventable diseases are not common causes of viral meningitis.

What are the roles of the educator and the family?

- Report the infection to the staff member designated by the early childhood education program or school for decision-making and action related to care of ill children. That person, in turn, alerts possibly exposed family and staff members to watch for symptoms.
- In communication with health professionals and parents/guardians, distinguish between viral and bacterial meningitis, which may be important in

determining which close contacts need additional management.
- If it is bacterial meningitis, report the infection to the local health department. If the health professional who makes the diagnosis does not inform the local health department that the infected child is a participant in an early childhood education program or school, this could delay controlling the spread of some types of meningitis. Preventive antibiotic treatment may be appropriate for children who have been in contact with the ill child. Involve the Child Care Health Consultant.
- Prevent contact with respiratory secretions. Teach children and educators to cover their noses and mouths when sneezing or coughing with a disposable facial tissue, if possible, or with an upper sleeve or elbow if no facial tissue is available in time. Teach everyone to remove any mucus or debris on skin or other surfaces and perform hand hygiene right after using facial tissues or having contact with mucus to prevent the spread of disease by contaminated hands. Change or cover clothing with mucus on it.
- Dispose of facial tissues that contain nasal secretions after each use.
- Use good hand-hygiene technique at all the times listed in Chapter 2.

Exclude from educational setting?

Yes, as soon as it is suspected.

Readmit to educational setting?

Yes, when all the following criteria are met:
- When the child is cleared to return by a pediatric health professional
- When the child is able to participate and staff members determine they can care for the child without compromising their ability to care for the health and safety of the other children in the group

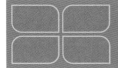

Molluscum Contagiosum

What is molluscum contagiosum?

A skin disease caused by a virus, somewhat similar to warts

What are the signs or symptoms?

Small, flesh-colored bumps on the skin, often with a tiny, hard, indented, seedlike center

What are the incubation and contagious periods?

- Incubation period: Usually between 2 and 7 weeks but may be as long as 6 months
- Contagious period: Unknown

How is it spread?

- Person to person through close contact
- Through sharing of inanimate objects, such as dress-up clothing, or direct contact

How do you control it?

- Perform hand hygiene after touching the bumps.
- Do not share clothing or other skin contact articles.
- Do not scratch the bumps because that may cause further spread of the virus to another site (autoinoculation).
- Usually goes away on its own in 6 to 12 months as the person develops antibodies to the virus; however, may last for years.
- In some cases, treatments may be used to destroy the bumps. However, the treatments may involve painful scraping, freezing, burning, or chemically damaging the bumps. These treatments may cause scars.
- Cover the lesions where possible with clothing or a watertight bandage when close skin-to-skin contact or water activities involve skin where the bumps are present.
- Although molluscum contagiosum bumps represent a viral infection, they are very mildly contagious and most often are spread to other areas of the affected child's body rather than to other children.

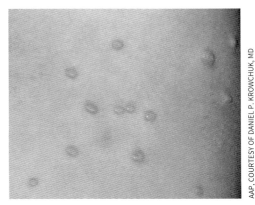

Small raised bumps, sometimes with a tiny indentation in the center, are typical of molluscum contagiosum.

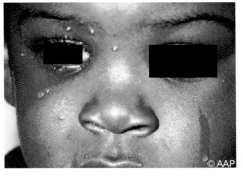

Molluscum contagiosum bumps may appear white or flesh-colored on darker-skinned individuals.

What are the roles of the educator and the family?

- Perform hand hygiene after touching the bumps.
- Do not let children pick at their bumps because this may cause an opening in the skin, which promotes bacterial infection or further spread of the viral infection.

Exclude from educational setting?

No.

Comment

To prevent spread, try to address skin disruption from scratching. Fingernails should be kept short. To reduce scratching at school or at home, use cold compresses (a small plastic bag of ice wrapped in a towel).

American Academy of Pediatrics

DEDICATED TO THE HEALTH OF ALL CHILDREN®

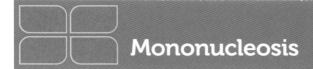

Mononucleosis

What is mononucleosis?

A disease most commonly caused by the Epstein-Barr virus (also called EBV or human herpesvirus 4) and sometimes by other viruses such as cytomegalovirus (human herpesvirus 5) and roseola (human herpesvirus 6); the illness is commonly known as mono.

What are the signs or symptoms?

- Usually mild or no signs or symptoms, especially in young children.
- Fever.
- Sore throat.
- Fatigue.
- Swollen lymph nodes.
- Enlarged liver and spleen.
- Rash may occur with those treated with amoxicillin or other penicillin.

What are the incubation and contagious periods?

- Incubation period: Estimated to be 30 to 50 days for EBV.
- Contagious period: Virus is excreted for many months after infection, and virus excretion can occur intermittently throughout life.

How is it spread?

Person-to-person contact
- Kissing on the mouth
- Sharing objects contaminated with saliva (eg, toys, toothbrushes, cups, bottles)
- May be spread by blood transfusion or organ transplantation

How do you control it?

- Hand hygiene.
- Avoid transfer or contact with saliva (ie, through kissing or sharing respiratory secretions directly or through contact with objects like food utensils, cups, soda cans, and bottles of water).
- People with signs and symptoms of mononucleosis should not donate blood.

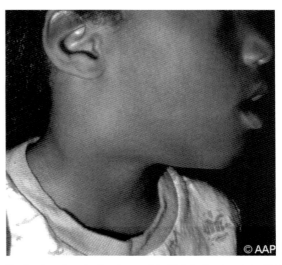

Swollen lymph nodes in a 7-year-old with infectious mononucleosis.

What are the roles of the educator and the family?

- Use good hand-hygiene technique at all the times listed in Chapter 2.
- Clean and sanitize toys and utensils before they are shared (ie, after each child has used them).
- Ensure all children have their own toothbrushes, cups, and eating utensils.
- Prevent children from sharing food
- Avoid kissing children on the mouth.

Exclude from educational setting?

No, unless
- The child is unable to participate and staff members determine they cannot care for the child without compromising their ability to care for the health and safety of the other children in the group.
- The child meets other exclusion criteria (see Conditions Requiring Temporary Exclusion in Chapter 4).

Readmit to educational setting?

Yes, when all the following criteria are met:

- When exclusion criteria are resolved, the child is able to participate, and staff members determine they can care for the child without compromising their ability to care for the health and safety of the other children in the group.
- School-aged children should avoid contact sports if they have an enlarged spleen until the spleen is no longer enlarged.

Comments

- Most people get the infection in early childhood when signs or symptoms are mild and the disease goes undiagnosed. However, rarely, the disease can be severe, particularly in adolescents.
- General exclusion of those with mononucleosis is not practical.

American Academy of Pediatrics

DEDICATED TO THE HEALTH OF ALL CHILDREN®

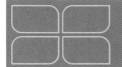

Mosquito-borne Diseases

What are mosquito-borne diseases?

- Diseases spread by infected mosquitoes—in the United States, most are caused by viruses.
- Examples of viruses spread by mosquitoes include West Nile virus, eastern equine encephalomyelitis (EEE), St Louis encephalitis (SLE), La Crosse encephalitis, western equine encephalomyelitis (WEE), dengue, chikungunya, and Zika virus.
- In children, most of these infections produce no signs or symptoms or mild headache and fever. More severe illness (including central nervous system involvement) can occur, especially among adults.
- Malaria is a mosquito-borne disease caused by a parasite that occurs commonly in tropical areas of the world. It is extremely uncommon in the United States, except among international travelers.
- Dengue and chikungunya are mosquito-borne viruses that have recently been introduced into the United States. Dengue has caused illness in certain southern states in recent years and is common in Puerto Rico, the Virgin Islands, and American Samoa, where children may vacation with parents. Chikungunya is another recent virus spread by mosquitos that has come to the United States. Hundreds of cases are reported in the United States each year, nearly all from international travelers.
- Zika is a mosquito-borne disease that usually causes mild illness that lasts from several days to a week. Outbreaks of Zika have occurred in Africa, Southeast Asia, the Pacific Islands, and the Americas but have been spreading to new areas of the world. Zika infection can be transmitted from mosquito bites, sexual contact, and an infected pregnant mother to her fetus. Most cases in the United States occur from travelers returning from affected areas, but small numbers of locally acquired infection from mosquitoes in the United States began in 2016 in Florida and Texas. For the most recent information, visit the Centers for Disease Control and Prevention (CDC) Zika website at https://www.cdc.gov/zika. When Zika virus infects a pregnant woman, it can spread to her fetus and cause microcephaly and other brain defects. The CDC recommends pregnant women consider putting off travel to areas where Zika virus is spreading, use repellents and other measures to avoid mosquito bites if they do travel to these areas, and use condoms for sexual activity of any type while pregnant.

What are the signs or symptoms?

- Many people have few signs or symptoms.
- Fever.
- Headache.
- Body aches.
- Nausea.
- Vomiting.
- Rash.
- Convulsions.
- Coma.
- Paralysis (in West Nile disease, paralysis of the facial muscles [Bell palsy] has been noted).
- Joint pain and conjunctivitis (pinkeye or red eyes) for Zika.

What are the incubation and contagious periods?

- Incubation periods
  - West Nile virus   2 to 14 days
  - EEE   3 to 10 days
  - SLE   4 to 14 days
  - La Crosse encephalitis   5 to 15 days
  - WEE   2 to 10 days
  - Zika   2 to 14 days
- Contagious period: These infections are not contagious except Zika virus, which can be transmitted from person to person; the virus has been detected in blood, urine, saliva, and semen for weeks after initial infection.

How are they spread?

Through the bite of an infected mosquito. West Nile and Zika virus may also be spread by blood transfusion and organ donation. Zika virus can also be transmitted from a pregnant mother to a fetus and through sexual contact with an infected individual.

How do you control them?

- By avoiding mosquito bites and getting rid of standing water where mosquitoes lay their eggs.
- Do not wear products that have an odor. They attract mosquitoes.
- Protect the skin by wearing clothing that puts a barrier over the skin, like long sleeves, long pants, socks, shoes, and hats.
- Use insect repellents containing diethyltoluamide (DEET). Repellents make the user unattractive to mosquitoes. They do not kill the insects.

- DEET is safe and is the most studied and effective mosquito repellent. Generally, higher concentrations of DEET provide longer protection times, but concentrations of more than 50% provide minimal additional benefit. The CDC recommends 20% to 30% DEET concentrations, which provide at least 3 hours of protection.

- DEET should not be used in a product that combines the repellent with a sunscreen. Sunscreens are often applied repeatedly because they can be washed off. DEET is not water-soluble and will last up to 8 hours. Repeated application of this combination product may increase the potential toxic effects of DEET.

- DEET may be applied to exposed intact skin according to CDC instructions (www.cdc.gov/westnile/faq/repellent.html) and the US Environmental Protection Agency (EPA) (www.epa.gov/insect-repellents/deet).

- Apply DEET sparingly on exposed skin; do not use under clothing. If repellent is applied to clothing, wash or dry-clean treated clothing before wearing again.

- Do not use DEET on the hands of young children; avoid getting DEET in the eyes and mouth, as DEET irritates these tissues. According to the EPA, there is no age restriction for DEET use. However, it is prudent to carefully comply with the precautions listed herein when using DEET in this age-group.

- Do not use DEET over cuts, wounds, or irritated skin. Wash treated skin with soap and water after returning indoors; wash treated clothing.

- Avoid spraying in enclosed areas; do not use DEET near food.

- Non-DEET products containing picaridin or icaridin and IR3535 have been shown to be effective mosquito repellents, although less so than DEET. Some plant-based products, such as oil of lemon, eucalyptus, and citronella, show some benefit, although they are not as effective as DEET.

- Many other products claim they prevent mosquito bites, but objective evaluation of them finds they are of little or no value. Among the products that have been found to be ineffective in objective tests are catnip oil, essential plant oils, garlic, vitamin B_1, wearing sound-producing devices, or wearing impregnated wristbands.

- Mosquito traps, bug zappers, ultrasonic repellers, and other devices to prevent mosquito bites are not very effective. Spatial repellent devices that release a repellent material into an area in the form of a vapor are becoming widely available. These products release volatile active ingredients, such as pest repellents metofluthrin and allethrin, and are approved by the EPA for use outdoors. Although many of these products have documented repellent activity, their ability to provide protection from mosquito bites has not been evaluated thoroughly.

- If possible, stay inside during dusk and dawn, when mosquitoes are most active. When outside at these times, wear long sleeves and long pants.

- Check windows to make sure there are no holes in the screens to allow mosquitoes to get indoors.

- Empty or remove standing water from wading pools, buckets, pet dishes, flowerpots, areas where gutter drains leave standing water, and other sources that can attract mosquitoes.

- Some mosquitoes that spread certain viral diseases are active during the day (eg, Zika virus, which can damage a pregnant woman's fetus). Where Zika is known to be spreading, pregnant women should use the measures described herein to prevent mosquito bites at any time of day.

What are the roles of the educator and the family?

- Follow public health recommendations about preventing mosquito bites.
- Share information about the disease.

Exclude from educational setting?

No, unless

- The child is unable to participate and staff members determine they cannot care for the child without compromising their ability to care for the health and safety of the other children in the group.
- The child meets other exclusion criteria (see Conditions Requiring Temporary Exclusion in Chapter 4).

Readmit to educational setting?

Yes, when all the following criteria are met:

When exclusion criteria are resolved, the child is able to participate, and staff members determine they can care for the child without compromising their ability to care for the health and safety of the other children in the group

Comments

- Mosquitoes become infected with West Nile virus after biting infected birds. If you find a dead bird (especially blue jays, crows, or wrens), report it to your local health department and ask for instructions on disposing of the bird's body. Do not handle the body with your bare hands.
- Most cases of mosquito-borne infection are caused by West Nile virus. West Nile virus infections in children are usually mild.

- Resources
  - AAP Family Readiness Kit: https://www.aap.org/en-us/Documents/disasters_family_readiness_kit.pdf
  - Zika Virus: What Parents Need to Know: https://www.healthychildren.org/English/ages-stages/prenatal/Pages/Zika-Virus.aspx
  - Zika Virus: Pediatrician Advice for Families: https://downloads.aap.org/HC/ZIKA_FAMILY_HANDOUT_Infographic_2017.pdf

American Academy
of Pediatrics

DEDICATED TO THE HEALTH OF ALL CHILDREN®

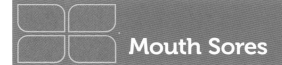

Mouth Sores

What are the causes of mouth sores?

Herpes simplex, canker sores, hand-foot-and-mouth disease, and thrush

What is herpes simplex?

- A virus that can cause a variety of infections in different age-groups.
- In early childhood, most commonly causes blister-like sores (vesicles) in the mouth, around the lips, and on skin that is in contact with the mouth, such as a sucked thumb or finger.
- Virus may be shed by children and adults with no signs or symptoms.
- Herpesviruses stay in the body without symptoms after initial infection; recurrent disease may occur because of a variety of triggers, such as stress, cold, or sunlight.
- See Herpes Simplex (Cold Sores) Quick Reference Sheet for more details.

What are canker sores?

- Shallow ulcers in the mouth and inside of lips and gums.
- The cause is not known but may be related to trauma from biting the inside of the cheek or lip or from injury to mouth tissues while brushing teeth.
- These sores are not contagious.

What is hand-foot-and-mouth disease?

- A virus (enterovirus) that can cause a rash on the hands and feet and shallow ulcers on the inside of the mouth.
- See Hand-Foot-and-Mouth Disease Quick Reference Sheet for more details.

What is thrush?

- White patches on the inside of the cheeks, gums, and tongue caused by a fungus/yeast called *Candida*.
- See Thrush (Candidiasis) Quick Reference Sheet for more details.

What are the signs or symptoms?

- Herpes is the most severe of these conditions, and a primary or initial infection may result in
  - Fever
  - Irritability
  - Tender, swollen lymph nodes
  - Painful, small, fluid-filled blisters (vesicles) in the mouth and on the gums and lips
  - Vesicles that weep clear fluid, bleed, and are slow to crust over
- Canker sores and hand-foot-and-mouth disease may cause pain with eating and swallowing. Some children will drool excessively because it hurts to swallow the saliva.
- Thrush does not usually cause discomfort unless the infection is severe.

What are the incubation and contagious periods?

See individual Quick Reference Sheets for herpes simplex, hand-foot-and-mouth disease, and thrush. Canker sores are not known to be contagious.

How is it spread?

See individual Quick Reference Sheets for herpes simplex, hand-foot-and-mouth disease, and thrush.

How do you control it?

See individual Quick Reference Sheets for herpes simplex, hand-foot-and-mouth disease, and thrush. There is no cure for canker sores. They must run their course for 1 or 2 weeks. Pain medication, such as acetaminophen (eg, Tylenol) or ibuprofen (eg, Advil, Motrin), may be used.

What are the roles of the educator and the family?

- Report these conditions to the staff member designated by the early childhood education program or school for decision-making and action related to care of ill children. That person, in turn, alerts possibly exposed family and staff members to watch for symptoms.
- Stress the importance of good hand hygiene and other measures aimed at controlling the transmission of infected secretions (eg, saliva, tissue fluid, fluid from a skin sore).
- Wash and sanitize mouthed toys, bottle nipples, and utensils that have come into contact with saliva or have been touched by children who are drooling and put fingers in their mouths.
- Avoiding touching cold sores with hands. This is difficult but should be attempted. When sores have been touched, careful hand hygiene should follow immediately.

Exclude from educational setting?

No, unless

* The child has mouth ulcers and blisters and does not have control of drooling. (*Exception:* For hand-foot-and-mouth disease with drooling, children do not need to be excluded.)
* The child is unable to participate and staff members determine they cannot care for the child without compromising their ability to care for the health and safety of the other children in the group.
* The child meets other exclusion criteria (see Conditions Requiring Temporary Exclusion in Chapter 4).

Note: Children and educators with recurrent infection (ie, cold sores without drooling) do not need to be excluded.

Readmit to educational setting?

Yes, when all the following criteria are met:

* When no drooling or exposed open sores
* When the child is able to participate and staff members determine they can care for the child without compromising their ability to care for the health and safety of the other children in the group

American Academy of Pediatrics

DEDICATED TO THE HEALTH OF ALL CHILDREN®

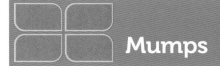

Mumps

What is mumps?

- A viral illness with swelling of 1 or more of the salivary glands
- Uncommon in children with up-to-date immunizations

What are the signs or symptoms?

- Swollen glands in front of and below the ear or under the jaw (no swelling or symptoms in one-third of infections).
- Fever.
- Headache.
- Earache.
- In teenaged boys, painful swelling of the testicles may occur. Girls may have swelling of the ovaries, which may cause abdominal pain.
- Complications include meningitis, deafness (usually permanent), glomerulonephritis (kidney inflammation), and inflammation of joints.

What are the incubation and contagious periods?

- Incubation period: Usually 16 to 18 days but may be up to 12 to 25 days after exposure
- Contagious period: From several days before to 5 days after onset of swelling of glands

How is it spread?

- Respiratory (droplet) route: Contact with large droplets that form when a child talks, coughs, or sneezes. These droplets can land on or be rubbed into the eyes, nose, or mouth. The droplets do not stay in the air; they usually travel no more than 3 feet and fall onto the ground.
- Contact with the respiratory secretions from or objects contaminated by children who carry the mumps virus.

How do you control it?

- Mumps is a vaccine-preventable infection. Immunize according to the current schedule—when a child is 12 to 15 months of age and with a second dose at 4 to 6 years of age.
- Review immunization status of all children.

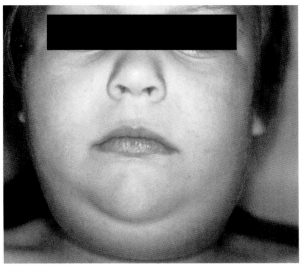

Child with mumps

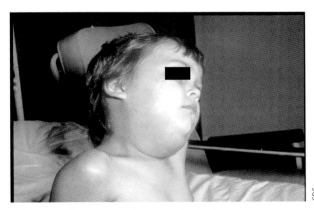

Child very swollen under the jaw and in the cheeks due to mumps

- Unlike some infections, such as measles, mumps vaccine given after an unimmunized child is already exposed to mumps has not been shown to prevent infection. However, vaccinating nonimmune contacts of a child with mumps may prevent ongoing transmission and stop a possible outbreak.

What are the roles of the educator and the family?

- Report the infection to the staff member designated by the early childhood education program or school for decision-making and action related to care of ill children. That person, in turn, alerts possibly exposed family and staff members and parents of unimmunized children to watch for symptoms and notifies the Child Care Health Consultant.
- Report the infection to the local health department. If the health professional who makes the diagnosis does not inform the local health department that the infected child is a participant in an early childhood education program or school, this could delay controlling the spread.
- Refer to the individual's health professional and involve the Child Care Health Consultant to provide education to staff members and families.
- Ensure up-to-date immunization of children, staff members, volunteers, and family members, according to the current immunization schedule.

Exclude from educational setting?

Yes.

- Mumps is a highly communicable illness for which routine exclusion of infected children is warranted.
- Exclusion of unimmunized children may be considered in consultation with local public health authorities. If unimmunized, exposed children are excluded for this reason, they may be readmitted on receiving mumps immunization. If they remain unimmunized, they should be excluded until at least 26 days after onset of swelling in the last case.

Readmit to educational setting?

Yes, when all the following criteria are met:

- Five days after onset of swelling
- When the child is able to participate and staff members determine they can care for the child without compromising their ability to care for the health and safety of the other children in the group

Comment

Most cases of mumps now occur in young adults.

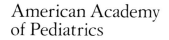

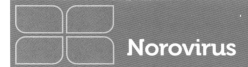

Norovirus

What is norovirus?

- A virus that causes diarrhea and vomiting.
- Currently, the leading cause of diarrhea outbreaks in the United States.
- Disease occurs more frequently in cooler months (ie, late autumn to early spring) than other times of the year.
- Common cause of foodborne and cruise ship outbreaks.

What are the signs or symptoms?

- Fever.
- Non-bloody, watery diarrhea.
- Nausea.
- Abrupt onset of vomiting.
- Muscle ache.
- Headache.
- Dehydration in severe cases.
- Generally lasts 1 to 5 days but may be longer in young children.
- Some children may have very mild or no symptoms.

What are the incubation and contagious periods?

- Incubation period: 12 to 48 hours.
- Contagious period: Virus may be present before vomiting or diarrhea begins and can persist for 4 weeks or more.

How is it spread?

- Fecal-oral route: Contact with feces or vomit of children or adults who are infected. This generally involves an infected person contaminating their own fingers and then touching an object that another person touches. The person who touched the contaminated surface then puts their fingers into their own mouth or another person's mouth.
- Water or food contaminated by human feces.

How do you control it?

- Use good hand-hygiene technique at all the times listed in Chapter 2, especially after toilet use or handling soiled diapers and before anything to do with food preparation or eating. For norovirus, washing hands with soap and water is better than alcohol-based hand sanitizer, which does not adequately kill the virus. Norovirus is highly contagious.
- Ensure proper surface disinfection that includes cleaning and rinsing of surfaces that may have become contaminated with stool (feces) with detergent and water and application of a US Environmental Protection Agency–registered disinfectant according to the instructions on the product label.
- Ensure proper cooking and storage of food.
- Exclude infected staff members who handle food.
- Exclude children and adults who have specific symptoms (see the section Exclude from educational setting?).

What are the roles of the educator and the family?

- Usually, educators will not know that a child has a norovirus infection because the condition is not distinguishable from other common forms of watery diarrhea. The following recommendations apply for a child or staff member with diarrhea from any cause (see Diarrhea Quick Reference Sheet):
  - Report the condition to the staff member designated by the early childhood education program or school for decision-making and action related to care of ill children and staff members. That person, in turn, alerts possibly exposed family and staff members to watch for symptoms and notifies the Child Care Health Consultant.
  - Ensure staff members follow the control measures listed in the section How do you control it?
  - Report outbreaks of diarrhea (more than 2 children and/or staff members in the group) to the Child Care Health Consultant, who may report to the local health department.
- If a child or staff member has a known norovirus infection, follow these steps.
  - Follow the advice of the child's or staff member's health professional.
  - Report the infection to the local health department, as the health professional who makes the diagnosis may not report that the infected child or staff member is a participant in an early childhood education program or school, and this could lead to delay in controlling the spread of the disease.
  - Reeducate staff members to ensure strict and frequent handwashing, diapering, toileting, food handling, and cleaning and disinfection procedures.
  - In an outbreak, follow the direction of the local health department.

Exclude from educational setting?

Yes, if

- The local health department determines if exclusion is needed to control an outbreak.
- Stool is not contained in the diaper for diapered children.
- Diarrhea is causing "accidents" for toilet-trained children or for adults (ie, failing to reach the toilet without having some stool leakage).
- Stool frequency exceeds 2 stools above normal for that child during the time the child is in the program because this may cause too much work for educators and make it difficult for them to maintain sanitary conditions.
- There is blood or mucus in stool.
- The ill child's stool is all black.
- The child has a dry mouth, no tears, or no urine output in 8 hours (suggesting the child's diarrhea may be causing dehydration).
- The child is unable to participate and staff members determine they cannot care for the child without compromising their ability to care for the health and safety of the other children in the group.
- The child meets other exclusion criteria (see Conditions Requiring Temporary Exclusion in Chapter 4).

Readmit to educational setting?

Yes, when all the following criteria are met:

- Once diapered children have their stool contained by the diaper (even if the stools remain loose) and when toilet-trained children do not have toileting accidents
- Once stool frequency is no more than 2 stools above normal for that child during the time the child is in the program, even if the stools remain loose
- When the child is able to participate and staff members determine they can care for the child without compromising their ability to care for the health and safety of the other children in the group

American Academy of Pediatrics

DEDICATED TO THE HEALTH OF ALL CHILDREN®

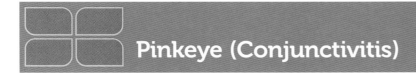

Pinkeye (Conjunctivitis)

What is conjunctivitis?

Inflammation (ie, redness, swelling) of the thin tissue covering the white part of the eye and the inside of the eyelids

What are the signs or symptoms?

There are several kinds of conjunctivitis, including
- Bacterial
  - Red or pink, itchy, painful eye(s).
  - More than a tiny amount of green or yellow discharge.
  - Infected eyes may be crusted shut in the morning.
  - May affect 1 or both eyes.
- Viral
  - Pink, swollen, watering eye(s) sensitive to light
  - May affect only 1 eye or both eyes.
- Allergic
  - Itching, redness, and excessive tearing, usually of both eyes
- Chemical
  - Red, watery eyes, especially after swimming in chlorinated water
- Immune mediated, such as that related to a systemic disease, like Kawasaki disease
  - Red eyes, no discharge, usually affects both eyes

What are the incubation and contagious periods?

Depending on the type of conjunctivitis, the incubation period varies.
- Bacterial
  - The incubation period is unknown because the bacteria that cause it are commonly present in most individuals and do not usually cause infection.
  - The contagious period ends when the course of medication is started or when the symptoms are no longer present.
- Viral
  - Sometimes occurs early in the course of a viral respiratory tract disease that has other signs or symptoms.
  - One type of viral conjunctivitis, caused by adenovirus, may be contagious for weeks after the appearance of signs or symptoms. Children with adenovirus infection are often ill with fever, sore throat, and other respiratory tract symptoms. This virus may uncommonly cause outbreaks in early childhood education and school settings.

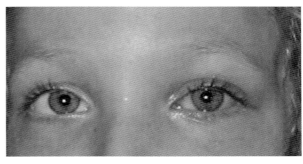

Child with pinkeye

MARK PETER HUGHES

Antibiotics for this condition do not help the patient or reduce spread.
  - The contagious period continues while the signs or symptoms are present.
- Allergic
  - Occurs in response to contact with the agent that causes the allergic reaction. The reaction may be immediate or delayed for many hours or days after the contact.
  - No contagious period.
- Chemical
  - Usually appears shortly after contact with the irritating substance
  - No contagious period
- Immune mediated
  - Occurs in response to a condition that stimulates the immune system of the body, often accompanied by other symptoms
  - No contagious period

How is it spread?

Hands become contaminated by direct contact with discharge from an infected eye or by touching other surfaces that have been contaminated by respiratory tract secretions and then touching the child's eyes.

How do you control it?

- Consult a health professional for diagnosis and possible treatment. The role of antibiotics in preventing spread of bacterial conjunctivitis is unclear. Antibiotics shorten the course of pinkeye only minimally, if at all. Most children with pinkeye get better after 5 or 6 days without antibiotics.
- Careful hand hygiene before and after touching the eyes, nose, and mouth.
- Careful sanitation of objects that are commonly touched by hands or faces, such as tables, doorknobs, telephones, cots, cuddle blankets, and toys.

What are the roles of the educator and the family?

- Report the infection to the staff member designated by the early childhood education program or school for decision-making and action related to care of ill children. That person, in turn, alerts possibly exposed family and staff members to watch for symptoms.
- Notify child's parent/guardian to consult with the child's health professional about diagnosis and treatment by telephone or office visit. Documentation from the child's health professional is not required.
- Seek advice from the local health department or the program's Child Care Health Consultant about how to prevent further spread if 2 or more children in 1 room have red eyes with watery discharge.
- Review hand-hygiene techniques and sanitation routines.
- Complete course of medication, if prescribed (not required), for bacterial conjunctivitis.

Exclude from educational setting?

No, unless
- The child is unable to participate and staff members determine they cannot care for the child without compromising their ability to care for the health and safety of the other children in the group.
- The child meets other exclusion criteria (see Conditions Requiring Temporary Exclusion in Chapter 4).
- There is a recommendation from the local health department or the child's health professional.

Readmit to educational setting?

Yes, when all the following criteria are met:
- When exclusion criteria are resolved, the child is able to participate, and staff members determine they can care for the child without compromising their ability to care for the health and safety of the other children in the group.
- Antibiotics are not required to return to care.

Comments

- It is helpful to think of bacterial conjunctivitis like the common cold. Both conditions may be passed on to other children but resolve without treatment. We do not exclude for the common cold. Bacterial conjunctivitis generally results in less symptoms of illness than the common cold. The best method for preventing spread is good hand hygiene.
- One form of viral conjunctivitis, caused by adenovirus, can cause epidemics. As indicated in the third bullet in the section What are the roles of the educator and the family? if 2 or more children in an educational setting develop conjunctivitis in the same period, seek the advice of the program's Child Care Health Consultant.

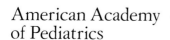

American Academy
of Pediatrics

DEDICATED TO THE HEALTH OF ALL CHILDREN®

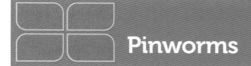

Pinworms

What are pinworms?
Small, white, threadlike worms (0.25–0.5" long) that live in the large intestine

What are the signs or symptoms?
- Most people have no signs or symptoms.
- Itching and irritation around the anal or vaginal area.

What are the incubation and contagious periods?
- Incubation period: 1 to 2 months or longer from the time of ingesting the pinworm egg until an adult worm migrates to the anal area
- Contagious period: As long as the female worms are discharging eggs to the skin around the anus

How are they spread?
- Fecal-oral route: Contact with feces of children who are infected. This generally involves an infected child contaminating their own fingers and then touching an object that another child touches. The child who touched the contaminated surface then puts their fingers into their own mouth or another person's mouth.
- By sharing toys, bedding, clothing, toilet seats, or baths. The eggs are light and float in the air.
- Pinworm eggs remain infective for 2 to 3 weeks in indoor environments.
- Infestation with pinworms commonly clusters within families.

How do you control them?
- Use good hand-hygiene technique at all the times listed in Chapter 2.
- Keep the child's fingernails short.
- Treatment with oral medication once or repeated in 2 weeks may be necessary for the whole family and the group of children who share a common environment.

What are the roles of the educator and the family?
- Report the infection to the staff member designated by the early childhood education program or school for decision-making and action related to care of ill children. That person, in turn, alerts possibly exposed family and staff members to watch for symptoms.

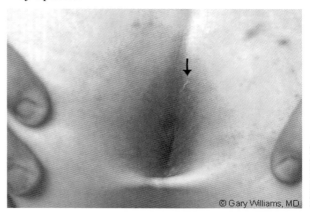

© Gary Williams, MD

GARY WILLIAMS, MD

Adult pinworm in the area around the anus. Inspection 2 to 3 hours after the child goes to sleep may reveal pinworms that have migrated outside of the intestinal tract to lay their eggs on the skin around the anus.

- Suspect pinworms if a child has intense itching around the anal or vaginal area.
- Refer the person with the infection to a health professional for treatment recommendations.
- Bathe the child in the morning to remove a large proportion of eggs that are laid at night.
- Avoid shaking bedding or underwear to prevent spreading ova through the air.
- Wash children's hands directly after using the toilet and before hands are involved with putting something into their mouths.
- Wash toys frequently.
- Clean and sanitize surfaces used for eating, toileting, hand hygiene, food preparation, and diapering.

Exclude from educational setting?
No.

Comments

- Pinworms are not dangerous.
- Pinworms are relatively common among preschool and school-aged children and easily shared within these groups.
- In the past, pinworms were found in 5% to 15% of the US population, but prevalence has since decreased.

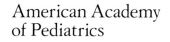

American Academy of Pediatrics

DEDICATED TO THE HEALTH OF ALL CHILDREN®   American Academy of Pediatrics website—www.HealthyChildren.org

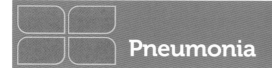

Pneumonia

What is pneumonia?

An inflammation of the lungs primarily caused by a viral or, less commonly, bacterial infection. Infection of the lungs often is secondary to an infection that starts in the nose and throat area (ie, the upper portion of the respiratory tract) and then spreads to the lungs (ie, the lower portion of the respiratory tract).

What are the signs or symptoms?

- Cough
- Fast, difficult breathing
- Fever
- Muscle aches
- Loss of appetite
- Lethargy

What are the incubation and contagious periods?

- Incubation period: Pneumonia is a condition caused by a variety of types of germs; therefore, incubation periods will vary depending on the germ causing the pneumonia.
- Contagious period: Depends on the germ causing the pneumonia.

How is it spread?

Pneumonia does not spread. The germ that causes pneumonia can spread if the person is still infectious at the time the pneumonia develops. Most of the germs that cause pneumonia spread by direct or close contact with mouth and nose secretions and touching contaminated objects.

How do you control it?

- Good hand-hygiene techniques and reducing crowding by ensuring space and ventilation meet the requirements in national standards.

- Prevent contact with respiratory secretions. Teach children and educators to cover their noses and mouths when sneezing or coughing with a disposable facial tissue, if possible, or with an upper sleeve or elbow if no facial tissue is available in time. Teach everyone to remove any mucus or debris on skin or other surfaces and perform hand hygiene right after using facial tissues or having contact with mucus to prevent the spread of disease by contaminated hands. Change or cover clothing that has mucus on it.
- Dispose of facial tissues that contain nasal secretions after each use.
- Sanitize surfaces that are touched by hands frequently, such as toys, tables, and doorknobs, according to the Routine Schedule for Cleaning, Sanitizing, and Disinfecting in Chapter 8.

What are the roles of the educator and the family?

- Immunizations against *Haemophilus influenzae* type b, *Streptococcus pneumoniae* (pneumococcus), and pertussis prevent some of the bacterial infections that cause pneumonia. Influenza vaccine may prevent pneumonia that sometimes occurs as a complication of influenza infection.
- Ensure all immunizations are up to date, including annual influenza immunization for all people older than 6 months. See the most recent immunization schedule at www.cdc.gov/vaccines.

Exclude from educational setting?

No, unless
- The child is unable to participate and staff members determine they cannot care for the child without compromising their ability to care for the health and safety of the other children in the group.
- The child meets other exclusion criteria (see Conditions Requiring Temporary Exclusion in Chapter 4).

Readmit to educational setting?

Yes, when all the following criteria are met:
When exclusion criteria are resolved, the child is able to participate, and staff members determine they can care for the child without compromising their ability to care for the health and safety of the other children in the group

Comments

- Pneumonia is most common during the fall, winter, and early spring, when children spend more time indoors in close contact with others.
- Although most pneumonias are caused by viruses, pediatric health professionals cannot always tell the difference between viral and bacterial pneumonia at the time of diagnosis. Sometimes a child who actually has a viral pneumonia will be given an antibiotic to cover bacteria, just in case.

American Academy of Pediatrics

DEDICATED TO THE HEALTH OF ALL CHILDREN®

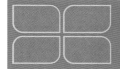

Respiratory Syncytial Virus (RSV)

What is respiratory syncytial virus?

- A virus that causes the common cold and other respiratory signs or symptoms, mostly in children younger than 2 years
- Most common in winter and early spring; one of the most common diseases of early childhood (younger than 4 years)

What are the signs or symptoms?

- Cold-like signs or symptoms (runny nose, congestion, cough) for most children.
- Very young infants also can exhibit
  – Irritability
  – Poor feeding
  – Lethargy
  – Apnea (ie, brief periods of no breathing)
  – Cyanosis (Skin or mucous membranes turn blue, usually when coughing with respiratory syncytial virus [RSV].)
- Respiratory problems include
  – Bronchiolitis (ie, wheezing from narrowed airways in the lungs)
  – Pneumonia
  – Wheezing and asthma attack in children who already have asthma
- Children with weakened immune systems, preterm birth, or heart or lung problems have greater difficulty when ill with this infection compared with otherwise healthy children. Very young infants (<6 months) have higher risk of hospitalization due to RSV.

What are the incubation and contagious periods?

- Incubation period: 2 to 8 days; 4 to 6 days is most common.
- Contagious period: The virus can be shed for 3 to 8 days (3–4 weeks in young infants, usually beginning a day or so before signs or symptoms appear).

How is it spread?

- Respiratory (droplet) route: Contact with large droplets that form when a child talks, coughs, or sneezes. These droplets can land on or be rubbed into the eyes, nose, or mouth. The droplets do not stay in the air; they usually travel no more than 3 feet and fall onto the ground.
- Contact with the respiratory secretions from or objects contaminated by children who carry RSV.
- The virus can live on surfaces for many hours and 30 minutes or more on hands.
- Before signs or symptoms appear, the infected person starts to shed virus that may infect others.

How do you control it?

- Use good hand-hygiene technique at all the times listed in Chapter 2.
- Prevent contact with respiratory secretions. Teach children and educators to cover their noses and mouths when sneezing or coughing with a disposable facial tissue, if possible, or with an upper sleeve or elbow if no facial tissue is available in time. Teach everyone to remove any mucus or debris on skin or other surfaces and perform hand hygiene right after using facial tissues or having contact with mucus to prevent the spread of disease by contaminated hands. Change or cover clothing with mucus on it.
- Dispose of facial tissues that contain nasal secretions after each use.
- Several infection control measures may be considered:
  – Make sure handwashing facilities or alcohol-based hand sanitizers are nearby to encourage hand hygiene (see Chapter 2), especially before and after any activity involving food or touching the mouth, nose, and eyes.
  – Sanitize commonly touched surfaces more frequently during the winter and early spring when outbreaks can be expected.

What are the roles of the educator and the family?

- Report the infection to the staff member designated by the early childhood education program or school for decision-making and action related to care of ill children. That person, in turn, alerts possibly exposed family and staff members to watch for symptoms.
- Practice control measures at home and educational settings.
- Promote breastfeeding, which helps protect infants from RSV.

Exclude from educational setting?

No, unless

- Child exhibits rapid or labored breathing or cyanotic (blue) episodes. (Immediately refer a child with these symptoms to a health professional.)
- The child is unable to participate and staff members determine they cannot care for the child without compromising their ability to care for the health and safety of the other children in the group.
- The child meets other exclusion criteria (see Conditions Requiring Temporary Exclusion in Chapter 4).

Readmit to educational setting?

Yes, when all the following criteria are met:

When exclusion criteria are resolved, the child is able to participate, and staff members determine they can care for the child without compromising their ability to care for the health and safety of the other children in the group

Comments

- Respiratory syncytial virus is a very common cause of hospitalization, especially in infants in the first 12 months after birth. The infection can be fatal, especially in high-risk groups (eg, weakened immune systems, preterm birth, heart abnormalities, lung disease).
- Almost all children are infected at least once with RSV by 2 years of age. Reinfection during life is common. Respiratory syncytial virus infection is usually milder in older children. It can be very severe in the elderly.
- Certain infants and young children at high risk (eg, extremely preterm birth, heart or chronic lung disease related to preterm birth) may benefit from a monthly injection of antibody to RSV throughout the RSV season.
- All children should be protected from exposure to tobacco smoke, and special efforts to avoid tobacco smoke (directly or indirectly [eg, clothes]) are warranted for children who are at risk for serious disease from RSV.
- Children with RSV may wheeze like children with asthma. However, inhaler medications are not effective for most children with RSV who do not also have asthma.
- Cough from RSV often lasts as long as 3 weeks.

American Academy of Pediatrics

DEDICATED TO THE HEALTH OF ALL CHILDREN®

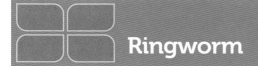

Ringworm

What is ringworm?

A fungal infection of the skin of the body, feet, or scalp

What are the signs or symptoms?

- Skin of the body or feet
  - Red, circular patches with raised edges and central clearing
  - Cracking and peeling of skin between toes
- Scalp
  - Patchy areas of dandruff-like scaling with or without hair loss
  - Redness and scaling of scalp with broken hairs or patches of hair loss

What are the incubation and contagious periods?

- Incubation period: 1 to 3 weeks but can be shorter.
- Contagious period: A child with ringworm of the skin is infectious as long as the fungus remains present in the skin lesion. The fungus is no longer present when the lesion starts to shrink. Spores of the fungus that cause ringworm of the scalp are found on objects in the environment and on people who have no obvious lesions. Once the child begins treatment with a medication taken by mouth, the child is no longer considered infectious.

How is it spread?

Contact with infected humans, animals (eg, cats, dogs), or contaminated surfaces or objects, such as combs, brushes, towels, clothing, or bedding

How do you control it?

- Early treatment of infected people.
- Examination of siblings and other household contacts.
- Not sharing ribbons, combs, or hairbrushes. Launder ribbons and dress-up clothes between users. Do not permit sharing of bike helmets without wiping the contact surfaces of the helmet between users with a cloth dampened with water. Do not use anything other than water to clean the surface of a helmet because some products contain chemicals that make the impact-absorbing materials and straps less safe.
- Covering skin lesions.

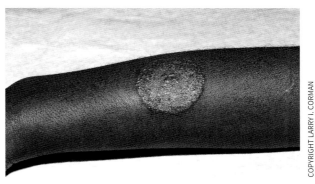

Tinea corporis in a 4-year-old with an enlarging lesion on the right arm

COPYRIGHT LARRY I. CORMAN

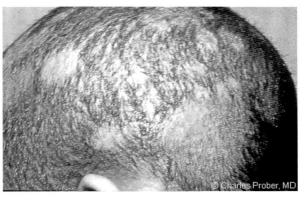

CHARLES PROBER, MD

A patient with ringworm of the scalp, tinea capitis, due to an infection caused by *Microsporum canis*

What are the roles of the educator and the family?

- Report the infection to the staff member designated by the early childhood education program or school for decision-making and action related to care of children with ringworm. That person, in turn, alerts possibly exposed family and staff members to watch for symptoms.
- Give medication as prescribed.
- On arrival and by observation while the child is in care, note any areas of the skin or scalp that might be infected.
- Do not permit the sharing of bike helmets, hats, combs, brushes, barrettes, scarves, clothing, bedding, or towels without washing these items between users. Wash helmets between users with a cloth dampened with water. Do not use anything other than water to clean the surface of a helmet because some products contain chemicals that make the impact-absorbing materials and straps less safe.

- Restructure dress-up corner to make sure an outfit is laundered before a second child wears it or by having and making sure children use and properly discard disposable outfits.

Exclude from educational setting?

At the end of the day, the child should consult a pediatric health professional and, if ringworm is confirmed, the child should start treatment before returning. If treatment is started before the next day, no exclusion is necessary. However, the child may be excluded until treatment has started.

Readmit to educational setting?

Yes, when all the following criteria are met:

Once treatment is started. Athletes with ringworm of the body (tinea corporis) in sports with person-to-person contact cannot participate in matches for 72 hours after starting treatment unless area can be covered.

Comments

- This infection is only mildly contagious.
- Extreme measures of shaving the head or wearing a cap are unnecessary.
- Ringworm of the scalp occurs most commonly in children between 3 and 9 years of age. This infection of the scalp requires about 6 weeks of oral antifungal medicine. Antifungal cream can be used for ringworm of the skin of the body or feet. Sometimes, the fungus can produce a reaction, causing the scalp to swell and be painful (kerion).
- One type of fungus that can cause ringworm of the body and scalp can be transmitted to humans from animals, especially dogs. These animals should be treated.

American Academy of Pediatrics

DEDICATED TO THE HEALTH OF ALL CHILDREN®

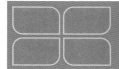

Roseola (Human Herpesvirus 6 and 7)

What is roseola?

A viral infection causing fever or rash in infants and children that primarily occurs between 6 and 24 months of age

What are the signs or symptoms?

- High fever (temperature above 103 °F [39.4 °C] measured orally, axillary, or rectally) lasting 3 to 7 days.
  - Often, the child is not very ill when fever is present.
- Red, raised rash lasting from hours to several days that becomes apparent the day the fever breaks (usually the fourth day).
- Not every infected child will have fever and the rash; in fact, many children have no symptoms at all.

What are the incubation and contagious periods?

- Incubation period: 9 to 10 days
- Contagious period: After infection, the virus is present in the saliva on and off for the rest of a person's life.

How is it spread?

- Respiratory (droplet) route: Contact with large droplets that form when a child talks, coughs, or sneezes. These droplets can land on or be rubbed into the eyes, nose, or mouth. The droplets do not stay in the air; they usually travel no more than 3 feet and fall onto the ground.
- Nearly all children have had human herpesvirus 6 infection by the time they are 2 years old; human herpesvirus 7 infection may occur later in childhood.
- Most likely source of transmission to children is healthy adults. Saliva from three-fourths of adults without symptoms contains infectious virus.

How do you control it?

Use good hand-hygiene technique at all the times listed in Chapter 2.

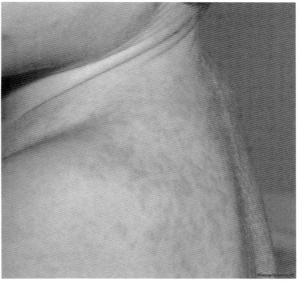

A 13-month-old developed high fever that persisted for 4 days without any apparent cause. The child appeared relatively well and the fever went away, followed by the appearance of a slightly raised pink rash that began on the child's trunk and spread to the child's face and extremities. This is a typical course for roseola.

What are the roles of the educator and the family?

- Report the infection to the staff member designated by the early childhood education program or school for decision-making and action related to care of ill children. That person, in turn, alerts possibly exposed family and staff members to watch for symptoms.
- Inform parents/guardians about the nature of the illness and that, while the fever phase of the illness can cause concern, once the rash appears, the child is in the recovery phase.

Exclude from educational setting?

No, unless

- The child is unable to participate and staff members determine they cannot care for the child without compromising their ability to care for the health and safety of the other children in the group.
- The child meets other exclusion criteria (see Conditions Requiring Temporary Exclusion in Chapter 4).

Readmit to educational setting?

Yes, when all the following criteria are met:

When exclusion criteria are resolved, the child is able to participate, and staff members determine they can care for the child without compromising their ability to care for the health and safety of the other children in the group

American Academy of Pediatrics

DEDICATED TO THE HEALTH OF ALL CHILDREN®

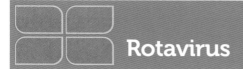

Rotavirus

What is rotavirus?

- A virus that causes diarrhea and vomiting.
- Before the vaccine was released in 2006, the most common cause of diarrhea in children younger than 2 years.
- Disease occurs more frequently in cooler months (ie, late autumn to early spring).
- Nearly all children have been infected by the time they reach 3 years of age.
- Children can get infected more than once because the virus has many types.

What are the signs or symptoms?

- Fever.
- Non-bloody diarrhea.
- Nausea.
- Vomiting.
- Dehydration in severe cases.
- Generally lasts 3 to 7 days.
- Some children may have very mild or no symptoms.

What are the incubation and contagious periods?

- Incubation period: 1 to 3 days.
- Contagious period: Virus is present several days before diarrhea begins and can persist for more than a week after the illness.

How is it spread?

Fecal-oral route: Contact with feces of children who are infected. This generally involves an infected child contaminating their own fingers and then touching an object that another child touches. The child who touched the contaminated surface then puts their fingers into their own mouth or another person's mouth.

How do you control it?

- Rotavirus is vaccine preventable. Follow the most recent immunization schedule. Unlike other vaccines, rotavirus vaccine must be started by 4 months of age and can't be given past 8 months of age.
- Use good hand-hygiene technique at all the times listed in Chapter 2, especially after toilet use or handling soiled diapers and before anything to do with food preparation or eating.
- Ensure proper surface disinfection that includes cleaning and rinsing of surfaces that may have become contaminated with stool (feces) with detergent and water and application of a US Environmental Protection Agency–registered disinfectant according to the instructions on the product label.
- Ensure proper cooking and storage of food.
- Exclude infected staff members who handle food.
- Exclusion for specific types of symptoms (see the section Exclude from educational setting?).

What are the roles of the educator and the family?

- Usually, educators will not know a child has a rotavirus infection because the condition is not distinguishable from other common forms of watery diarrhea. The following recommendations apply for a child with diarrhea from any cause (see Diarrhea Quick Reference Sheet):
  - Report the condition to the staff member designated by the early childhood education program or school for decision-making and action related to care of ill children and staff members. That person, in turn, alerts possibly exposed family and staff members to watch for symptoms and notifies the Child Care Health Consultant.
  - Ensure staff members follow the control measures listed in the section How do you control it?
  - Report outbreaks of diarrhea (more than 2 children and/or staff members in the group) to the Child Care Health Consultant, who may report to the local health department.
- If a child has a known rotavirus infection, follow these steps.
  - Follow the advice of the child's or staff member's health professional.
  - Report the infection to the local health department, as the health professional who makes the diagnosis may not report that the infected child is a participant in an early childhood education program or school, and this could lead to delay in controlling the spread of the disease.
  - Reeducate staff members to ensure strict and frequent handwashing, diapering, toileting, food handling, and cleaning and disinfection procedures.
  - In an outbreak, follow the direction of the local health department.
- Encourage breastfeeding because it helps to protect infants against rotavirus.

Exclude from educational setting?

Yes, if

- The local health department determines exclusion is needed to control an outbreak.
- Stool is not contained in the diaper for diapered children.
- Diarrhea is causing "accidents" for toilet-trained children.
- Stool frequency exceeds 2 stools above normal for that child during the time the child is in the program because this may cause too much work for educators and make it difficult for them to maintain sanitary conditions.
- There is blood or mucus in stool.
- The ill child's stool is all black.
- The child has a dry mouth, no tears, or no urine output in 8 hours (suggesting the child's diarrhea may be causing dehydration).

- The child is unable to participate and staff members determine they cannot care for the child without compromising their ability to care for the health and safety of the other children in the group.
- The child meets other exclusion criteria (see Conditions Requiring Temporary Exclusion in Chapter 4).

Readmit to educational setting?

Yes, when all the following criteria are met:

- Once diapered children have their stool contained by the diaper (even if the stools remain loose) and when toilet-trained children do not have toileting accidents
- Once stool frequency is no more than 2 stools above normal for that child during the time in the child is in the program, even if the stools remain loose
- When the child is able to participate and staff members determine they can care for the child without compromising their ability to care for the health and safety of the other children in the group

American Academy of Pediatrics

DEDICATED TO THE HEALTH OF ALL CHILDREN®

Single copies of this Quick Reference Sheet may be made for noncommercial, educational purposes. The information contained in this publication should not be used as a substitute for the medical care and advice of a pediatric health professional. There may be variations in treatment that a pediatric health professional may recommend based on individual facts and circumstances.

The American Academy of Pediatrics is an organization of 67,000 primary care pediatricians, pediatric medical subspecialists, and pediatric surgical specialists dedicated to the health, safety, and well-being of all infants, children, adolescents, and young adults.

American Academy of Pediatrics website—www.HealthyChildren.org   © 2023 American Academy of Pediatrics. All rights reserved.

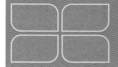

Rubella (German Measles)

What is rubella?

A mild viral infection usually lasting 3 days that is now rare in the United States because of routine immunization

What are the signs or symptoms?

- Many children have no signs or symptoms.
- Red or pink rash appearing first on the face and then spreading downward over the body.
- Swollen glands behind ears.
- Slight fever.
- May experience joint aches or pain (rare in children; more common in adults).

What are the incubation and contagious periods?

- Incubation period: 14 to 21 days; usually 16 to 18 days.
- Contagious period: May be spread 7 days before to 14 days after the rash; however, children are most contagious from 3 to 4 days before rash starts until 7 days after the rash.

How is it spread?

- Respiratory (droplet) route: Contact with large droplets that form when a child talks, coughs, or sneezes. These droplets can land on or be rubbed into the eyes, nose, or mouth. The droplets do not stay in the air; they usually travel no more than 3 feet and fall onto the ground.
- Contact with the respiratory secretions from or objects contaminated by children who carry the rubella virus.

How do you control it?

- Rubella is a vaccine-preventable infection. Immunize according to the current schedule—when a child is 12 to 15 months of age and with a second dose at 4 to 6 years of age.
- Review immunization status of all children.
- Unimmunized children should be excluded from educational settings if there is an outbreak.

What are the roles of the educator and the family?

- Report the infection to the staff member designated by the early childhood education program or school for decision-making and action related to care of ill children. That person, in turn, alerts possibly exposed family and staff members and parents of unimmunized children to watch for symptoms and notifies the Child Care Health Consultant.
- Report the infection to the local health department. The health professional who makes the diagnosis may not report that the infected child is a participant in an early childhood education program or school, and this could delay controlling the spread of the disease.
- Staff members of childbearing age who care for children should have rubella immunity documented because rubella infection during pregnancy can result in miscarriage, fetal death, or severe abnormalities in the fetus, including developmental delays.

Exclude from educational setting?

Yes.

- Rubella is a highly contagious illness for which routine exclusion of infected children is warranted.
- For outbreaks, exclude exposed children who have not been immunized (or, if older than 4–6 years, have received fewer than 2 doses of vaccine) or who lack evidence of rubella immunity by laboratory methods until they become immunized, or if they are not immunized because of an accepted exemption. Continue to exclude them until the local health department determines it is safe for them to return. Unimmunized or nonimmune children need to be excluded until 21 days after onset of the rash in the last case.

Readmit to educational setting?

Yes, when all the following criteria are met:

- Seven days after onset of rash
- When the child is able to participate and staff members determine they can care for the child without compromising their ability to care for the health and safety of the other children in the group

Comment

There is a congenital form of rubella. *Congenital* means babies are born with it, infected from their mothers during pregnancy. Babies with congenital rubella should be considered contagious for at least 1 year, unless the infant is 3 months or older and has 2 specimen results obtained 1 month apart that are negative for rubella virus. If female caregivers of these infected infants are themselves not immune to rubella, the caregivers should be made aware of a potential infectious risk to their unborn babies should they become pregnant.

American Academy of Pediatrics

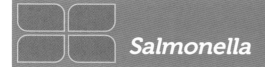

Salmonella

What is *Salmonella*?

- Bacteria that can infect intestines.
- Typhoid fever is caused by a type of *Salmonella* infection that is more serious and can cause outbreaks but is uncommon in the United States.

What are the signs or symptoms?

- Diarrhea
- Fever
- Abdominal cramps and tenderness
- Nausea or vomiting
- Sometimes blood or mucus in stool

What are the incubation and contagious periods?

- Incubation period: 6 to 48 hours (for nontyphoidal *Salmonella* strains, those strains most commonly responsible for diarrhea in the United States).
- Contagious period: About half of children younger than 5 years still have *Salmonella* in their feces/stool 12 weeks after having this infection.

How is it spread?

- Fecal-oral route: Contact with feces of infected children and animals, especially reptiles, amphibians, and poultry, but also birds, rodents, other small mammals, farm animals, and even dogs and cats (see the specific list of animals in the section How do you control it?). This generally occurs when children touch a contaminated surface and then put their contaminated fingers in their own mouth and/or touch an object or put their contaminated fingers in the mouth of another person.
- Ingestion of contaminated food, water, meats, eggs, and unpasteurized milk.
- Contact with fecal material transferred to food preparation or other surfaces or objects contaminated by children or animals with *Salmonella*.

How do you control it?

- Use good hand-hygiene technique at all the times listed in Chapter 2, especially after toilet use or handling soiled diapers and before anything to do with food preparation or eating.
- Ensure proper surface disinfection that includes cleaning and rinsing of surfaces that may have become contaminated with stool (feces) with detergent and water and application of a US Environmental Protection Agency–registered disinfectant according to the instructions on the product label.
- Animals that are known to carry *Salmonella* should not be allowed in an early childhood education (ECE) program or school facility. *Salmonella* is a normal bacterial inhabitant of the intestinal tract of many animals without making the animals sick. Cages and all surfaces involved in the care of these animals should be considered contaminated with *Salmonella*. These objects are a common source of spread of *Salmonella* infection to children in educational settings. The animals most known to commonly spread *Salmonella* to humans include reptiles (turtles, lizards, and snakes), amphibians (frogs and toads), poultry (chicks, chickens, ducklings, ducks, geese, and turkeys).
- Use proper sanitation methods for food processing, preparation, and service. Special attention is necessary to avoid contamination by raw poultry of surfaces such as cutting boards and utensils.
- Eggs and other foods of animal origin, especially poultry, should be cooked thoroughly.
- Exclude infected staff members who handle food.
- Exclusion for specific types of symptoms (see the section Exclude from educational setting?).

What are the roles of the educator and the family?

- A child or staff member with *Salmonella* may have bloody diarrhea. Bloody diarrhea should trigger a medical evaluation.
- There are multiple causes of bloody diarrhea. Until the cause of the diarrhea is identified, apply the recommendations for a child or staff member with diarrhea from any cause (see Diarrhea Quick Reference Sheet).
  - Report the condition to the staff member designated by the ECE program or school for decision-making and action related to care of ill children or staff members. That person, in turn, alerts possibly exposed family and staff members to watch for symptoms and notifies the Child Care Health Consultant.
  - Ensure staff members follow the control measures listed in the section How do you control it?
  - Report outbreaks of diarrhea (more than 2 children and/or staff members in the group) to the Child Care Health Consultant, who may report to the local health department.

- If you know a child in the program has *Salmonella*
  - Follow advice from the child's health professional and care for the ill child.
  - Report the infection to the local health department, as the health professional who makes the diagnosis may not report that the infected child is a participant in an ECE program or school, and this could delay controlling the spread of the disease.
  - Reeducate staff members to ensure strict and frequent handwashing, as well as proper diapering, toileting, food handling, cleaning, and disinfection procedures.
  - In an outbreak (rare), follow the directions of the local health department.
- Prevent contact of young children with animals known to spread *Salmonella* to humans and the habitat of these animals (see the section How do you control it?). Pet dogs and cats should be tested to be sure they are not carriers of *Salmonella* before allowing these animals into the ECE program or school facility. (Ensure immediate hand hygiene if there has been any contact with any of these animals.)

Exclude from educational setting?

Yes, if

- The local health department determines exclusion of an infected child or staff member is needed to control an outbreak.
- Stool is not contained in the diaper for diapered children.
- Diarrhea is causing "accidents" for toilet-trained children.
- Stool frequency exceeds 2 stools above normal for that child during the time the child is in the program because this may cause too much work for educators and make it difficult for them to maintain sanitary conditions.
- There is blood or mucus in stool of the child or of a staff member with diarrhea.
- The ill child's stool is all black.

- The child has a dry mouth, no tears, or no urine output in 8 hours (suggesting the child's diarrhea may be causing dehydration).
- The child is unable to participate and staff members determine they cannot care for the child without compromising their ability to care for the health and safety of the other children in the group.
- The child meets other exclusion criteria (see Conditions Requiring Temporary Exclusion in Chapter 4).

Readmit to educational setting?

Yes, when all the following criteria are met:

- Most types of *Salmonella* (exception is serotype Typhi) do not require negative test results from stool cultures.
- Three negative test results from stool cultures are needed for children with S Typhi.
- Once diapered children have their stool contained by the diaper (even if the stools remain loose) and when toilet-trained children do not have toileting accidents.
- Once stool frequency is no more than 2 stools above normal for that child during the time the child is in the program, even if the stools remain loose.
- When the child is able to participate and staff members determine they can care for the child without compromising their ability to care for the health and safety of the other children in the group.
- When an infected staff member is judged by health department staff to no longer pose a risk to others in the facility.

Comments

- Despite the presence of *Salmonella* in the stool for prolonged periods after infection, outbreaks in educational settings are rare.
- Antibiotics usually are not indicated because they do not shorten duration of diarrheal disease and may prolong the time *Salmonella* is in the stool after the symptoms of infection have resolved.

American Academy of Pediatrics

DEDICATED TO THE HEALTH OF ALL CHILDREN®

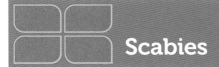

Scabies

What is scabies?

An infestation of the skin by small insects called *mites*

What are the signs or symptoms?

- Rash, severe itching (increased at night).
- Itchy red bumps or blisters found on skinfolds between the fingers, toes, wrists, elbows, armpits, waistline, thighs, genital areas, abdomen, and lower buttocks.
- Children younger than 2 years are likely to be infested on the head, neck, palms, and soles of feet or in a diffuse distribution over the body.

What are the incubation and contagious periods?

- Incubation period
  - Four to 6 weeks for those who have never been infected
  - One to 4 days for those who have been previously infected and sensitized. (Repeated exposures tend to be milder but produce symptoms earlier after exposure.)
- Contagious period: Until the insect infestation is treated

How is it spread?

Prolonged and close person-to-person contact

How do you control it?

- Treatment of the affected child and family by a health professional, usually with a cream containing 5% permethrin.
- Launder bedding and clothing (hot water and hot drying cycle) worn next to skin during the 3 days before start of treatment.
- Items that cannot be laundered should be placed in plastic bags for at least 4 days. Scabies mites cannot survive away from humans for more than 4 days.

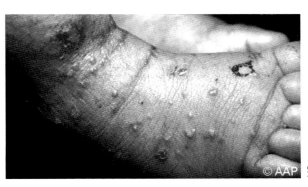

Rash of scabies, which is a widespread area of irritation, often with pink to red bumps along lines and tracks where the insects have burrowed—blisters and pimple-like lesions called pustules

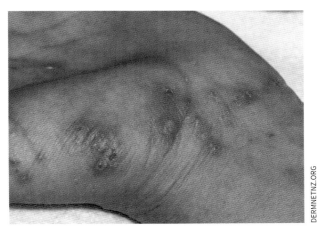

Pustules on wrist and base of thumb

What are the roles of the educator and the family?

- Report the infection to the staff member designated by the early childhood education program or school for decision-making and action related to care of ill children. That person, in turn, alerts possibly exposed family and staff members to watch for symptoms.
- Contact the child's health professional if itching continues for several weeks after treatment. This could represent a reinfestation.
- Family members and very close contacts should be treated at the same time as the child, even if no signs or symptoms are present.

Exclude from educational setting?

At the end of the day, the child should consult a pediatric health professional and, if scabies is confirmed, the child should start treatment before returning. If treatment is started before the next day, no exclusion is necessary.

Readmit to educational setting?

Yes, when treatment has been completed (usually overnight)

Comments

- Scabies affects people from all socioeconomic levels without regard to sex, age, or personal hygiene.
- Itching is related to an allergic reaction to the mites and often goes on for weeks after effective treatment.

American Academy
of Pediatrics

DEDICATED TO THE HEALTH OF ALL CHILDREN®

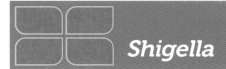

Shigella

What is *Shigella*?

Bacteria that cause an intestinal infection

What are the signs or symptoms?

- Loose, watery stools with blood or mucus
- Fever
- Headache
- Convulsions
- Abdominal pain

What are the incubation and contagious periods?

- Incubation period: 1 to 7 days; average is 1 to 3 days.
- Contagious period: Untreated, *Shigella* persists in stool for up to 4 weeks.

How is it spread?

- Fecal-oral route: Contact with feces of children who are infected. This generally involves an infected child contaminating their own fingers and then touching an object that another child touches. The child who touched the contaminated surface then puts their fingers into their own mouth or another person's mouth.
- Very small numbers of organisms can cause infection.
- Children 5 years or younger, adults who care for young children, and others living in crowded conditions are at increased risk of becoming infected with *Shigella*.

How do you control it?

- Use good hand-hygiene technique at all the times listed in Chapter 2, especially after toilet use or handling soiled diapers and before anything to do with food preparation or eating.
- Ensure proper surface disinfection that includes cleaning and rinsing of surfaces that may have become contaminated with stool (feces) with detergent and water and application of a US Environmental Protection Agency–registered disinfectant according to the instructions on the product label.
- When one or more staff members or children have *Shigella* diarrhea in an early childhood education (ECE) setting, the local health department should be contacted and may recommend that children or staff members with diarrhea be referred to their health professional for stool culture and antibiotic treatment if their culture test result is positive for *Shigella*. While most *Shigella* infections will resolve in 2 to 3 days without antibiotics, antibiotics are effective in shortening the duration of diarrhea and eliminating the *Shigella* bacteria from the stool.
- Exclude infected staff members who handle food.
- Exclusion for specific types of symptoms (see the section Exclude from educational setting?).

What are the roles of the educator and the family?

- A child or staff member with bloody diarrhea should have a medical evaluation.
- There are multiple causes of bloody diarrhea. Until the cause of the diarrhea is identified, apply the recommendations for a child or staff member with diarrhea from any cause (see Diarrhea Quick Reference Sheet).
  - Report the condition to the staff member designated by the ECE program or school for decision-making and action related to care of ill children or staff members. That person, in turn, alerts possibly exposed family and staff members to watch for symptoms and notifies the Child Care Health Consultant.
  - Ensure staff members follow the control measures listed in the section How do you control it?
  - Report outbreaks of diarrhea (more than 2 children and/or staff members in the group) to the Child Care Health Consultant, who may report to the local health department.
- If you know a child has *Shigella*
  - Follow appropriate pediatric health professional advice and care for the ill child.
  - Report the infection to the local health department, as the health professional who makes the diagnosis may not report that the infected child is a participant in an ECE program or school, and this could delay controlling the spread of the disease.
  - Reeducate staff members to ensure strict and frequent handwashing, diapering, toileting, food handling, and cleaning and disinfection procedures.
  - In an outbreak, follow the direction of the local health department.

Exclude from educational setting?

Yes, if

- The local health department determines exclusion is needed to control an outbreak.
- Stool is not contained in the diaper for diapered children.
- Diarrhea is causing "accidents" for toilet-trained children.
- Stool frequency exceeds 2 stools above normal for that child during the time the child is in the program because this may cause too much work for educators and make it difficult for them to maintain sanitary conditions.
- There is blood or mucus in stool.
- The ill child's stool is all black.
- The child has a dry mouth, no tears, or no urine output in 8 hours (suggesting the child's diarrhea may be causing dehydration).
- The child is unable to participate and staff members determine they cannot care for the child without compromising their ability to care for the health and safety of the other children in the group.
- The child meets other exclusion criteria (see Conditions Requiring Temporary Exclusion in Chapter 4).

Readmit to educational setting?

Yes, when all the following criteria are met:

- Individuals with *Shigella* can return once treatment is complete and at least 1 stool culture result is negative. (Some states may require more than 1 negative stool culture result.)
- A pediatric health professional must clear child for readmission for all cases of *Shigella*.
- Once diapered children have their stool contained by the diaper (even if the stools remain loose) and when toilet-trained children do not have toileting accidents.
- Once stool frequency is no more than 2 stools above normal for that child during the time the child is in the program, even if the stools remain loose.
- When the child is able to participate and staff members determine they can care for the child without compromising their ability to care for the health and safety of the other children in the group.

Comment

Compared with other bacterial causes of diarrhea, *Shigella* is the most likely to cause outbreaks in ECE or school settings. Such outbreaks may spread to family members and other close contacts of affected children.

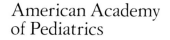

American Academy of Pediatrics

DEDICATED TO THE HEALTH OF ALL CHILDREN®

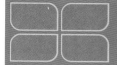

Shingles (Herpes Zoster)

What is shingles?

An infection caused by the reactivation of varicella-zoster (chickenpox) virus within the body of someone who previously had chickenpox or, less commonly, someone who received the chickenpox vaccine in the past

What are the signs or symptoms?

Appearance of clusters of blisters (vesicles), usually in a narrow area on one side of the body. The rash may be itchy or painful.

What are the incubation and contagious periods?

- Incubation period: The virus remains in the body in an inactive state for life after the original chickenpox infection. Shingles may occur when the virus (varicella zoster) reactivates many years after having chickenpox or the chickenpox vaccine.
- Contagious period: Until the vesicles are covered by scabs.

How is it spread?

The virus in the shingles rash can spread by direct contact to a person who has never been vaccinated or had chickenpox. In this circumstance, the virus will cause chickenpox (not shingles) in that person.

How do you control it?

- Use good hand-hygiene technique at all the times listed in Chapter 2.
- Cover skin rash.

What are the roles of the educator and the family?

- Report the infection to the staff member designated by the early childhood education program or school for decision-making and action related to care of ill children. That person, in turn, alerts possibly exposed family and staff members to watch for symptoms.
- Inform others of the greater risk to
  - Susceptible adults and children (ie, those who neither had chickenpox nor were adequately vaccinated)
  - Children or adults with impaired immune systems

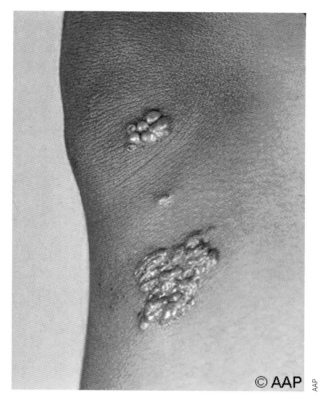

Herpes zoster (shingles) lesions in a child

Exclude from educational setting?

No, unless

- The rash cannot be covered.
- The child is unable to participate and staff members determine they cannot care for the child without compromising their ability to care for the health and safety of the other children in the group.
- The child meets other exclusion criteria (see Conditions Requiring Temporary Exclusion in Chapter 4).

Readmit to educational setting?

Yes, when all the following criteria are met:

- When rash can be covered or when all lesions have crusted
- When the child is able to participate and staff members determine they can care for the child without compromising their ability to care for the health and safety of the other children in the group

Comment

The virus that causes shingles is the virus that causes chickenpox. Vaccination of susceptible individuals is the best way to prevent or decrease the severity of infection with this virus. A vaccine is currently available to boost immunity to the virus and prevent shingles in individuals who previously had chickenpox. It is recommended for use only in those 50 years and older.

American Academy of Pediatrics

DEDICATED TO THE HEALTH OF ALL CHILDREN®

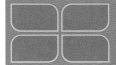
Staphylococcus aureus (Methicillin-Resistant [MRSA] and Methicillin-Sensitive [MSSA])

What is *Staphylococcus aureus*?

- *Staphylococcus aureus* are bacteria that primarily cause skin infections, although, less commonly, these bacteria can cause pneumonia and bone, joint, and blood infections. The "resistant" or "sensitive" part of the name refers to how effectively these bacteria can be treated with methicillin or related antibiotics, such as penicillin, amoxicillin, and cephalosporins.
- Having a methicillin-resistant *Staphylococcus aureus* (MRSA) skin infection is no more serious than other staphylococcal skin infections. Either type can sometimes cause severe infections.
- Although community acquired MRSA is resistant to some antibiotics, there are other effective antibiotics that can be given by intravenous and oral routes.
- Most people who have *S aureus* bacteria living in their noses, on their skin, and around the anus do not become infected; rather, they are carriers (ie, they just carry the bacteria). These bacteria tend to be carried for months to years. Almost half of children carry some type of *S aureus*.

What are the signs or symptoms?

- Carriers have no signs or symptoms.
- With an infection, the signs and symptoms depend on the site of infection.
- When *S aureus* causes skin infections, there may be red bumps that progress to pus-filled pimples, boils, or abscesses.
- Boils may spontaneously drain pus.
- Sometimes, boils and abscesses can progress to *cellulitis*, an enlarging, painful, red area of the skin that extends beyond the boil. Cellulitis may be associated with fever.
- Rarely, the infection spreads from the skin into the deeper tissues, causing a rapidly spreading, dangerous, and very painful infection called *fasciitis*.
- Symptoms of *S aureus* infection in areas other than the skin include fever, tiredness, pain and swelling of the joints or bones, and cough when the infection is in the lungs.

What are the incubation and contagious periods?

- Incubation period: Unknown.
- Contagious period: Children are contagious with *S aureus* when they have actively draining sores or boils. But children may also be contagious with *S aureus* without any symptoms (carriers).

How is it spread?

- Close skin-to-skin contact.
- Crowded conditions.
- Poor hygiene.
- Contact with open sores or boils.
- Contact with toys or surfaces that have been contaminated with the bacteria. A carrier who picks his or her nose could easily contaminate a toy or surface.

How do you control it?

- Use good hand-hygiene technique at all the times listed in Chapter 2.
- Any skin condition that may cause skin breaks, such as eczema, is a risk factor for having a skin infection (including *S aureus*) and passing this on to others. Educators with eczema on their hands or excessively dry skin should practice good eczema/dry skin control. Educators with cracked skin on their hands should wear gloves during activities that involve touching the skin of the children. For children and staff members who have eczema or excessively dry skin, work with the child's family, adults, and the affected people's health professionals to control the eczema/dry skin condition.
- Avoid sharing personal items, such as dress-up clothing.
- Cover open or draining sores or boils.
- Occasionally, *S aureus* may cause infections in multiple individuals in a family or early childhood education program.
- Infectious disease specialists may recommend special soaps and/or baths for individuals and families who get recurrent disease caused by *S aureus* infections; however, the infections may come back despite this treatment.
- Children infected with boils may occasionally have a culture taken; however, more commonly, the health professional may also choose to treat with antibiotics without taking a culture based on their knowledge of local antibiotic resistance patterns.
- Children who do not have symptoms of infection may be carrying *S aureus* but should not be cultured.

What are the roles of the educator and the family?

- Use good hand-hygiene technique at all the times listed in Chapter 2. Provide hand lotion to use following handwashing to reduce the drying effect of frequent hand hygiene.
- Review Standard Precautions, particularly hand hygiene.
- Identify children with red or draining skin lesions, cover the lesions, and report the problem to parents/guardians. Recommend seeking care from their child's health professional.

Exclude from educational setting?

No, unless

- The child is unable to participate and staff members determine they cannot care for the child without compromising their ability to care for the health and safety of the other children in the group.
- The child meets other exclusion criteria (see Conditions Requiring Temporary Exclusion in Chapter 4), or the lesions cannot be covered so that contact with others and surfaces with drainage does not occur.
- Having a MRSA or methicillin-sensitive *S aureus* (MSSA) infection or harboring MRSA or MSSA bacteria (carrier) is not a reason for exclusion unless other exclusion criteria are met.

Readmit to educational setting?

Yes, when all the following criteria are met:

When exclusion criteria are resolved, the child is able to participate, and staff members determine they can care for the child without compromising their ability to care for the health and safety of the other children in the group

American Academy of Pediatrics

DEDICATED TO THE HEALTH OF ALL CHILDREN®

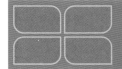

Strep Throat (Streptococcal Pharyngitis) and Scarlet Fever

What is strep throat?

A disease caused by group A *Streptococcus* bacteria

What is scarlet fever?

- A fine red rash that makes the skin feel like sand-paper. Scarlet fever is caused by a toxin produced by a strep infection of the throat or another area of the body. The rash is usually quite prominent in the armpits and groin area, often making the creases in the bend of the elbow and back of the knee pinker than usual. Sometimes, the area around the mouth has a pale appearance.
- Children who have scarlet fever are generally not any sicker than children with strep throat.

What are the signs or symptoms?

- Some of the following symptoms may be present:
  - Sore throat
  - Fever
  - Stomachache
  - Headache
  - Swollen lymph nodes in neck
  - Decreased appetite
- Strep throat is much less likely if there is
  - Runny nose
  - Cough
  - Congestion
- Children younger than 3 years with group A strep-tococcal infection rarely have a sore throat. Most commonly, these children have a persistent nasal discharge (which may be associated with a foul odor from the mouth), fever, irritability, and loss of appetite.

What are the incubation and contagious periods?

- Incubation period: 2 to 5 days.
- Contagious period: The risk of spread is reduced when a person who is ill with strep throat is treated with antibiotics. Up to 25% of asymptomatic school-children and a small number of adults carry the bacteria that cause strep throat in their nose and throat and are not ill. In outbreaks, a higher propor-tion of children with no symptoms of illness may be carriers. The risk of transmission from someone who is not sick but is carrying the bacteria is low.

Note: The bacteria that cause strep throat also can cause impetigo.

How is it spread?

- Respiratory (droplet) route: Contact with large droplets that form when a child talks, coughs, or sneezes. These droplets can land on or be rubbed into the eyes, nose, or mouth. The droplets do not stay in the air; they usually travel no more than 3 feet and fall onto the ground.
- Contact with the respiratory secretions from or objects contaminated by children who carry strep bacteria.
- Close contact helps the spread of the infection.

How do you control it?

- Use good hand-hygiene technique at all the times listed in Chapter 2.
- Have a health professional evaluate individuals with a severe sore throat with a rash and those who have only a severe sore throat that lasts longer than 24 hours.
- If cough/runny nose are major symptoms, strep is unlikely and testing for strep is not indicated.
- Testing for strep in children/adults who are not hav-ing symptoms is not indicated.

What are the roles of the educator and the family?

- Report the infection to the staff member designated by the early childhood education program or school for decision-making and action related to care of ill children. That person, in turn, alerts possibly exposed family and staff members to watch for symptoms.
- Antibiotics for infected individuals.

Exclude from educational setting?

Yes.

Readmit to educational setting?

Yes, when all the following criteria are met:

- At least the first 12 hours of antibiotic treatment has been given. Research has shown that children infected with strep do not pose a risk to others once they have received their first 12 hours of antibiotic treatment.
- When the child is able to participate and staff members determine they can care for the child without compromising their ability to care for the health and safety of the other children in the group.

Comments

- Most frequent cause of sore throat in children is viral infection, not strep throat.
- A throat culture or rapid strep test is the only way to be certain of the diagnosis of strep throat.
- Even if untreated, most children and adults with group A streptococcal infections recover on their own. Some who are not treated develop complications, including ear infections, sinusitis, abscesses in the tonsils, infection of the lymph nodes (ie, tender and warm swollen glands) or a rare kidney disease called post-streptococcal glomerulonephritis. Indications for testing include a sudden development of sore throat, fever, headache, pain on swallowing, abdominal pain, nausea, vomiting, and enlarged, tender lymph nodes in the front part of the neck without a runny nose.
- A more rare but very serious complication of strep throat is the development of rheumatic heart disease, a condition that affects the valves and function of the heart. Children younger than 3 years are very unlikely to get strep throat infection or develop rheumatic heart disease. Therefore, testing these younger children is generally not recommended, especially if they show signs of a viral illness like runny nose or cough.

American Academy
of Pediatrics

DEDICATED TO THE HEALTH OF ALL CHILDREN®

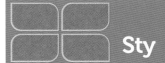

Sty

What is a sty?

A mild infection of a gland in the eyelid at the base of the eyelashes. Also called *hordeolum*.

What are the signs or symptoms?

- Mild pain and a red bump at or near the edge of the eyelid.
- Sties may enlarge and burst and spontaneously drain.
- Sties differ from chalazions. *Chalazions* are caused by inflammation or an infection of an oil gland in the eyelid. Chalazions are not typically red or tender, do not spontaneously drain, and may persist for months.

What are the incubation and contagious periods?

- Incubation period: Unknown.
- Contagious period: Sties may drain pus that contains bacteria. This could be contagious to others, but the drainage period is usually brief.

How is it spread?

It does not spread from one person to another.

How do you control it?

- Use good hand-hygiene technique at all the times listed in Chapter 2.
- Avoid rubbing, which may spread the infection to the other eye.
- Sties will resolve most quickly by applying a warm compress (eg, a wet paper towel wrapped around a plastic bag of warm water) for 10 minutes, 3 or 4 times daily. This usually results in spontaneous drainage.
- Occasionally, a sty may progress to a more widespread infection, called *cellulitis*, indicated by surrounding redness and swelling of the lid. Any spreading redness and swelling of the eyelid requires immediate medical attention.

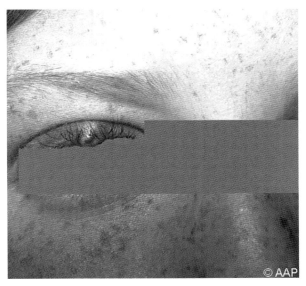

Sty

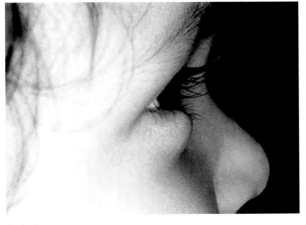

Chalazion

What are the roles of the educator and the family?

- Use good hand-hygiene technique at all the times listed in Chapter 2.
- Review Standard Precautions, particularly hand hygiene.
- Identify children with red or draining eye lesions. Report this to parents/guardians and recommend they seek care from their child's health professional.

Exclude from educational setting?

No, unless

- The eye is actively draining. It is impractical to cover the eye for an extended period.
- The child is unable to participate and staff members determine they cannot care for the child without compromising their ability to care for the health and safety of the other children in the group.
- The child meets other exclusion criteria (see Conditions Requiring Temporary Exclusion in Chapter 4).

Readmit to educational setting?

Yes, when all the following criteria are met:

When exclusion criteria are resolved, the child is able to participate, and staff members determine they can care for the child without compromising their ability to care for the health and safety of the other children in the group

American Academy of Pediatrics

DEDICATED TO THE HEALTH OF ALL CHILDREN®

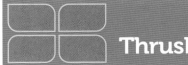

Thrush (Candidiasis)

What is thrush?

A yeast infection predominately produced by *Candida albicans*, causing mouth infections in young infants

What are the signs or symptoms?

- White patches on the inside of cheeks and on gums and the tongue
- Usually causes no other signs or symptoms

What are the incubation and contagious periods?

- Incubation period: Unknown.
- Contagious period: The yeast that causes thrush is widespread in the environment, normally lives on the skin, and is found in the mouth and stool. Mild infection of the lining of the mouth is common in healthy infants. Thrush can occur during or after antibiotic use. Repetitive or severe thrush could signal immune problems.

How is it spread?

- *C albicans* is present in the intestinal tract and mucous membranes of healthy people.
- A warm environment (eg, mouth) fosters growth and spread.
- Person-to-person transmission (although very rare) may occur from a mother to her baby when the mother has a vaginal yeast infection and from breastfeeding babies to their mothers when babies with thrush infect mothers' nipples.

How do you control it?

- Use good hand-hygiene technique at all the times listed in Chapter 2.
- Treatment of individuals who have an infection so the quantity of fungus in any area is reduced to levels the body can control.
- Wash and sanitize toys, bottles, and pacifier nipples after they have been mouthed. Do not allow sharing of mouthed objects between children without first washing and sanitizing them.

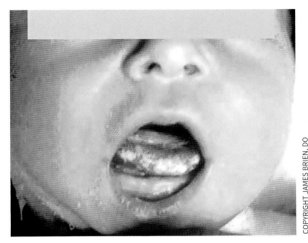

COPYRIGHT JAMES BRIEN, DO

Candida (thrush) infection in a 1-week-old

What are the roles of the educator and the family?

- Report the infection to the staff member designated by the early childhood education program or school for decision-making and action related to care of ill children. That person, in turn, alerts the parents/guardians for treatment of the child.
- Administer prescribed medication as instructed by the child's health professional.

Exclude from educational setting?

No.

American Academy of Pediatrics

DEDICATED TO THE HEALTH OF ALL CHILDREN®

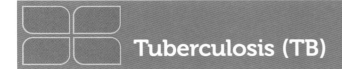

Tuberculosis (TB)

What is tuberculosis?

A disease caused by an infection with the bacteria *Mycobacterium tuberculosis* that usually involves the lungs but could affect other parts of the body

What are the signs or symptoms?

- Most children and adults initially infected with the bacteria do not have signs or symptoms of disease. That is why tuberculosis (TB) testing is necessary when children are in situations with increased risk of exposure to TB and staff need initial screening when starting to work in early childhood education (ECE) programs and schools.
- Tuberculin testing is only indicated for children at risk (eg, family member with TB or positive tuberculin skin test [TST] result, born in or traveled to a high-risk country). Testing should occur 8 to 12 weeks after the last known exposure because it takes some time for the body to develop an immune reaction to TB that the tests can detect.
- Children who are at risk for TB as described previously and who are younger than 2 years should have the TST to detect TB infection. Children at risk for TB infection who are 2 years and older and at-risk adults can have a TST or a blood test called *interferon-gamma release assay* (IGRA). Some children and staff who come from other countries may have received an immunization against TB called the BCG vaccine. For these children and adults, IGRA is a better test.
- All children and adults with a positive TB test result need a chest radiograph (x-ray).
  - If the chest radiograph result is negative and the person has no symptoms or signs of disease, the person is said to have TB infection. If there are no findings of infection in a child's or staff member's body other than the positive TB test result, the child or staff member usually requires only 1 antibiotic.
  - If the chest radiograph result is abnormal, this is called *active disease*. The child or adult may require multiple antibiotics.
- If an infected child or adult does develop signs or symptoms of TB, it most often occurs 1 to 6 months after the initial infection and may include
  - Chronic cough
  - Weight loss
  - Fever
  - Growth delay
  - Night sweats
  - Chills

What are the incubation and contagious periods?

- Incubation period: 2 to 10 weeks after the initial infection. The risk of disease after infection is highest in the first 2 years, but the bacteria can be carried in the body for many years before active disease develops. Most infected people never develop active disease. They remain with latent infection.
- Contagious period: Individuals with latent infection (do not have active disease) are not contagious. Generally, infants and children younger than 12 years with active TB disease are not contagious either. This is because they do not form cavities in their lungs with secretions that contain TB bacterium. When they cough, they do not create enough force to expel large numbers of TB germs into the air. Adults and some adolescents who have active TB spread the bacteria by coughing and contaminating the environment, which is how infants and young children can get infected. Usually, a person with active disease will remain contagious until treated.

How is it spread?

- Infection in children is nearly always the result of close contact with an adult who has TB.
- Airborne route: Breathing small particles containing these bacteria floating in the air. These particles first come from a infected person's respiratory secretions as droplets after a cough or sneeze. The infected person is usually an adult. These germ-containing particles dry out quickly in the air or fall onto surfaces and then dry out and attach to dust particles, which become suspended again in the air. These particles travel along air currents and can infect people in another room. People are only contagious when there is active disease in their lungs or throat.
- It is not spread through clothes, dishes, floors, or furniture.

How do you control it?

- Assessment of the risk of individuals for TB and their need for TB testing should be part of the routine health assessment of all adults who work in the ECE program or school. Each staff member should be tested once on entering the education field. Further testing is based on risk level. Risk is determined by assessing whether the staff member is in a group or exposed to individuals in groups who have higher rates of TB disease. Specific groups with greater TB disease rates include immigrants, international adoptees, and refugees from or travelers to high-prevalence regions (ie, Asia, Africa, Latin America, and countries of the former Soviet Union); homeless people; and residents of correctional facilities.

- TB testing of all contacts of adults with active disease. TB testing of children and staff members may be necessary if there has been an exposure to TB.
- Exclusion and treatment of educators with active disease.

What are the roles of the educator and the family?

- Report the infection to the staff member designated by the ECE program or school for decision-making and action related to care of ill children. That person, in turn, alerts possibly exposed family and staff members to watch for symptoms and notifies the Child Care Health Consultant.
- Immediate notification of local or state health authorities of suspected cases involving children or staff members. If the health professional who makes the diagnosis does not inform the local health department that the infected child or staff member is a participant in an ECE program or school, this could delay controlling the spread.
- Ensure children and staff members take all prescribed medication. Directly observed treatment, performed by clinical or public health staff, may be necessary for active disease and is often advised by the local public health department. For latent TB infection, directly supervised medication taking is not usually used.
- Staff members with previously positive TB testing results, especially those who were not treated, should be evaluated by their health professionals anytime they develop a disease that involves fever, night sweats, weight loss, or persistent coughing to assess their need for treatment and any risk of contagion related to their TB status.

Exclude from educational setting?

Yes, if there is active (infectious) TB disease.

Readmit to educational setting?

Yes, when all the following criteria are met:

- As soon as effective therapy has been started, adherence to medication is documented, and the person is considered noninfectious
- When the child or staff member is approved to return and considered noninfectious to others by local health officials
- When the child is able to participate and staff members determine they can care for the child without compromising their ability to care for the health and safety of the other children in the group

Comment

Some children may develop enlarged lymph nodes, usually in the neck, and be diagnosed with a nontuberculous lymph node infection. These infections are caused by bacteria referred to as *nontuberculous mycobacteria*. Nontuberculous mycobacteria are not considered contagious and no restrictions apply to participation in ECE and school settings.

American Academy of Pediatrics

DEDICATED TO THE HEALTH OF ALL CHILDREN®

Single copies of this Quick Reference Sheet may be made for noncommercial, educational purposes. The information contained in this publication should not be used as a substitute for the medical care and advice of a pediatric health professional. There may be variations in treatment that a pediatric health professional may recommend based on individual facts and circumstances.

The American Academy of Pediatrics is an organization of 67,000 primary care pediatricians, pediatric medical subspecialists, and pediatric surgical specialists dedicated to the health, safety, and well-being of all infants, children, adolescents, and young adults.

American Academy of Pediatrics website—www.HealthyChildren.org   © 2023 American Academy of Pediatrics. All rights reserved.

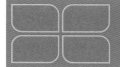

Upper Respiratory Infection (Common Cold)

What is an upper respiratory infection?

The term *upper respiratory infection* usually refers to a viral infection of the upper respiratory tract (ie, nose, throat, ears, and eyes). Upper respiratory infections are common among infants in child care (10–12 per year) but become less common as children mature. Older children and adults have an average of 4 upper respiratory infections per year.

What are the signs or symptoms?

- Cough
- Sore or scratchy throat or tonsillitis
- Runny nose
- Sneezing
- Watery eyes
- Headache
- Fever
- Earache

What are the incubation and contagious periods?

- Incubation period: 2 to 14 days.
- Contagious period: Usually a few days before signs or symptoms appear and while signs and symptoms are present. The presence of green or yellow discharge from the nose is common. Darker or greener nasal discharge does not mean the child is more ill or contagious or has a greater need for antibiotics.

How is it spread?

- Respiratory (droplet) route: Contact with large droplets that form when a child talks, coughs, or sneezes. These droplets can land on or be rubbed into the eyes, nose, or mouth. The droplets do not stay in the air; they usually travel no more than 3 feet and fall onto the ground.
- Contact with the respiratory secretions from or objects contaminated by children who carry these viruses.

How do you control it?

- Use good hand-hygiene technique at all the times listed in Chapter 2.
- Prevent contact with respiratory secretions. Teach children and educators to cover their noses and mouths when sneezing or coughing with a disposable facial tissue, if possible, or with an upper sleeve or elbow if no facial tissue is available in time. Teach everyone to remove any mucus or debris on skin or other surfaces and perform hand hygiene right after using facial tissues or having contact with mucus to prevent the spread of disease by contaminated hands. Change or cover clothing with mucus on it.
- Dispose of facial tissues that contain nasal secretions after each use.
- Sanitize or disinfect surfaces that are touched by hands frequently, such as toys, tables, and doorknobs (see Routine Schedule for Cleaning, Sanitizing, and Disinfecting in Chapter 8).
- Ventilate the facility with fresh outdoor air when possible and maintain temperature and humidity conditions as described in *Caring for Our Children: National Health and Safety Performance Standards; Guidelines for Early Care and Education Programs* Standard 5.2.1.2 (https://nrckids.org/CFOC).
  - Winter months: 68 °F to 75 °F (20.0 °C–23.9 °C) with 30% to 50% relative humidity.
  - Summer months: 74 °F to 82 °F (23.3 °C–27.8 °C) with 30% to 50% relative humidity.
  - Air quality: Have a contractor assess and recommend what should be done to have the air quality in the facility meet the current American Society of Heating, Refrigerating, and Air-Conditioning Engineers standards (https://www.ashrae.org/technical-resources/standards-and-guidelines) or US Environmental Protection Agency standards for air quality in schools (https://www.epa.gov/iaq-schools).

What are the roles of the educator and the family?

Exclusion of children with signs or symptoms has no benefit in reducing the spread of common respiratory infections. Viruses that cause upper respiratory infections are often spread by children who do not have signs or symptoms (ie, before they get sick or after they recover) or who never develop symptoms.

Exclude from educational setting?

No, unless

- The child is unable to participate and staff members determine they cannot care for the child without compromising their ability to care for the health and safety of the other children in the group.
- The child meets other exclusion criteria (see Conditions Requiring Temporary Exclusion in Chapter 4).

Readmit to educational setting?

Yes, when all the following criteria are met:

When exclusion criteria are resolved, the child is able to participate, and staff members determine they can care for the child without compromising their ability to care for the health and safety of the other children in the group

American Academy of Pediatrics

DEDICATED TO THE HEALTH OF ALL CHILDREN®

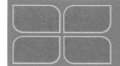

Urinary Tract Infection

What is a urinary tract infection?

An infection of 1 or more parts of the urinary system. The urinary system includes the kidneys, tubes that join the kidneys to the bladder (ureters), bladder, and tube that leads from the bladder to the outside (the urethra).

What are the signs or symptoms?

- Pain when urinating or in the abdomen
- Increased frequency of urinating
- Fever
- Vomiting
- Irritability in preverbal children
- Loss of toilet training after the child has had good control of urine for a period, especially when loss of control occurs in the daytime, with little warning

What are the incubation and contagious periods?

- Incubation period: Usually a few days.
- Contagious period: Urinary tract infections are not contagious.

How is it spread?

Infection usually occurs from bacteria from feces on the skin that enter the urethra, particularly in girls. Urinary tract infection is more common in children with constipation and who do not fully empty their bladders during voiding. Less commonly, it is caused by bacteria from the bloodstream entering the kidneys in young infants. Urinary tract infection is not passed from one person to another.

How do you control it?

- Have the child evaluated and treated by a pediatric health professional.
- Many people believe it is wise to teach young girls to wipe from front to back to avoid spreading fecal bacteria from the rectal into the urinary and vaginal area. No scientific evidence is available that shows the direction of wiping matters for healthy girls. However, when fecal material is present, it is usually easier to remove it by cleaning from front to back.

What are the roles of the educator and the family?

Children with signs or symptoms of urinary tract infection should be evaluated by a pediatric health professional. Educators and the family should implement the advice of the health professional, which may include offering fluids frequently, giving prescribed medication, and gentle wiping after using the toilet.

Exclude from educational setting?

No, unless

- The child is unable to participate and staff members determine they cannot care for the child without compromising their ability to care for the health and safety of the other children in the group.
- The child meets other exclusion criteria (see Conditions Requiring Temporary Exclusion in Chapter 4).

The Urinary Tract

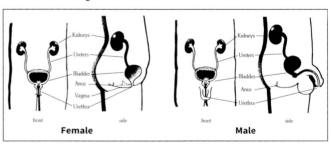

Readmit to educational setting?

Yes, when all the following criteria are met:

When exclusion criteria are resolved, the child is able to participate, and staff members determine they can care for the child without compromising their ability to care for the health and safety of the other children in the group

Comment

A pediatric health professional should see a child with symptoms of a urinary tract infection for a diagnosis and proper treatment. Ignoring urinary tract symptoms can lead to damage to the kidneys, even if the symptoms seem to go away without treatment.

American Academy of Pediatrics

DEDICATED TO THE HEALTH OF ALL CHILDREN®

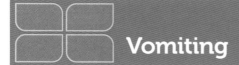

Vomiting

What is vomiting?

- The exit of stomach contents through the mouth.
- Vomiting may have many causes and is not always from an infection. For example, children with gastroesophageal reflux have frequent spit-ups and vomiting episodes that are neither contagious nor necessarily abnormal. A child who has fallen may vomit because of a head injury.

What are the signs or symptoms?

- Children with vomiting from an infection often have diarrhea and, sometimes, fever.
- Prolonged or severe vomiting can result in children becoming dehydrated (dry mouth, no tears, no urine).

What are the incubation and contagious periods?

If vomiting is associated with an infection, the incubation and contagious periods depend on the type of germ causing the infection.

How is it spread?

Direct contact with vomit can result in the spread of certain infections.

How do you control it?

- Use good hand-hygiene technique at all the times listed in Chapter 2.
- Clean and disinfect surfaces that have been contaminated with body fluids.
- Exclude children with vomiting who do not have a known reason and care plan for it. Reflux is an example of a condition that does not require exclusion because it is a known reason for the vomiting.

What are the roles of the educator and the family?

- Use good hand-hygiene technique at all the times listed in Chapter 2.
- Review Standard Precautions, particularly hand hygiene.
- Report the condition to the staff member designated by the early childhood education program or school for decision-making and action related to care of ill children. That person, in turn, alerts possibly exposed family and staff members to watch for symptoms.
- Suggest the family consult the child's health professional if vomiting continues or the child develops other symptoms.

Exclude from educational setting?

Yes, if

- Vomited more than 2 times in 24 hours and vomiting is not from a known condition for which the child has a care plan.
- Vomiting and fever.
- Vomit that appears green or bloody.
- No urine output in 8 hours.
- Recent history of head injury.
- Child looks or acts very ill.
- The child is unable to participate and staff members determine they cannot care for the child without compromising their ability to care for the health and safety of the other children in the group.

Readmit to educational setting?

Yes, when all the following criteria are met:

- When vomiting has resolved
- When other exclusion criteria are resolved, the child is able to participate, and staff members determine they can care for the child without compromising their ability to care for the health and safety of the other children in the group

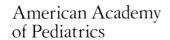

American Academy of Pediatrics

DEDICATED TO THE HEALTH OF ALL CHILDREN®

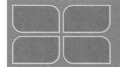

Warts (Human Papillomavirus)

What are warts?

Many different types of human papillomavirus (HPV) cause different types of warts. The most familiar are the common warts (often on the skin of the hands), anogenital warts (on the genitalia, anus, vagina, and cervix), and plantar warts (on the feet). Some members of this group of viruses can cause cancer in deeper tissues (cervix, vagina, vulva, penis, anus, back of the throat, base of the tongue, and tonsils).

What are the signs or symptoms?

- Dome-shaped growth inside the skin that may become a raised area with small bumps within it.
- Usually painless but may be painful when they occur on the feet.
- Often found on the hands and around or under fingernails.
- Black dots may appear in the warts.

What are the incubation and contagious periods?

- Incubation period: Unknown but estimated to range from 3 months to several years
- Contagious period: Unknown but probably at least as long as the wart is present

How are they spread?

Person to person through close contact

How do you control them?

- Perform hand hygiene after touching the warts.
- Do not share articles in contact with the warts of an infected child or educator.
- Do not scratch warts. Scratching could cause bacterial infection or spread of virus to other sites.
- The body may make antibodies to the virus so that, over time, the wart spontaneously resolves.
- Tissue-destructive treatments, such as medicated tape and liquid nitrogen, may activate the body's immune response to the virus that causes the wart and hasten resolution of the warts. However, treated warts may return and often require re-treatment.

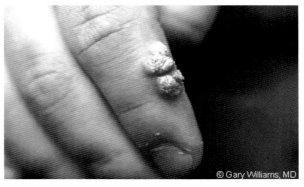

Child with wart on finger

GARY WILLIAMS, MD

- Although skin warts are caused by a viral infection, they are only mildly contagious. In children the skin wart virus most often spreads to other areas of the affected child's body rather than to other children. Warts do not need to be covered like shingles or other oozing sores. Treatment is a personal choice and is not required for infection control in an educational setting.

What are the roles of the educator and the family?

- After contact with the child's warts, use good hand hygiene technique.
- Do not let children pick at their warts because this may cause an opening in the skin, which may lead to bacterial infection.

Exclude from educational setting?

No.

Comments

- Many people have warts at some time in their lives.
- Children who are immunocompromised, including those with HIV infection, may have more severe and widespread wart lesions.
- Genital warts and cervical cancer are caused by different HPVs than the ones that cause skin warts. The HPV vaccine protects against HPVs that cause most cases of cervical cancer and genital warts. Refer to the childhood and adult immunization schedules (www.cdc.gov/vaccines) to find out the recommended age-groups for vaccinations.

American Academy of Pediatrics

DEDICATED TO THE HEALTH OF ALL CHILDREN®

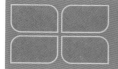

Whooping Cough (Pertussis)

What is whooping cough?

A contagious bacterial infection that causes a range of illnesses, from mild cough to severe disease

What are the signs or symptoms?

- Begins with cold-like signs or symptoms.
- Coughing that may progress to sudden, severe coughing, which may cause
  - Vomiting while coughing
  - Loss of breath; difficulty catching breath
  - Cyanosis (ie, blueness)
- Whooping (ie, high-pitched crowing) sound when inhaling after a period of coughing (may not occur in very young children).
- Coughing persists for weeks to months.
- Fever is usually absent or minimal.
- Symptoms more severe in infants (those younger than 12 months).
- Infants younger than 6 months may develop complications and often require hospitalization.

What are the incubation and contagious periods?

- Incubation period: 5 to 21 days; usually 7 to 10 days.
- Contagious period: From the beginning of symptoms until 3 weeks after the cough begins, depending on age, immunization status, previous episodes of infection with pertussis, and antibiotic treatment. An infant who has no pertussis immunizations may remain infectious for 6 weeks or more after the cough starts.

How is it spread?

Respiratory (droplet) route: Contact with large droplets that form when a child talks, coughs, or sneezes. These droplets can land on or be rubbed into the eyes, nose, or mouth. The droplets do not stay in the air; they usually travel no more than 3 feet and fall onto the ground.

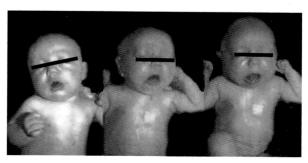

Coughing baby

BROWN UNIVERSITY

How do you control it?

- Whooping cough is a vaccine-preventable disease; however, protection is incomplete and decreases over time.
- Follow the most recent immunization schedule for children and adults. A booster immunization containing tetanus, diphtheria, and acellular pertussis (Tdap) should be given to all 11-year-olds and adults at the time of their next planned tetanus booster and to all who care for infants, regardless of how recently they had their last tetanus booster.
- Review immunization status of all children and staff members. Make sure all are up to date with their vaccine that protects against pertussis. All staff members should have received Tdap vaccine.
- Use good hand-hygiene technique at all the times listed in Chapter 2.
- Preventive antibiotic treatment for exposed household and other close contacts of an infected individual, including staff members, and exposed, incompletely immunized children in educational settings who have close or extensive contact with an individual with confirmed pertussis infection.
- Household members and close contacts who are incompletely immunized should complete their immunizations as well as receive the preventive antibiotic treatment.
- Testing staff members who develop respiratory symptoms after exposure to someone with confirmed pertussis may be recommended by the local health department.

What are the roles of the educator and the family?

- Report the infection to the staff member designated by the early childhood education program or school for decision-making and action related to care of ill children. That person, in turn, alerts possibly exposed family and staff members and parents of unimmunized children to watch for symptoms and notifies the Child Care Health Consultant.
- All adults who have contact with a child who has pertussis in educational settings also should be advised to seek testing if symptoms develop.
- Report the infection to the local health department. If the health professional who makes the diagnosis does not inform the local health department that the infected child is a participant in an early childhood education program or school, this could delay controlling the spread.
- Ensure all children have received their immunization series according to the current schedule.
- Encourage staff members without record of receiving Tdap vaccine to receive the vaccine unless contraindicated.
- Monitor incompletely immunized children for respiratory signs or symptoms for 21 days after last contact with a person infected with pertussis.
- Monitor staff members for respiratory signs or symptoms and recommend treatment if cough develops within 21 days of exposure to pertussis.

Exclude from educational setting?

Yes.

- Pertussis is a highly contagious illness for which routine exclusion of infected children is warranted.
- Exclude close contacts (including educators) who are coughing until they receive appropriate evaluation and treatment.

Readmit to educational setting?

Yes, when all the following criteria are met:

- After 5 days of appropriate antibiotic treatment.
- Untreated children should be excluded from educational settings for 21 days after the onset of cough.
- When the child is able to participate and staff members determine they can care for the child without compromising their ability to care for the health and safety of the other children in the group.

Comment

Older children, adolescents, and adults are most responsible for spreading pertussis because their immunity from the pertussis vaccine lessens over time. A cough present longer than 2 weeks, especially with vomiting after coughing, should raise suspicion of a pertussis infection.

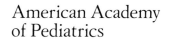

American Academy of Pediatrics

DEDICATED TO THE HEALTH OF ALL CHILDREN®

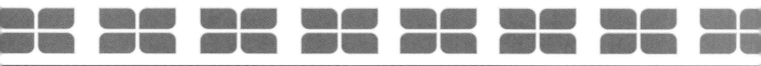

CHAPTER 7

Emergencies and Disasters

Infectious Disease Outbreaks, Epidemics, Pandemics, and Bioterrorism

Emergencies and Disasters: Infectious Disease Outbreaks, Epidemics, Pandemics, and Bioterrorism

Why Children Are Especially Vulnerable

Children are particularly vulnerable to rapid spread of infectious diseases and exposure to toxic substances for several reasons. Young children, especially infants and toddlers, have a natural curiosity that leads to frequent and wide-ranging handling of objects and surfaces. Their developmentally appropriate behaviors include self-soothing by mouthing their hands and other objects. Also, many young children have not completed their series of immunizations for most vaccine-preventable diseases. Until they complete their immunizations, they are more vulnerable to these infectious diseases. Because their immune systems are still developing, they may be more susceptible to other non–vaccine-preventable infectious diseases too. Children can get sicker from smaller numbers of germs because of their immature immune systems and smaller size.

Children breathe faster than adults and therefore can inhale larger doses of toxic agents in the air. This makes them more susceptible to aerosolized biological or chemical agents than adults. Additionally, children spend much of their time closer to the ground or floor than adults. Because many toxic agents are heavier than air, the agents are more concentrated in the breathing zone of children, again putting young children at greater risk than older children and adults.

Children are more vulnerable to agents that act on or through the skin because they have a larger skin surface to body mass ratio than adults and their top skin layer is thinner. Children have lower body fluid reserves compared to adults and are at higher risk of dehydration from biological agents that cause vomiting and diarrhea.

Children are dependent on others for their care. Young children may have difficulty communicating the symptoms they are experiencing. They need to receive vigilant direct supervision by sight and sound. This is especially important during and after an outbreak of disease or exposure to toxic substances.

Children with special health care needs, including developmental disabilities or technology dependence, require focused planning and extra consideration. Thinking ahead of an event about which children may be at increased or even highest risk in a specific disaster or emergency will allow development of plans based on rational setting of priorities and necessary actions. The rapid spread of H1N1 influenza across the population in 2009 and the COVID-19 pandemic that began in early 2020 are examples of situations that would have benefitted from more advanced planning about what to do in a pandemic.

Planning

Before any emergency or disaster occurs, early childhood education (ECE) programs and schools should prepare a written disaster or emergency plan that addresses all relevant risks.

Programs caring for children must assess the types of emergencies and disasters most likely to occur based on the geographic region. Examples of disasters that are based on geography include weather-related phenomena (eg, tornadoes, ice storms), earthquakes, or flooding. Programs must then develop a specific procedure to prepare, respond, and then recover after each emergency. Consultations with local emergency and disaster experts is highly recommended. Plans and procedures must include practicing and revising the response yearly. Children's emergency contacts must be routinely updated, as parent's/caregivers' cell phone contacts may change or children's health professionals may change periodically. Programs should have emergency contact and identification cards of children (for examples, see https://www.savethechildren.org/content/dam/usa/reports/emergency-prep/emergency-contact-cards.pdf). Programs also need to have an emergency kit with supplies to last at least 72 hours (including formula, diapers, and blankets) if there is a need to shelter in place. Plans must include accommodations for any children with special medical needs and chronic health conditions, including an emergency supply of required medications or formulas. Particular attention must be paid to children with technology dependence, as life-sustaining equipment may rely on electricity or require specific formula or other nutritional considerations. Each facility should have an emergency and disaster preparedness staff member who makes certain that policies and procedures are updated, routinely communicates and updates families, confirms that staff receive yearly training, and can act as a liaison with community emergency experts (eg, local sheriff, fire). Early childhood education programs should also update local emergency response authorities related to their location and how many children they have on-site, as these authorities may not be aware the program exists.

Risks of disaster and emergencies include
- Infectious disease
- Artificial disasters/emergencies (bioterrorism, security, presence of threatening individuals, acts of violence)
- Environmental health emergencies (eg, chemical spills, gas leak).
- Natural disasters (floods, tornadoes, ice, earthquakes)
- Facility damage or fire

Several free toolkits exist to help ECE programs prepare for emergencies and disasters.
- Emergency Preparedness Manual for Early Childhood Programs, from the Head Start Early Childhood Learning & Knowledge Center (https://eclkc.ohs.acf.hhs.gov/safety-practices/emergency-preparedness-manual-early-childhood-programs/emergency-preparedness-manual-early-childhood-programs)
- *Do the Prep Steps! Preschool: Five 30-Minute Emergency Preparedness Lessons*, from Save the Children (https://www.savethechildren.org/content/dam/usa/reports/emergency-prep/GRGS-PREPSTEP-PRESCHOOL.PDF)
- *Are You Prepared for Disasters? Family Readiness Kit*, from the American Academy of Pediatrics (https://www.aap.org/en/patient-care/disasters-and-children/resources-for-families)

The plan should specify procedures for conducting regular drills related to each risk that include
- Mechanisms for communicating with parents/legal guardians and public officials in the event of an emergency, including if typical communication mechanisms (phone, internet) are not working (eg, using short message service [SMS] text messaging).
- Evacuation and safe transport procedures
- Primary and secondary meeting places for reunification of parents/legal guardians with their children
- Mechanisms for tracking and caring for children until parents/legal guardians can accept responsibility for their care
- Procedures for sheltering in place
- Care for children and adult workers with special needs
- Procedures for record maintenance, recovery, or preservation of health and other essential documents
- Education of staff members and parents/legal guardians about these emergency procedures

For specific plans to have in place for emergencies or disasters and seasonal and pandemic influenza, see *Caring for Our Children*, Standards 9.2.4.3 and 9.2.4.4 (https://nrckids.org/CFOC).

Types of Infectious Disease Emergencies

When an unexpected or unknown type of illness occurs or an unusually high number of individuals develop an illness or symptom, the situation may be an outbreak, epidemic, pandemic, environmental issue, or incident of bioterrorism. If a suspected reportable illness occurs in a person at an ECE program or school, the ill person's health professional should be involved in the identification, diagnosis, and reporting to public health authorities. However, the designated staff person in the ECE facility or school should also contact the health department about any unusual situation because reporting from the person's health professional may be delayed. The designated staff member may be the director, another administrative staff person, or the facility's health advocate. As part of the planning process to prepare for an emergency, the designated staff member should obtain information from the local health department about how to report and what type of illnesses of children or staff members should be reported. These may vary by state or locality within a state. If a designated staff person quickly realizes an outbreak of an illness or symptom is occurring, prompt action may reduce the number of people who become ill. A good immediate response to a suspected outbreak of infectious disease is to pay special attention to hand hygiene and sanitation practices. Sheltering in place or temporary closure of children's facilities and suspension of activities may be necessary.

Outbreak

An *outbreak* is a sudden rise in the number of cases of a disease. Most outbreaks are expected and are not emergencies, such as those associated with influenza, hand-foot-and-mouth disease, and bronchiolitis, which occur seasonally each year. A designated staff member (eg, health advocate, director, principal) should report to public health authorities any outbreak or unusual symptoms of illness among staff members or children. This allows public health officials to track these situations to determine if they are expected or if they indicate an unusual disease for which they may suggest control measures and facilitate accurate communication among health professionals, EC educators, administrators, and families.

The term *outbreak* might be used when one or more cases of an unusual disease or severe illness occurs. An outbreak of an unusual or severe illness should be reported to the local public health authorities immediately. For example, if any child or adult in the facility develops symptoms of fever, neck pain, and rapidly spreading dark purple or red rash, this should be reported immediately because it could indicate a dangerous form of meningitis that can spread rapidly. The Quick Reference Sheets in Chapter 6 specify when an outbreak of an infectious disease should be reported. Additionally, ECE programs and schools can serve as important communication links between public health officials and involved families.

Epidemic

The occurrence of more cases of disease than would be expected in a community or region during a given period is called an *epidemic.* The term is similar to outbreak. However, epidemic describes an unexpected increase in frequency of illness in a group of people that is not explained by normal seasonal increases.

Pandemic

An epidemic that spreads through human populations worldwide is called a *pandemic.* For example, influenza causes seasonal epidemics annually. Infrequently, the influenza virus has enough of a shift in its genetic makeup to evade a population's immunity, causing rapid global spread or a pandemic. Coronaviruses are one cause of the common cold. However, in 2019 a coronavirus (SARS-CoV-2) emerged that was so different from previous versions that no one was immune. This was the cause of the COVID-19 pandemic (ie, coronavirus disease 2019). Aside from influenza virus and coronavirus, there are other infectious diseases that have the potential to cause a pandemic. Public health officials are engaged in ongoing efforts to prepare for and reduce the effects of a pandemic, but it is also important that ECE programs and schools have a pandemic plan in place. As demonstrated during the COVID-19 pandemic, these viruses can have a significant effect on the function of ECE programs and schools and so planning ahead can help decrease disruptions when outbreaks occur.

Bioterrorism

Intentional release of a biological agent to cause illness is *bioterrorism.* The biological agent involved in bioterrorism may be a living germ or a poison from a germ, such as anthrax, ricin, or botulism toxin. If a group of children and adults becomes ill with similar symptoms at the same time, public health authorities should be notified.

Closure of Educational Facilities

During an infectious disease emergency, the decision to close educational facilities should be based on recommendations from national, state, or local public health officials. Closures may involve individual classrooms or entire centers or schools. Health officials must tailor the response depending on how the infectious disease spreads (eg, air, food, direct contact) and weigh the benefit of closure in reducing the spread against the negative effects that prolonged closure of ECE programs and schools has on children and families. Chiefly, these closures affect the social-emotional well-being of children and youth. Additionally, closures impair the ability of parents to earn income and hold their job, disrupting the economy. Early childhood education program closures for longer than 2 weeks can result in permanent closure due to lack of revenue to pay rent and staff. Also, when a closure occurs, some families are likely to put their children in other ECE settings in the area and, thus, contribute to the spread of the problem in the community. Administrators of ECE programs or schools may elect to suspend operations voluntarily when illness among staff and students reaches levels that exceed their ability to operate safely or efficiently.

Every ECE program and school should have a disaster plan that specifies procedures for possible program closure. These plans should be updated and tested routinely (eg, drills, discussing disaster scenarios at staff meetings). The written plans should also be easily accessible, so staff can find them quickly. Educators, parents/legal guardians, Child Care Health Consultants, and public health officials should be involved in this planning.

Symptom Records

Conducting daily health checks and keeping symptom records for each child on a regular basis is a good way for educators to identify possible infectious disease outbreaks, epidemics, or emergencies within a group. Early childhood education and school facilities typically document enrollment and attendance, yet not all perform regular health checks and track the symptoms of the children in their care. Some programs use a sign-in sheet, which is completed when the child is brought to the facility for the day. This is usually kept at the entrance to the facility or at the entrance to the shared space; others have a classroom log. See Chapter 8 for the Enrollment/Attendance/Symptom Record, a tool to easily track key information for a month about individual children who receive care together in a space in the facility.

Tracking Procedure

Quick and appropriate response to unusual circumstances is critical. Every day, someone should look at the records of symptoms for individual groups of children in the facility to detect patterns of illness promptly within each group of children and in the facility overall. If the records suggest an emerging pattern of illness, fewer people may become ill if staff members become more vigilant about performing sanitation and hygiene routines.

In addition, someone on the staff should review the daily illness symptom records about once a month, noting differences in patterns within and among groups of children in the facility. Such differences might indicate a need to increase infection control and prevention procedures.

Corrective Action

When children in a group seem to have similar symptoms that suggest a contagious disease or toxic exposure, the program staff should consult with the program's Child Care Health Consultant or public health professional to develop a plan of action. The plan of action might include
- Environmental assessment to determine the scope and nature of the problem
- Immediate education of educators, other staff members, and families about risks, what to watch for, and what to do if symptoms occur
- Enhancement of routine hygiene and sanitation practices, such as monitoring hand hygiene performance to be sure it is done correctly and when appropriate
- Implementation of symptom or screening guidelines
- Modified guidelines related to exclusion and separation of groups in the facility
- Use of medicines that can prevent disease if indicated and other precautionary measures
- On-site immunization clinics (and checking or verifying immunization records show up-to-date status for all staff and enrolled children)
- Other mitigation strategies, such as masking if recommended by the public health department

Parent/Legal Guardian Notification

Providing clear, accurate, and helpful information to families at enrollment and as soon as possible when an emergency occurs is crucial. As part of the preparation for enrollment, the program should talk with parents/legal guardians and give them written information about routine practices (eg, hand hygiene, sanitation, symptom monitoring). The preenrollment preparation should let families know how they will receive information about illness or other health problems that might involve their child. Periodic reminders about the procedures the facility follows will help prepare families to respond appropriately to information when such a situation occurs. It is challenging to notify families about their child's exposure to a potential infection, outbreak, or epidemic without causing

alarm or prompting inappropriate action. The content of such communications will depend on the situation. Sometimes, it will be necessary to provide information to families before the cause of certain symptoms is known or a diagnosis has been made. Families need clear and accurate information about what to do for their own child as well as what actions are unnecessary. The Quick Reference Sheets in Chapter 6 and sample forms in Chapter 8 can help staff members provide needed information once the cause of the exposure to a potential infection, outbreak, epidemic, or pandemic is known. Depending on the scope of the risk, notification may need to be conducted with assistance from local and state public health officials.

Additional Resources

The following resources offer additional information and useful materials about preventing and managing influenza for ECE programs, preschools, and K–12 schools:
- Centers for Disease Control and Prevention information about seasonal and pandemic influenza specifically for ECE programs and and schools (https://www.cdc.gov/flu/school/index.htm)
- American Academy of Pediatrics
  - Preparing Child Care Programs for Pandemic Influenza (strategies, *Caring for Our Children* standards, and other resources related to managing influenza in child care) (https://www.aap.org/en/patient-care/disasters-and-children/disaster-management-resources-by-topic/influenzapandemics)
  - "Pandemic Influenza Preparedness Among Child Care Center Directors in 2008 and 2016" (https://doi.org/10.1542/peds.2016-3690)
  - *Red Book® Online* provides up-to-date information and resource links on current infectious disease outbreaks affecting the pediatric population (https://publications.aap.org/redbook/resources/17748)
- Early Childhood Disaster-Related Resources for Early Childhood Education Policymakers and Providers, from the US Health and Human Services Office of Child Care (https://www.acf.hhs.gov/occ/training-technical-assistance/child-care-resources-disasters-and-emergencies)
- Child Care Emergency Preparedness Training Workbook, from Save the Children (https://oregonearlylearning.com/wp-content/uploads/2017/02/Child-Care-Emergency-Preparedness-Workbook.pdf)
- Crisis and Disaster Resources, from Child Care Aware of America (www.childcareaware.org/our-issues/crisis-and-disaster-resources)

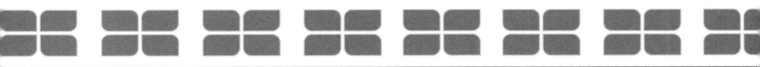

CHAPTER 8

Sample Letters, Forms, and Relevant Resources

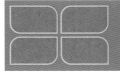

Sample Letters, Forms, and Relevant Resources

See earlier chapters for how these forms can be used and strategies for using them.

Copy or adapt these sample letters and forms to facilitate communication among parents/legal guardians, educators, administrators, and pediatric health professionals. No permission is necessary to make single copies for noncommercial, educational purposes.

Child Health Assessment Form

Parent/legal guardian and educators fill in this part.

CHILD'S NAME (LAST)	(FIRST)	PARENT'S/LEGAL GUARDIAN'S NAME (Last, First)	
DATE OF BIRTH	HOME PHONE	ADDRESS	
EARLY CHILDHOOD EDUCATION PROGRAM NAME		WORK PHONE/MOBILE PHONE	
FACILITY PHONE	COUNTY	EMAIL ADDRESS	

To parents/legal guardians: Be sure to sign a consent form for your child's educators and one for your child's health professional to share information about your child's health with one another.

This facility requires that children who are enrolled in a group care setting have received age-appropriate preventive health services, including screenings and immunizations that meet the current recommendations of the American Academy of Pediatrics. This schedule of required health services is available at www.aap.org/periodicityschedule.

PERTINENT INFORMATION IN HEALTH HISTORY, MEDICAL CONCERNS, RESULTS OF SCREENINGS, FAMILY STRESS[a] INFORMATION PERTINENT TO ROUTINE CHILD CARE AND EMERGENCIES (DESCRIBE, IF ANY)—ATTACH ADDITIONAL SHEETS TO PROVIDE HELPFUL DETAILS. ☐ NONE **ALLERGIES TO FOOD OR MEDICINE (DESCRIBE, IF ANY)** ☐ NONE	DATE OF MOST RECENT WELL-CHILD EXAMINATION This form may be updated (instead of completing a new form) at each checkup by the child's health professional. Updates may be dated, initialed notes or an attached printout of an electronic medical record note.

[a] Name of screening tools if any were used, date, and results of developmental/behavioral screening used by the early childhood education program and pediatric health professional (if any):

Parents/legal guardians may write immunization dates; pediatric health professionals should verify and complete all data on this form or via a printout of an electronic medical record–generated form.

LENGTH/HEIGHT	WEIGHT	BMI	BLOOD PRESSURE
_____ (circle one: cm inch), % _____	_____ (circle one: kg pound), % _____	_____, % _____	(Beginning at age 3)
PHYSICAL EXAMINATION	**✓ if NORMAL**	**COMMENTS**	
HEAD/EARS/EYES/NOSE/THROAT			
TEETH			
CARDIORESPIRATORY			
ABDOMEN/GI			
GENITALIA/BREASTS			
EXTREMITIES/JOINT/BACK/CHEST			
SKIN/LYMPH NODES			
NEUROLOGIC, DEVELOPMENT, & BEHAVIOR			

Child Health Assessment Form (continued)

VACCINES[b]	DATE	DATE	DATE	DATE	DATE	COMMENTS
HEP B						
ROTAVIRUS						
DTaP						
HIB						
PCV13						
IPV						
INFLUENZA						
MMR						
VARICELLA						
HEPATITIS A						
MENINGOCOCCAL						
Tdap						
HPV						
PNEUMOCOCCAL POLYSACCHARIDE PPSV$_{23}$						
COVID-19						

SCREENINGS	DATE TEST DONE	NOTE HERE IF RESULTS ARE PENDING, NORMAL, OR ABNORMAL
LEAD		
ANEMIA (HGB/HCT)		
BEHAVIOR/DEVELOPMENT		
HEALTHY WEIGHT PER BMI		
HEARING		
VISION		
PROFESSIONAL DENTAL EXAMINATION		NAME OF CHILD'S DENTIST

HEALTH PROBLEMS OR SPECIAL NEEDS, RECOMMENDED TREATMENT/MEDICATIONS/SPECIAL CARE (ATTACH ADDITIONAL SHEETS TO PROVIDE HELPFUL DETAILS)

☐ NONE   NEXT APPOINTMENT—MONTH/YEAR:

PRINT HEALTH PROFESSIONAL NAME (PEDIATRICIAN, FAMILY PRACTICE PHYSICIAN, PEDIATRIC/FAMILY PRACTICE NURSE PRACTITIONER, OR PHYSICIAN ASSISTANT)	SIGNATURE OF PHYSICIAN, NURSE PRACTITIONER, OR PHYSICIAN ASSISTANT	
ADDRESS		
PHONE	LICENSE NUMBER	DATE COMPLETED OR UPDATED

[b] Vaccine list from "Table 1. Recommended Child and Adolescent Immunization Schedule for ages 18 years or younger, United States, 2022" (https://www.cdc.gov/vaccines/schedules/hcp/imz/child-adolescent.html).

For information updated every January/February about recommended vaccines by age and condition, see https://www.cdc.gov/vaccines/schedules.

Other useful forms for collecting health information that early childhood education programs should review and retain are on the website of WellCareTracker, an online system maintained by the Pennsylvania Chapter of the American Academy of Pediatrics for educators to document and track routine preventive health care services for enrolled children. To access WellCareTracker and the forms in the following 3 bullets, go to https://www.wellcaretracker.org:

• Letter to doctors requesting health record information

• Letter to parents about providing up-to-date health record information

• Letter to parents describing preventive health services

Special Care Plan Form

Care Plan for a Child With Special Needs in Early Childhood Education   Today's Date _____

First and Last Name of Child	Birth Date	Child's Present Weight
Parent's/Legal Guardian's First and Last Name	Cell/Home/Work Phone #	Signature for Consent[a]
Name of first person to contact about the child's care in an emergency	Cell/Home/Work Phone #	Relationship to child
Primary Health Care Professional	Emergency Phone #	HIPAA Authorization for Release of Information Form completed? ☐ N/A ☐ Yes ☐ No
Specialty Care Providers (For each provider, give type of specialty, phone numbers, and a HIPAA consent form signed by the child's parent/legal guardian for the educator to ask the specialty care provider for additional information.)	Emergency Phone #s	Emergency Information Form for Children With Special Needs completed? ☐ N/A ☐ Yes ☐ No

Allergies   ☐ No   ☐ Yes   If yes, please specify.

Medical/Behavioral/Family Concerns

Needed Accommodations (Please describe accommodation and why it is necessary. Attach additional pages if needed to provide complete information.)

Meals/Snacks/Diet/Feeding	Toileting
Playing Alone or in Group Activities	Outdoor or Field Trips
Nap/Sleep	Transportation

Special Care Plan Form (continued)

Recommended Treatment		
Medications to Be Given at Early Childhood Education Program Specify medications on Medication Administration Forms.	☐ No ☐ Yes	If yes, Medication Administration Forms completed? ☐ No ☐ Yes
Medications Given at Home	☐ No ☐ Yes	If yes, please list in additional information section or attach information.
Special Equipment/Medical Supplies	☐ No ☐ Yes	If yes, please list in additional information section or attach information.
Special Staff Training Needed	☐ No ☐ Yes	If yes, please list in additional information section or attach information.
Special Emergency Procedures	☐ No ☐ Yes	If yes, please list in additional information section or attach information.
Specialists Working With This Child	☐ No ☐ Yes	If yes, please list and indicate the role(s) of specialists who are working with the child and the child's family.
Parent/Legal Guardian Signature Acknowledging Review of Above Information		
Additional Information/Comments on Child, Family, or Medical Issues		Additional Information Attached ☐ No ☐ Yes
Pediatric Health Professional's Signature		Pediatric Health Professional's Name Printed

ᵃ Consent for pediatric health professional to communicate with my child's educators to discuss information relating to this care plan has been completed and filed with pediatric health professional.

For alternative special care forms, see https://cchp.ucsf.edu/sites/g/files/tkssra181/f/9-18-SpecialHealthCareForm.pdf and *Managing Chronic Health Needs in Child Care and Schools*, 2nd Edition, American Academy of Pediatrics (2018).

Other useful forms are on the website of WellCareTracker, an online system maintained by the Pennsylvania Chapter of the American Academy of Pediatrics for early childhood education programs to document and track routine preventive health care services for enrolled children. In addition to demonstration of how to access and use WellCareTracker the following forms are posted at https://www.wellcaretracker.org:

• Letter to doctors requesting health record information

• Letter to parents about providing up-to-date health record information

• Letter to parents describing preventive health services

Medication Administration Packet

Authorization to Give Medicine

PAGE 1—TO BE COMPLETED BY PARENT/LEGAL GUARDIAN

CHILD'S INFORMATION

Name of Facility/School _____

Today's Date ____/____/____

Name of Child (First and Last) _____

Date of Birth ____/____/____

Name of Medicine _____

Reason medicine is needed during school hours _____

Dose _____ Route _____

Time to give medicine _____

Additional instructions _____

Date to start medicine ____/____/____   Stop date ____/____/____

Known side effects of medicine _____

Plan of management of side effects _____

Child allergies _____

PRESCRIBER'S INFORMATION

Prescribing Health Professional's Name _____

Signature _____

Prescriber's Phone Number _____

Date Medication Was Prescribed _____

Note: Medication prescriptions/instructions are acceptable for one (1) year from the written date.

PERMISSION TO GIVE MEDICINE

I hereby give the facility/school permission to administer medicine as prescribed above. **I also give permission for (insert name)** _____**, the school staff person who is authorized to give my child medication, to contact the prescribing health professional about the administration of this medicine. I have administered at least one (1) dose of medicine to my child without adverse effects.**

Parent/Legal Guardian Name (Print) _____

Parent/Legal Guardian Signature _____

Address _____

Home Phone Number _____   Work Phone Number _____   Cell Phone Number _____

Adapted with permission from the NC Division of Child Development to the Department of Maternal and Child Health at the University of North Carolina at Chapel Hill, American Academy of Pediatrics, Connecticut Department of Public Health, Healthy Child Care Pennsylvania, and Healthy Child Care Colorado, 2011. Updated 2022.

Medication Administration Packet (continued)

Receiving Medication

PAGE 2—TO BE COMPLETED BY STAFF PERSON WHO WILL GIVE MEDICATION TO THE CHILD NAMED BELOW

Name of child _____ (first name) _____ (last name)

Name of medicine _____

Date medicine was received _____ /_____/_____

Safety Check

☐   1. Child-resistant container.

☐   2. Original prescription or manufacturer's label with the name and strength of the medicine.

☐   3. Name of child on container is correct (first and last names).

☐   4. Current date on prescription/expiration label covers period when medicine is to be given.

☐   5. Name and phone number of licensed health professional who ordered medicine is on container or on file.

☐   6. Copy of Child Health Record is on file.

☐   7. Instructions are clear for dose, route, and time to give medicine.

☐   8. Instructions are clear for storage (eg, temperature), and medicine has been safely stored.

☐   9. Child has had a previous trial dose.

Y ☐   N ☐   10. Is this a controlled substance? If yes, special storage and log may be needed.

(Print name of facility staff person authorized to give medication) _____

to (Print name of child) _____

Staff Person's Signature _____

Medication Log

PAGE 3—TO BE COMPLETED BY STAFF MEMBER GIVING MEDICATION

First Name _____ Last Name _____ of child receiving

Name of medication _____ Weight of child _____

	Monday	Tuesday	Wednesday	Thursday	Friday
Medicine					
Date	/ /	/ /	/ /	/ /	/ /
Actual time given	AM	AM	AM	AM	AM
	PM	PM	PM	PM	PM
Dose given					
Route (eg, mouth, ear, eye)					
Staff initials or signature					

	Monday	Tuesday	Wednesday	Thursday	Friday
Medicine					
Date	/ /	/ /	/ /	/ /	/ /
Actual time given	AM	AM	AM	AM	AM
	PM	PM	PM	PM	PM
Dose given					
Route (eg, mouth, ear, eye)					
Staff initials or signature					

Describe error/problem in detail in a Medical Incident Form. Observations can be noted here.

Date	Error/problem/reaction to medication	Action taken	Name of parent/guardian notified and time/date	Staff initials or signature

RETURNED to parent/guardian	Date	Parent/guardian signature	Educator signature
	/ /		
DISPOSED of medicine	Date	Educator signature	Witness signature
	/ /		

Medication Administration Packet (continued)

Medication Incident Report

Date of report _____ School/center _____

Name of person completing this report _____

Signature of person completing this report _____

Child's name (first and last) _____

Child's date of birth _____ Classroom/grade _____

Date incident occurred _____ Time _____

Person administering medication _____

Prescribing health professional _____

Name of medication _____

Dose _____ Scheduled time _____

Describe the incident and how it occurred (wrong child, medication, dose, time, or route?):

_____

_____

_____

Action taken/intervention: _____

Parent/legal guardian notified?   Yes _____ No _____ Date/Time _____

Name of the parent/legal guardian who was notified _____

Follow-up and outcome: _____

Administrator's name (print) _____ Signature _____

Adapted with permission from Healthy Child Care Colorado.

Preparing to Give Medication

This is a checklist to use at your early childhood education program or school to ensure your program is ready to give medication.

1. Paperwork

☐ Parent authorization to give medications is signed.

☐ Health professional authorization or instructions are on file.

☐ Child Health Record is on file.

2. Medication checked when received

☐ Properly labeled.

☐ Proper container.

☐ Stored correctly.

☐ Instructions are clear.

☐ Disposal plan is developed.

3. Administering medication

☐ Area is clean and quiet.

☐ Staff is trained to administer medication for this child.

☐ Hands of staff administering medication are washed.

☐ The 6 rights are followed—right child, medication, dose, time, route, and documentation.

☐ Child is observed for side effects.

4. Documentation

☐ Medication log is completed fully and in ink.

Adapted with permission from the NC Division of Child Development to the Department of Maternal and Child Health at the University of North Carolina at Chapel Hill, American Academy of Pediatrics, Connecticut Department of Public Health, Healthy Child Care Pennsylvania, and Healthy Child Care Colorado, 2011. Updated 2022.

Letter to Staff About Occupational Health Risks

Dear Valued Staff Member,

As a program that educates and cares for young children, we do whatever we can to protect the health and safety of all the adults who work in our facility and interact with the children we serve. Every workplace presents some risks. We want to be sure you are aware of and have an opportunity to minimize potential risks of your work in our program. In this letter and on the Staff Health Assessment Form, we identify known occupational risks. We urge you to consult with your health professional <u>to determine the risks of your job to your health and how best to respond to those risks</u>. If your role requires documentation of periodic health assessments, please bring this letter with our program's Staff Health Assessment Form to your health professional. Return the signed letter and completed form

to _____.

Health and safety experts have identified some specific risks for adults who work with young children in programs like ours. These include (but are not limited to)

1. Exposure to infectious diseases from close interactions with groups of children and adults, such as common viruses that can cause respiratory and gastrointestinal illnesses, as well as seasonal influenza and COVID-19.
2. A special health risk for women of childbearing age for exposure during pregnancy to certain viruses (eg, cytomegalovirus, fifth disease, rubella) that can harm their fetus if the women are not already immune to the particular virus. This risk is associated with increased contact with body fluids—saliva, urine, and blood. Personal care routines with children, such as diapering, toileting, nose wiping, and care for children with injuries or illnesses, increase the possibility of such exposure.
3. Injuries related to lifting, squatting, and using child-sized furniture.
4. Reactions to frequent handwashing and/or to the use of cleaning, sanitizing, and disinfecting chemicals.
5. Stress related to high expectations for job performance or job schedule.

Your routine health assessment (checkup) should identify any accommodations required to carry out your duties per your job description. Your health professional needs to understand what you do in your job to identify any particular risks and accommodations you might need. Bring a copy of your job description and explain what you will be doing.

The Staff Health Assessment Form we ask you to have your health professional fill out is from 3 nationally approved publications distributed by the American Academy of Pediatrics. The form should be used with this letter. It lists some of the key elements that your health professional should address during your checkup. We have these nationally approved publications available for you to review at our facility. They are *Caring for Our Children: National Health and Safety Performance Standards* (https://nrckids.org/CFOC), *Model Child Care Health Policies* (https://ecels-healthychildcarepa.org), and *Managing Infectious Diseases in Child Care and Schools*. Our facility's written health and safety policies and procedures are adapted from these resources. Everyone involved with our program in any way is required to comply with our policies and procedures.

Please read the Safety Data Sheets for any products you are required to use. Manufacturers are required to provide them for distribution to users of their products. The ones for products you will be using are located _____.
Thank you.

Please sign below to confirm a) you understand the risks in your job listed in items 1 through 5 above, b) you know how to access the national publications from which we adopted our Staff Health Assessment Form, c) you agree to comply with our program's health and safety policies and procedures, d) you agree to consult with your personal health professional about what risk-reduction actions are best for you, e) you will review the Safety Data Sheets for products you are required to use, and f) you agree to report any significant health problem you may be having to your supervisor when such a problem occurs.

Your signature indicates that you will hold _____ harmless and assume sole responsibility
for management   (name of program)

of the health and safety risks based on the advice you seek from your health professional.

REVIEWED, UNDERSTOOD, AND AGREED TO BY

NAME _____ TITLE _____ DATE _____

Form updated 2022

Staff Health Assessment Form *CFOC* Standard 1.7.0.1

Employer should complete this section.

Name of person to be examined: _____

Employer for whom examination is being done: _____

Employer's location: _____ Phone number: _____

Purpose of examination: ☐ preemployment (with conditional offer of employment) ☐ annual reexamination

Type of activity on the job: ☐ lifting, carrying children ☐ close contact with young children ☐ food preparation

☐ desk work ☐ driver of vehicles ☐ facility maintenance

Parts I and II must be completed and signed by a licensed physician, certified registered nurse practitioner, or certified physician's assistant.

Based on a review of the medical record, health history, and physical examination, does this person have any of the following conditions or problems that might affect job performance or require accommodation?

Date of examination: _____

Part I: Health Problems Determined by Testing, Physical Examination, and Health History

(Circle and clarify any conditions that would require accommodation for the person's proposed work role.)

Visual acuity is at least 20/30 (both eyes, with lenses if needed)?	yes	no
Hearing thresholds are ≤20 dB at 500, 1,000, 2,000, 4,000 Hz?	yes	no
Respiratory problems (asthma, emphysema, airway allergies, current smoker, other)?	yes	no
Heart, blood pressure, or other cardiovascular problems?	yes	no
Gastrointestinal problems (ulcer, colitis, special dietary requirements, obesity, other)?	yes	no
Endocrine problems (diabetes, thyroid, other)?	yes	no
Emotional disorders or addiction (depression, drug or alcohol dependency, difficulty handling stress, other)?	yes	no
Neurologic problems (epilepsy, Parkinson disease, other)?	yes	no
Musculoskeletal problems (low back pain, neck problems, arthritis, limitations on activity)?	yes	no
Skin problems (eczema, rashes, conditions incompatible with frequent handwashing, other)?	yes	no
Immune system problems (from medication, illness, allergies, susceptibility to infection)?	yes	no
Need for more frequent health visits or sick days than the average person?	yes	no
Dental problems assessed in a dental examination within the past 12 months?	yes	no
Other special medical problem or chronic disease that requires work restrictions or accommodation?	yes	no

Staff Health Assessment Form (continued)

Part II: Infectious Disease Status

<u>Vaccines:</u> The following immunizations are recommended for adults in contact with children. (State regulations or program policies may require that certain workers have received some or all of these vaccines.) Please ensure the patient has received the vaccines listed below as well as any others currently recommended by the Centers for Disease Control and Prevention (CDC) at www.cdc.gov/vaccines:

Tdap (once, no matter when the most recent Td was given)	yes	no
MMR (2 doses for persons born after 1989; 1 dose for those born in or after 1957)	yes	no
Polio (OPV or IPV in childhood)	yes	no
Hepatitis B (3-dose series)	yes	no
Varicella (2 doses or had the disease)	yes	no
Influenza	yes	no
Pneumococcal vaccine (if older than 49 years)	yes	no
SARS-CoV-2 (COVID-19) immunization	yes	no
Other vaccines for special situations or risk factors (identify vaccines)	yes	no

<u>Other Infectious Disease Concerns</u>

Female of childbearing age who is caring for young children other than her own?	yes	no	
If the patient could get pregnant, has she been counseled about the risk to the fetus due to increased exposure to cytomegalovirus and parvovirus?[a]	yes	no	n/a
Evaluation of TB status shows a risk for communicable TB?	yes	no	

Check test used.   ☐ Tuberculin skin test (TST)   ☐ Interferon gamma release assay (IGRA) test

Test date _____   Result _____

The results and appropriate follow-up of a tuberculosis (TB) screening, using the TST or IGRA, is required once on entering into the early childhood education field with subsequent TB screening as determined by history of high risk for TB thereafter. Anyone with a previously positive TST or IGRA who has symptoms suggestive of active TB should have a chest radiograph. All newly positive TB skin or blood test results should be followed by radiographic evaluation.

Please attach additional sheets to explain all "yes" answers. Include the plan for follow-up.

Health professional who reviewed the data on this form and provided accompanying explanations

MD   DO   CRNP   PA-C

_____
DATE   SIGNATURE   PRINTED LAST NAME   TITLE

Phone number of licensed physician, physician assistant, or certified registered nurse practitioner: _____

I have read, understand, and accept the occupational health risks identified in my health assessment.

_____
DATE   PATIENT'S SIGNATURE

---

[a] Special concerns for women of childbearing age if they become pregnant and are providing care for groups of young children.

Refusal to Vaccinate Form

(NOTE: States determine immunization requirements and exemptions. Follow state laws regarding immunization forms and procedures.)

CHILD'S or ADULT WORKER'S FIRST AND LAST NAME

_____

CHILD'S PARENT'S/LEGAL GUARDIAN'S NAME (If refusal is for a child to receive a vaccine)

_____

I have had the opportunity to discuss my questions about the recommended vaccines and my refusal with my/my child's health professional. I have had the opportunity to review a list of reasons for vaccinating, possible health consequences of not vaccinating, possible side effects, and recommended schedule for receipt of each vaccine using links from the Centers for Disease Control and Prevention website, https://www.cdc.gov/vaccines/hcp/vis/index.html. The recommended vaccines from birth to 18 years of age are updated annually in January/February on the Centers for Disease Control and Prevention website, https://www.cdc.gov/vaccines/schedules/hcp/imz/child-adolescent.html.

I understand the following:
- The purpose and the need for the recommended vaccine(s).
- The risks and benefits of the recommended vaccine(s).
- Some vaccine-preventable diseases are common in other countries and unvaccinated people could easily get one of these diseases while traveling or from a traveler who comes to any place in my community.
- Without receiving the vaccine(s) according to the medically accepted schedule,
  - My child/I may be infected with the disease, possibly causing cancer, pneumonia, illness requiring hospitalization, death, brain damage, paralysis, meningitis, seizures, and deafness, as well as other severe and permanent effects.
  - My child/I may have to quarantine (stay home and cannot come to the early childhood education program) for up to 3 weeks if exposed to another person infected with the disease my child/I is/am not vaccinated against.
  - My child/I may spread the disease my child/I is/am not vaccinated against to others (including those too young to be vaccinated or those with immune problems), possibly requiring that those who are under-immunized or who get the disease to stay at home for a prolonged time.

I still decline the following nationally recommended vaccinations:

Name of Vaccine	Check if Recommended for Age and Risk	Declined or Delayed; Initials and Date
Hepatitis B		
Diphtheria, tetanus, acellular pertussis (DTaP or Tdap)		
Diphtheria, tetanus (DT or Td)		
Haemophilus influenzae type b (Hib)		
Pneumococcal conjugate or polysaccharide		
Inactivated poliovirus (IPV)		
Measles-mumps-rubella (MMR)		
Varicella (chickenpox)		
Influenza (flu)		
Meningococcal conjugate or polysaccharide		
Hepatitis A		
Rotavirus		
Human papillomavirus (HPV)		
SARS-CoV-2 (COVID-19)		
Other		

Refusal to Vaccinate Form (continued)

I agree to tell all health and all educators in all settings what vaccines I/my child have/has not received. Lacking immunization may require isolation or immediate medical evaluation and tests that might not be necessary if the vaccines had been given.

I know that I may revisit this issue with my (child's) health professional at any time and that I may change my mind and accept vaccination any time in the future.

I acknowledge that I have read this document in its entirety and fully understand it.

ADULT WORKER OR PARENT/GUARDIAN SIGNATURE	DATE
WITNESS NAME (PRINT)	
WITNESS SIGNATURE	DATE

Reliable Immunization Resources for Educators and Parents/Legal Guardians

Websites

1. **American Academy of Pediatrics (AAP)**
   Information for providers and parents
   www.aap.org/immunization
2. **Immunize.org (formerly Immunization Action Coalition [IAC])**
   Immunize.org works to increase immunization rates by creating and distributing educational materials for health professionals and the public that enhance the delivery of safe and effective immunization services. The "Unprotected People Stories" are case reports, personal testimonies, and newspaper and journal articles about people who have suffered or died from vaccine-preventable diseases.
   www.immunize.org/reports
3. **Centers for Disease Control and Prevention (CDC) National Immunization Program**
   Information about vaccine safety. Provide possible health consequences of non-vaccination and possible side effects of each vaccine.
   www.cdc.gov/vaccines/parents/index.html
   https://www.cdc.gov/vaccines/hcp/vis/index.html
4. **Vaccine Education Center at Children's Hospital of Philadelphia**
   Information for parents includes vaccine safety frequently asked questions and "A Look at Each Vaccine."
   www.vaccine.chop.edu
5. **Why Immunize Your Child (updated 2021)**
   Answers to some common questions about vaccination.
   https://www.healthychildren.org/English/safety-prevention/immunizations/Pages/Why-Immunize-Your-Child.aspx
6. **Institute for Vaccine Safety, Johns Hopkins Bloomberg School of Public Health**
   Provides an independent assessment of vaccines and vaccine safety to help guide decision-makers and educate physicians, the public, and the media about key issues surrounding the safety of vaccines
   www.vaccinesafety.edu
7. **Pennsylvania Immunization Coalition (PAIC), Pennsylvania Chapter of the AAP**
   Includes answers to common vaccine questions and topics, such as addressing vaccine safety concerns, evaluating anti-vaccine claims, sources of accurate immunization information on the web, and talking with parents about vaccine safety.
   https://www.immunizepa.org
8. **Immunize Canada**
   Immunize Canada aims to meet the goal of eliminating vaccine-preventable disease through education, promotion, advocacy, and media relations. It includes resources for parents and health professionals.
   https://www.immunize.ca

Handout

1. Immunization Action Coalition. Reliable sources of immunization information: where parents can go to find answers! Published May 2019. Accessed September 7, 2022. http://www.immunize.org/catg.d/p4012.pdf

Books

1. Myers MG, Pineda D. *Do Vaccines Cause That?! A Guide for Evaluating Vaccine Safety Concerns*. Immunizations for Public Health; 2008
2. Offit PA. *Autism's False Prophets: Bad Science, Risky Medicine, and the Search for a Cure*. Columbia University Press; 2008. https://doi.org/10.7312/offi14636
3. Offit PA. *Deadly Choices: How the Anti-Vaccine Movement Threatens Us All*. Basic Books; 2011
4. Mnookin S. *The Panic Virus: A True Story of Medicine, Science, and Fear*. Simon and Schuster; 2011
5. Offit PA, Moser CA. *Vaccines and Your Child: Separating Fact from Fiction*. Columbia University Press; 2011

Routine Schedule for Cleaning, Sanitizing, and Disinfecting

Surface/Area	Method			Timing				Comments
	Clean	Sanitize	Disinfect	Before Each Use	After Each Use	Daily (end of day)	Weekly	
Food Preparation and Meal Service Areas								
Use an EPA-registered product that is safe for surfaces that touch food.								
Food preparation surfaces and countertops *Caring for Our Children*, Standards 4.9.0.9, 4.9.0.10	X	X		X	X			• Use a microfiber cloth or disposable paper towels. • Do not use sponges.
Eating utensils and dishes *Caring for Our Children*, Standards 4.5.0.2, 4.9.0.11, 4.9.0.12, 4.9.0.13	X	X			X			• Wash, rinse, and sanitize by hand OR • Use dishwasher; set on sanitize setting.
Bottle-feeding equipment *Caring for Our Children*, Standard 4.3.1.10	X	X			X			• Wash, rinse, and sanitize by hand OR • Use dishwasher; set on sanitize setting. • Squeeze water through nipple hole to be sure it is clean.
High chair trays *Caring for Our Children*, Standards 4.5.0.2, 9.2.3.12	X	X		X	X			• Also, clean legs and frame when soiled.
Mixed-use tables *Caring for Our Children*, Standard 4.9.0.9	X	X		X	X			• Also, clean legs and frame when soiled.
Food preparation equipment *Caring for Our Children*, Standard 4.9.0.9	X	X			X			• Wash, rinse, and sanitize by hand OR • Use dishwasher; set on sanitize setting.
Child Care/Classroom Areas								
Pacifiers *Used by one child* *Caring for Our Children*, Standard 3.1.4.3	X			X	X			• Sanitize if dirty or used by another child. — Use sanitizer safe for food contact OR — Boil for 1 minute and air-dry OR — Use dishwasher. • Squeeze water through nipple hole to be sure it is clean.

Surface/Area	Method			Timing				Comments
	Clean	Sanitize	Disinfect	Before Each Use	After Each Use	Daily (end of day)	Weekly	

Mouthed toys
Used by one child
Caring for Our Children, Standard 3.3.0.2
	X			X	X			• Sanitize if used by another child.
								  – Use sanitizer safe for food contact OR
								  – Use dishwasher.

Washable cloth toys *Used by one child* *Caring for Our Children*, Standard 3.3.0.2	X						X	• Machine wash and dry completely before use by another child.
Classroom toys *Caring for Our Children*, Standards 3.3.0.2, 5.3.1.4, 6.4.2.2	X						X	• Follow label directions for cleaning of wooden toys.
Play activity centers *Caring for Our Children*, Standard 5.3.1.4	X					X		
Counters and shelves *Caring for Our Children*, Standard 5.3.1.4	X					X		
Mixed-use tables for activities *Caring for Our Children*, Standard 5.3.1.4	X				X			• Sanitize if used for food preparation, meals, or toothbrushing.
Dress-up clothes (washable)	X						X	• Machine wash and dry completely. • Machine wash if soiled with body fluids.
Drinking fountains *Caring for Our Children*, Standard 5.2.6.10	X		X			X		• Clean frequently throughout the day. • Disinfect at the end of the day.
Water tables and water equipment *Caring for Our Children*, Standard 6.2.4.2	X		X		X			• Staff/children wash hands before/after use. • Change water, clean, then disinfect water table and toys before a new group begins water play or at the end of the day. • Children with open cuts or sores should not join in water play. • Do not use during illness outbreak.

Routine Schedule for Cleaning, Sanitizing, and Disinfecting (continued)

Surface/Area	Method			Timing				Comments
	Clean	Sanitize	Disinfect	Before Each Use	After Each Use	Daily (end of day)	Weekly	
Animal areas: feeders, fish tanks, or animal cages *Caring for Our Children,* Standard 3.4.2.3	X		X					• Disinfect these areas after cleaning activity is finished.
Floors *Caring for Our Children,* Standards 5.3.1.6, 5.6.0.4	X					X		• Sweep or vacuum, then damp mop. • Microfiber mops – Launder after use. • Cotton mopheads – Turn upside down to dry. • Disinfect if soiled with body fluids.
Carpets: Washable area rugs are a safer choice than wall-to-wall carpeting. *Caring for Our Children,* Standard 5.3.1.4	X						Clean area rugs.	• Vacuum daily (with HEPA filter). • Steam clean carpets every 3–6 months. – Spot clean if soiled with body fluids.
High-Touch Surfaces: May need to sanitize or disinfect more often during illness outbreaks. **Refer to state, local, tribal, or territorial health authorities and child care licensing for more information.**								
Doorknobs, handles, and light switches	X					X		• Clean often throughout the day with a microfiber cloth or disposable paper towels.
Shared computer keyboards, phones	X					X		• Clean often throughout the day. • Use silicone keyboard cover.
Sleeping Areas								
Sheets, blankets, and pillowcases *Used by one child* *Caring for Our Children,* Standards 3.3.0.4, 5.4.5.1	X						X	• Label and store each child's sleep items separately from other children. • Follow laundry detergent instructions. • Wash laundry at warmest temperature setting, and dry completely. • If soiled with body fluids, launder with non-chlorine bleach (preferred), or bleach and dry completely.

Surface/Area	Method			Timing				Comments
	Clean	Sanitize	Disinfect	Before Each Use	After Each Use	Daily (end of day)	Weekly	
Cribs, cots, and mats *Used by one child* *Caring for Our Children*, Standard 5.4.5.1	X				X		X	• Use fitted sheet to cover sleep surface. • Clean sleep surface regularly with a microfiber cloth or disposable paper towels. • Disinfect surface if soiled with body fluids. • Follow manufacturer's instructions.
Cribs, cots, and mats *Used by more than one child* *Caring for Our Children*, Standard 5.4.5.1	X				X			• Use fitted sheet to cover sleep surface. • Clean sleep surface with a microfiber cloth or disposable paper towels after use by another child. • Disinfect surface if soiled with body fluids. • Follow manufacturer's instructions.
Toilet and Diapering Areas								
Changing tables *Caring for Our Children*, Standards 3.2.1.4, 3.2.1.5, 5.4.2.6	X		X		X			• Allow the surface to air-dry between uses.
Diaper pails *Caring for Our Children*, Standard 5.4.1.8	X		X			X		
Toilets *Caring for Our Children*, Standards 5.4.1.7, 5.4.1.8	X		X			X		• Disinfect after use if soiled.
Sinks and faucets *Caring for Our Children*, Standards 5.4.2.2, 5.4.2.3	X		X			X		
Countertops	X		X			X		
Floors *Caring for Our Children*, Standard 5.6.0.4	X		X			X		• Use separate mops/mopheads for toilet/diapering areas and other areas. • Use microfiber mops with split bucket (cleaning/rinsing system).

Adapted with permission from Appendix K of American Academy of Pediatrics, American Public Health Association, National Resource Center for Health and Safety in Child Care and Early Education. *Caring for Our Children: National Health and Safety Performance Standards; Guidelines for Early Care and Education Programs*. Updated July 25, 2022. Accessed September 7, 2022. https://nrckids.org/files/appendix/AppendixK.pdf

Selecting an Appropriate Sanitizer or Disinfectant

COVID-19 Modification: Resources to Choose Sanitizing and Disinfecting Products

- Cleaning and Disinfecting Best Practices During the COVID-19 Pandemic (EPA): https://www.epa.gov/sites/default/files/2021-04/documents/cleaning-disinfecting-one-pager.pdf
- About List N: Disinfectants for Coronavirus (COVID-19) (EPA): https://www.epa.gov/coronavirus/about-list-n-disinfectants-coronavirus-covid-19-0
- Infographic: Guidance for Cleaning & Disinfecting Public Spaces, Workplaces, Businesses, Schools and Home (EPA): https://www.epa.gov/sites/default/files/2020-04/documents/316485-b_reopeningamerica_combo_placard_infographic_4.19_6pm.pdf
- Safer Cleaning, Sanitizing and Disinfecting Strategies to Reduce and Prevent COVID-19 Transmission (OSHA – Washington): https://osha.washington.edu/sites/default/files/documents/FactSheet_Cleaning_Final_UWDEOHS_0.pdf

Cleaning, sanitizing, and/or disinfecting surfaces are important steps in reducing the risk of spreading infectious diseases to children, staff, and visitors in early childhood education programs. In most situations, routine cleaning with soap and water is enough to remove dirt and some germs from surfaces. Sanitizing and/or disinfecting may be needed after cleaning to further reduce the risk of spreading illness. Sanitizers and disinfectants need to be applied to a clean surface to work effectively at killing germs. You can find specific information on the label on how to use the product.

Activity	Type of Product	Method	Comments
Clean	Soap/detergent and water, or all-purpose cleaners, to remove germs, dirt, oils, and sticky substances from surfaces or objects	Clean surfaces, preferably with a microfiber cloth/mop, rinse the surface thoroughly, and air-dry. Or dry with a paper towel or microfiber cloth.	If using a cleaner other than soap and water, choose a product that has safer chemical ingredients and is certified by a third party (Safer Choice, Green Seal, or UL ECOLOGO).
Sanitize	Chemical product that reduces the number of most germs on nonporous surfaces or objects to a safe level	Sanitize surfaces that touch food (dishes, cutting boards, or mixed-use tables) or objects that a child might place in their mouth (toys).	Choose a US Environmental Protection Agency (EPA)-registered product with directions for food-contact surfaces on the label.
Disinfect	Chemical product to kill bacteria and viruses on surfaces or objects	Disinfect equipment and surfaces that are used in toileting or diapering and in cleaning body fluids (blood). Allow disinfectant to sit on the surface and be visibly wet for the number of minutes listed on the product label.	Choose a disinfectant product certified by the EPA Design for the Environment program: https://www.epa.gov/pesticide-labels/dfe-certified-disinfectants.

Products Registered With the US Environmental Protection Agency (EPA)

Sanitizers are products that kill bacteria on surfaces, and disinfectants are products that kill bacteria and viruses on surfaces. Sanitizers and disinfectants are registered with the EPA as antimicrobial pesticides. A product with an EPA registration number on the label has been tested and is effective in reducing or killing germs.

Cleaners, sanitizers, and disinfectants are used for different purposes. It is important to choose the least hazardous and most effective chemical. Some products both sanitize and disinfect, with different concentrations and/or different amounts of time a product needs to sit on a surface to effectively kill germs.

Before choosing a cleaning or antimicrobial product, you will need to know whether the surface needs to be cleaned, sanitized, or disinfected. When choosing a product, pay careful attention to words on the label like *Warning* or *Danger* and labels that point out if there is a hazard in using the product. Follow the manufacturer's instructions for use and safe handling of products. This includes
1. How to clean before a sanitizer or cleaning product is used.
2. How long the product needs to stay visibly wet on the surface or item (contact or dwell time).
3. Whether the product should be diluted or used as is.
4. If rinsing is needed after the contact time or if it is allowed to air-dry.
5. How to apply the product to surfaces; carefully consider whether the early childhood program can follow all the precautions.

Note: Unless the product label specifically includes disinfection directions for fogging, fumigation, wide-area or electrostatic spraying, the EPA does not recommend using these methods to apply disinfectants. The EPA has not evaluated the product's safety and efficacy for methods that are not on the label.

Choosing Safer Products: Safety Data Sheet (SDS)

EPA-registered products have the SDS that gives instructions for safe use of the product, hazardous chemical ingredients, how to clean up spills, and first aid response to chemical exposure. The SDS also describes what type of personal protective equipment (PPE) is needed. PPE such as chemical-resistant gloves (nitrile and rubber are best), masks, and goggles may be needed while working with chemicals. It is safer to use products that need little or no PPE.

According to the Occupational Health and Safety Administration (OSHA) Hazard Communication Standard (see https://www.osha.gov/hazcom), employers must keep the SDS on site for all hazardous cleaning products, and the SDS must be available to employees when they ask for it. When they're hired and also once every year, all employees must be trained on how to use chemicals safely in their workplace. This is the law.

Labeling Requirements

All containers of cleaning products and chemicals must be labeled and include their contents and hazards. Original labels must be kept on the containers of cleaning products.

When you take a cleaning product out of the original container and put it into another container, such as a spray bottle, this is a *secondary container*. The secondary container products must be labeled with
- Name of the product and/or chemicals
- Warnings for health hazards (eye, ear, skin, and respiratory)
- Physical hazards (flammable)
- Name and address of chemical manufacturer

You can buy preprinted labels, which makes this task easier.

Indoor Air Quality and Ventilation

Cleaning, sanitizing, and disinfecting products can increase indoor air pollution. Mists, vapors, and other gases from cleaning chemicals can irritate the eyes, nose, throat, and lungs. It is important to make sure that the ventilation system is working properly to reduce the concentration of chemicals in indoor air. Ventilation also occurs naturally by opening windows or doors. Good ventilation also reduces the spread of airborne germs.

Protecting Staff and Children's Health

Children are more sensitive to chemicals than adults because their bodies and organs are still developing. Developmentally, children are at a higher risk for exposure to chemicals because they play on the floor, put toys in their mouths, and put their hands in their mouths. Other people may also be sensitive to chemicals, such as pregnant people and individuals with asthma or other respiratory issues. Exposure to some cleaning and disinfecting products has been shown to trigger asthma and can contribute to respiratory illnesses. Using products with safer ingredients helps reduce exposure and related health concerns such as damaged skin, cancer, and reproductive health harm. Safer products also protect the environment since toxic chemicals are often disposed in our waterways and soil.

Selecting an Appropriate Sanitizer or Disinfectant (continued)

Safer Products Options

The use of products that have safer (less toxic) chemicals helps reduce health and environmental concerns. Manufacturers may claim that their products are "green," "natural," or "earth friendly," but these claims are often misleading and might not be related to a chemical's safety.

Organizations now certify and label products that meet certain health and environmental standards.

For cleaning products, the main Third Party Certifications logos include

Cleaning Product	Logo	Website Link
Safer Choice is an EPA Pollution Prevention (P2) program (see https://www.epa.gov/p2) that recognizes more than 2,700 products, including cleaners, hand soaps, laundry detergents, and floor care products.		Safer Choice | US EPA: https://www.epa.gov/saferchoice
Green Seal certifies thousands of products (cleaners, hand soaps, paper products, and floor care products) that contain no harmful chemicals, are sustainably packaged, and are sold in concentrated form.		Standards | Green Seal: https://greenseal.org/green-seal-standards/our-standards
UL ECOLOGO certifies cleaners, floor care products, laundry detergents, hand soaps, paper products, and industrial wipes.		ECOLOGO Certification Program | UL: https://www.ul.com/resources/ecologo-certification-program#cleaning

For sanitizing and disinfecting products, the only certification logo is

EPA Design for the Environment (DfE) disinfectants program identifies antimicrobial products that are better for health and the environment. Sanitizers and disinfectants that meet EPA standards have ingredients such as hydrogen peroxide, lactic acid, citric acid, isopropanol, and ethanol.		DfE-Certified Disinfectant Pesticide Labels | US EPA: https://www.epa.gov/pesticide-labels/dfe-certified-disinfectants

Bleach Products

Early childhood programs often use bleach to sanitize and disinfect. EPA-registered bleach products are described as sanitizers and disinfectants. Make sure your bleach product's label has an EPA registration number. Bleach typically is sold in concentrations that have 5.25% to 8.25% sodium hypochlorite. Read the label to find the concentration of sodium hypochlorite in the product and follow instructions to prepare the bleach solution.

Care is needed to prepare and use bleach products safely. Bleach is toxic when swallowed and can lead to serious injury and even death. Bleach that is released into the air can both aggravate and trigger asthma and irritate the skin and eyes. Children are especially at risk of having their lungs irritated when bleach is in in the air they breathe, because their lungs are still developing.

To safely prepare bleach solutions
- Store bleach at room temperature of 70 °F (21.1 °C) or cooler and keep out of direct sunlight.
- Properly stored bleach has a shelf life of no more than 1 year from the manufacturing date.
- Never mix or store bleach with ANY other chemicals.
- Make sure the room is well ventilated.
- Choose a bottle made of opaque material.
- Choose pump sprays that have a stream option. Avoid aerosols and foggers; both can spread tiny particles that stay in the air long after being used and get deep into the lungs.
- Wear gloves and eye protection when preparing the bleach solution.
- Use a funnel to pour bleach.
- Add bleach to the water (rather than water to the bleach) to reduce fumes.
- Dilute bleach with cool water, and only use the recommended amount of bleach.
- Make a fresh bleach dilution <u>daily</u>; label the bottle with the contents and the date mixed. Bleach strength rapidly gets weaker in the presence of light and when mixed with water.

To safely use bleach solutions
- Use when children are not in the area.
- Clean the surface or items with soap and water; rinse and dry the surface before applying the bleach solution.
- Allow solution to stay wet on the surface for the contact time listed on the label.
- Ventilate area by allowing fresh air to circulate and allow surfaces to completely air-dry (or wipe dry) after the required contact time before allowing children back into the area.
- Safely store chemicals and be sure they will not tip or spill and are out of reach of children.

Using diluted bleach in a spray bottle creates droplets that can be inhaled. Using microfiber or cloths soaked in the bleach solution creates the least amount of bleach released into the air. People with asthma should avoid using bleach and areas where bleach is being used.

Selecting an Appropriate Sanitizer or Disinfectant (continued)

Tools and Tips for Cleaning, Sanitizing, and Disinfecting

Tools and Tips	Overview
Microfiber cloths and mops *Caring for Our Children*, Standard 5.6.0.4	• Ultra-fine, high-quality microfiber cleaning cloths and mops work well for removing dirt and germs from surfaces. • Wash microfiber cloths and mops by hand or machine. • Laundering microfiber cloths helps prevent the spread of germs from one surface to another. • Resource: What's So Great About Microfiber? (https://wspehsu.ucsf.edu/wp-content/uploads/2015/10/FactSheet_Microfiber.pdf)
Washing and sanitizing dishes and toys *Caring for Our Children*, Standards 3.3.0.2, 4.9.0.11, 4.9.0.13	Dishwasher • Make sure dishwasher has a "sanitizing cycle" or is set to heat dry. • Follow manufacturer's instructions for use. 3-sink method • Wash, rinse, and sanitize dishes and toys.
Washing machine and laundry *Caring for Our Children*, Standard 5.4.4.2	• Wash laundry at the warmest temperature setting, and dry completely.
Use of floor mats	• Place floor mats at entryways and teach children to wipe their feet. • Recommend that people remove their shoes when they come indoors. • Vacuum mats daily.
Vacuums with HEPA (high-efficiency particulate air) filters *Caring for Our Children*, Standard 5.3.1.4	• Vacuums with HEPA filters remove more dirt and germs than traditional vacuums. • Choose a vacuum with a "clean" light signal. • Vacuuming collects more dust and germs from floors than sweeping. • Vacuum each day after the children/staff leave.
Proper ventilation *Caring for Our Children*, Standard 5.2.1.1	• Be sure the ventilation system is working properly to reduce the concentration of chemicals in indoor air. • Ventilation occurs naturally by opening windows or doors. • Good ventilation reduces the spread of airborne germs. • Resource: Tips for Working with a Ventilation Consultant (https://eclkc.ohs.acf.hhs.gov/publication/tips-working-ventilation-consultant)
Carpeting tips *Caring for Our Children*, Standards 5.3.1.4, 5.3.1.6	• Carpets collect dust, dirt, pesticides, and germs. • Vacuum carpets every day. • Carpet steam cleaning is recommended every 3–6 months. • Smaller area rugs that can be removed for cleaning are a safer choice. • Remove shag carpets because they hold dust and pesticides over time.
Chemical-free cleaning systems	• Steam cleaners are used to sanitize and remove grease, dirt, and residues without chemicals. • Resource: Devices for Disinfecting Surfaces and Air (http://wspehsu.ucsf.edu/wp-content/uploads/2021/05/fs_devices_0429.pdf)

For additional resources related to green cleaning, use of bleach products, and safety when cleaning, sanitizing, and disinfecting, see *Caring for Our Children*, Appendix J (https://nrckids.org/CFOC).

Selecting an Appropriate Sanitizer or Disinfectant is adapted with permission from Appendix J of American Academy of Pediatrics, American Public Health Association, National Resource Center for Health and Safety in Child Care and Early Education. *Caring for Our Children: National Health and Safety Performance Standards; Guidelines for Early Care and Education Programs.* Updated July 25, 2022. Accessed September 7, 2022. https://nrckids.org/files/appendix/AppendixJ.pdf

Sample Health Information Consent Form

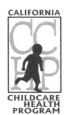

CALIFORNIA
CCHP
**CHILDCARE
HEALTH
PROGRAM**

Consent for Release of Information and Referral
From Child Care Health Consultant and/or Child Care Program
to Other Individuals/Programs/Agencies

I understand that information regarding my child is generally confidential and may not be given to employees of other schools, public agencies, or individual professionals in private practice without my consent or other legal requirement.

Consent for Release of Information

I, _____ , hereby consent to the release of the
(First and Last) NAME OF PARENT/LEGAL GUARDIAN

following information checked and initialed below, regarding my child _____
(First and Last) NAME OF CHILD

to _____   _____
FULL NAME OF INDIVIDUAL OR AGENCY/ADDRESS   (First and Last) NAME OF CHILD CARE HEALTH CONSULTANT

_____ ☐ Educational/Developmental Records
INITIAL

_____ ☐ Diagnostic Assessments/Evaluations (OCCUPATIONAL/PHYSICAL THERAPY, SPEECH AND LANGUAGE PATHOLOGY,
INITIAL   PSYCHOLOGICAL, SOCIAL-EMOTIONAL)

_____ ☐ Developmental/Health Screening(s): _____
INITIAL   and SPECIFY

_____ ☐ Medical   _____ ☐ Dental   _____ ☐ Immunization Records
INITIAL   INITIAL   INITIAL

_____ ☐ Other: _____
INITIAL   and SPECIFY

Consent for Referral

I also authorize communication and exchange of information between: _____
(First and Last) NAME OF INDIVIDUAL/AGENCY HOLDING RECORDS

and/or:

_____   _____
(First and Last) NAME OF CHILD CARE HEALTH CONSULTANT   or   NAME OF CHILD CARE PROGRAM

Further, _____
(First and Last) NAME OF CHILD CARE HEALTH CONSULTANT

is authorized to share the information gained with their supervisor(s) and/or child care health consulting staff working directly with them. Consent for release of information and authorization of communication shall be for the limited purpose of understanding and addressing my child's needs.

This consent is voluntary, and I understand that I can withdraw my consent for my child at any time. Unless I withdraw this consent, this

authorization will be effective for the period my child is continuously enrolled in the _____
NAME OF CHILD CARE PROGRAM

By signing below, I confirm that I have read, understood, and agreed to the above.

Name: _____   Signature: _____   _____
PRINT FULL PARENT/GUARDIAN NAME   PARENT/GUARDIAN SIGNATURE   DATE

NOTE: IN ACCORDANCE WITH THE HEALTH INSURANCE PORTABILITY AND ACCOUNTABILITY ACT (HIPAA) AND APPLICABLE STATE LAWS, ALL PERSONAL AND HEALTH INFORMATION IS PRIVATE AND MUST BE PROTECTED.

California Childcare Health Program • School of Nursing, University of California, San Francisco (UCSF) • https://cchp.ucsf.edu

Rev 03/19
Reprinted with permission from California Childcare Health Program (CCHP).

Sample Food Service Cleaning Schedule

Task	After each use	Before and after each use	Daily	Weekly	As necessary	Comment
RANGE/STOVE						
Clean grill and grease pans.	✓					
Clean burners.	✓					
Clean outside.			✓			
Wipe out oven.			✓	✓		
Clean edges around hood.				✓		
Clean hood screening and grease trap.				✓		
REFRIGERATOR AND FREEZER						Or when more than ¼-inch frost develops, or temperature exceeds 0 °F
Defrost freezer and clean shelves.					✓	
Wipe outside.			✓			
Dust top.				✓		
Clean inside shelves in order.				✓		
MIXER AND CAN OPENER						
Clean mixer base and attachments.	✓					
Clean and wipe can opener blade.	✓					
WORK SURFACES						
Clean and sanitize.		✓				
Organize for neatness.			✓			
WALLS AND WINDOWS						
Wipe if splattered or greasy.					✓	
Wipe window sills.					✓	
Wipe window screens.					✓	
SINKS						
Keep clean.	✓					
Scrub.			✓			
CARTS (if applicable)						
Wipe down.	✓					
Sanitize.			✓			
GARBAGE						Or more often, as needed
Take out.			✓			
Clean can.					✓	
TABLES AND CHAIRS						
Clean and sanitize.		✓				
LINENS						
Wash cloth napkins.	✓					
Wash tablecloths and place mats.	✓ if plastic		✓ if cloth			
Wash dishcloths.			✓			
Wash pot holders.				✓		
STORAGE AREAS						
Wipe shelves, cabinets, and drawers.					✓	

Graves DE, Suitor CW, Holt KA, eds. *Making Food Healthy and Safe for Children: How to Meet the National Health and Safety Performance Standards Guidelines for Out of Home Child Care Programs*. National Center for Education in Maternal and Child Health; 1997.

Diapering Poster

This poster is based on *Caring for Our Children*, 4th Edition, a publication of the American Academy of Pediatrics (AAP), American Public Health Association, and the National Resource Center for Health and Safety in Child Care and Early Education. It was created by CCA Global with guidance from the Early Childhood Education Linkage System of the Pennsylvania Chapter of the AAP.

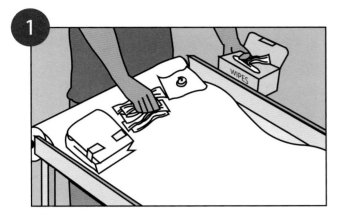

1

Cover surface with disposable paper.

Remove from containers and place on diapering surface **away from child's reach**:

- Wipes
- Clean diaper
- Dab of diapering cream on facial tissue
- Plastic bag for soiled clothes
- [Put on gloves if using]

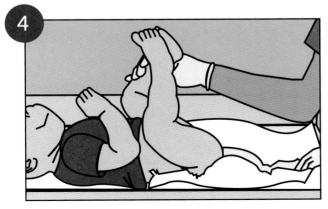

2

Place child on diapering surface. Always keep a hand on the child.

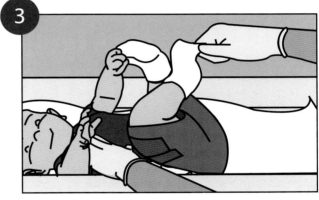

3

Remove bottom clothing including shoes & socks if feet cannot be kept from contacting soiled skin or surfaces. [If clothing is soiled, remove and place in plastic bag.]

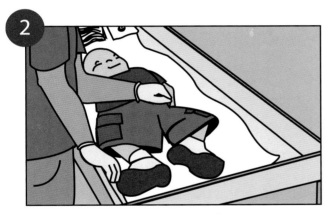

4

Unfasten diaper but keep soiled diaper under child's bottom.

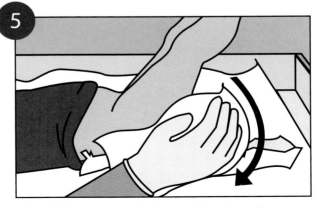

5

Lift child's legs and clean skin from front to back. Use fresh wipe each time.

Diapering Poster (continued)

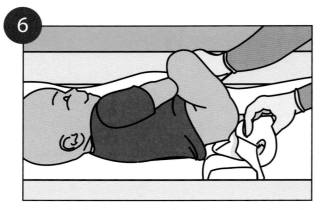

Put soiled wipes in soiled diaper or directly into a hands-free, plastic-lined can. Then, dispose of soiled diaper in the hands-free can.

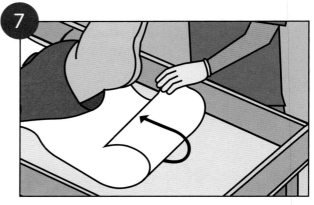

If paper is soiled, use corner to fold clean side of paper back under child's cleaned bottom.

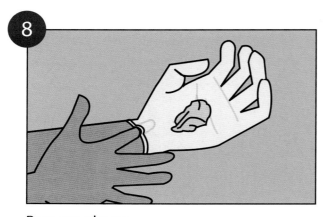

Remove gloves.
Dispose in hands-free can.

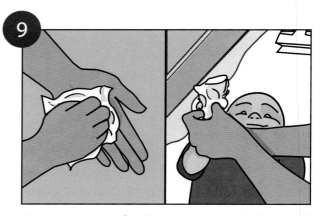

Use separate fresh wipe on adult's and child's hands. Dispose in hands-free can.

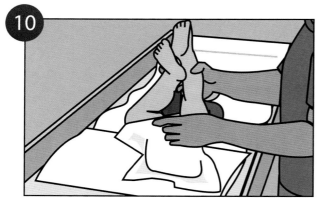

Put clean diaper under child's bottom.
[If using diaper cream, apply with facial/toilet tissue or glove, then discard in hands-free can.]

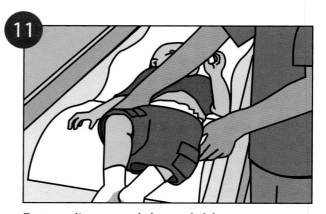

Fasten diaper and dress child.

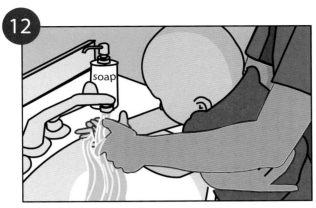

Wash child's hands at sink.*

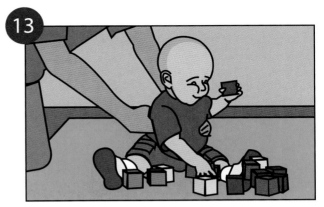

Return child to supervised area.

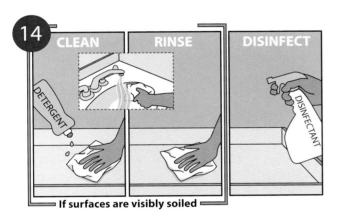

CLEAN · RINSE · DISINFECT

DETERGENT

DISINFECTANT

If surfaces are visibly soiled

A. Dispose of changing table paper.

B. If diapering surfaces are visibly soiled
   • Clean surfaces with detergent, water, and paper towels.
   • Rinse surfaces with water.

C. Wet all diapering surfaces with disinfectant solution.

D. Leave solution on for required contact time.

WASH HANDS*

If diapering surface is wet after required contact time, dry with clean paper towel before next change.

* Washing with soap and water is preferred. If this is not possible and hands are not visibly soiled, use of alcohol-based hand sanitizers according to the manufacturer's instructions on the product label is an acceptable alternative for adults and children.

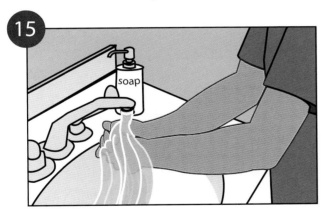

Record in Daily Report form for family
   • Time of diaper change
   • Diaper contents
   • Any problems such as loose stool, skin irritation, etc

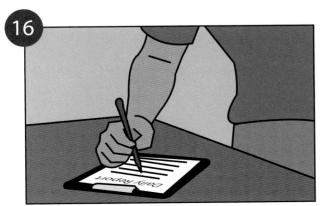

Cleaning Up Body Fluids

Treat urine, stool, vomit, blood, and body fluids, except for human milk, as potentially infectious. Spills of body fluid should be cleaned up and surfaces disinfected immediately. The federal US Occupational Safety and Health Administration (OSHA) blood-borne pathogens standard requires that staff who might come in contact with blood or body fluids that might contain blood-borne pathogens must have annual training specified by OSHA. The procedure to be used is

a. Wear gloves while cleaning. Although disposable gloves can be used, household rubber gloves are adequate for all spills except blood and bloody body fluids. Disposable gloves should be used when blood may be present in the spill.

b. For small amounts of urine and stool on smooth surfaces, wipe off and clean away visible soil with a little detergent solution. Then rinse the surface with clean water.

c. Apply a disinfectant following the manufacturer's instructions.

For larger spills on floors, or any spills on rugs or carpets

d. Take care to avoid splashing any contaminated material onto the mucous membranes of your eyes, nose, or mouth or into any open sores you may have.

e. Wipe up as much of the visible material as possible with disposable paper towels and carefully place the soiled paper towels and other soiled disposable material in a leakproof plastic bag that has been securely tied or sealed. Use a wet/dry vacuum on carpets if such equipment is available.

f. Immediately use a detergent or a combination detergent/disinfectant to clean the spill area. Then rinse the area with clean water. Additional cleaning by shampooing or steam cleaning the contaminated surface may be necessary.

g. For blood and body fluid spills on carpeting, blot to remove body fluids from the fabric as quickly as possible. Then disinfect by spot cleaning with a combination detergent/disinfectant and shampooing or steam cleaning the contaminated surface.

h. If directed by the manufacturer's instructions, dry the surface.

i. Clean and rinse reusable household rubber gloves, then apply disinfectant. Remove, dry, and store these gloves away from food or food surfaces. Discard disposable gloves.

j. Mops and other equipment used to clean up body fluids should be
   1. Cleaned with detergent and rinsed with water
   2. Rinsed with a fresh disinfectant solution
   3. Wrung as dry as possible
   4. Air-dried

k. Wash your hands afterward, even though you wore gloves.

l. Remove and bag clothing (yours and those worn by children) soiled by body fluids.

m. Put on fresh clothes after washing the soiled skin and hands of everyone involved.

See Selecting an Appropriate Sanitizer or Disinfectant earlier in this chapter for guidance on sanitizers and disinfectants.

Reference

1. American Academy of Pediatrics. *Red Book: 2021–2024 Report of the Committee on Infectious Diseases*. Kimberlin DW, Barnett ED, Lynfield R, Sawyer MH, eds. 32nd ed. American Academy of Pediatrics; 2021:116–133

Gloving

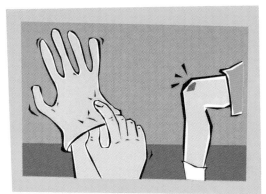

1. Put on a clean pair of gloves.

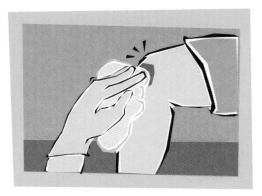

2. Provide appropriate care.

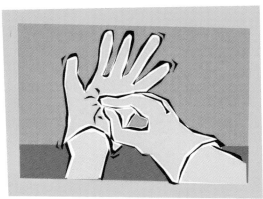

3. Remove each glove carefully. Grab the first glove at the palm and strip the glove off. Touch dirty surfaces only to dirty surfaces.

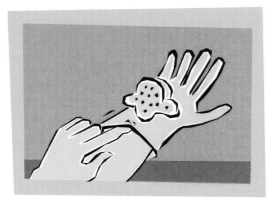

4. Ball up the dirty glove in the palm of the other gloved hand.

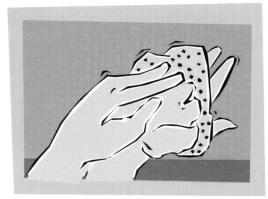

5. Remove the second glove without touching the outside of either dirty glove.

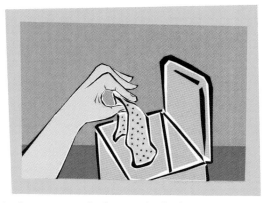

6. Dispose of the soiled glove in a covered trash receptacle. Always practice hand hygiene after the use of gloves.

Note that sensitivity to latex is a growing problem. If educators or children who are sensitive to latex are present at the facility, non-latex gloves should be used.

Adapted with permission from California Department of Education (CDE). Keeping Kids Healthy: Preventing and Managing Communicable Diseases in Child Care. CDE; 1995.

Infections Caused by Interactions of Humans With Pets and Wild Animals

What Infections Are Caused by Animal Contact?

Infections of animals can infect humans. The US Centers for Disease Control and Prevention (CDC) reports, "These germs can cause many different types of illnesses in people and animals ranging from mild to serious illness and even death. Some animals can appear healthy even when they are carrying germs that can make people sick."

Animals known to be associated with human infection include reptiles, amphibians, rodents (eg, aquatic frogs, iguanas, hedgehogs, hamsters, mice), poultry (ie, chicks, chickens, ducks, ducklings, geese, goslings, and turkeys), and ruminant livestock (ie, cattle, sheep, and goats), as well as kittens, mature cats, puppies, and mature dogs. Some animals pose a special risk because of their high asymptomatic carriage rates of germs that cause disease in humans. For example, *Salmonella* infections are commonly spread from seemingly well animals to humans this way. In addition to direct contact, indirect contact with animals and animal products can be a source of illness (eg, contact with water in a reptile tank, contaminated barriers or fencing used to contain animals, contact with certain foods).

An extensive list of diseases spread by animals is in Appendix VIII of *Red Book®: 2021–2024 Report of the Committee on Infectious Diseases.*

Nontraditional Pets and Wild Animals

Most imported, nonnative animal species are caught in the wild rather than bred in captivity. Exotic birds, Burmese pythons, iguanas, lionfish, and rhesus monkeys are examples of imported animals that have escaped captivity and are living in Florida. Nonnative animals are held and transported in close contact with multiple other species. This increases the risk of spreading germs that can cause disease for humans and domestic animals. Some nonnative animals are brought into the United States illegally, bypassing rules established to reduce the introduction of disease and potentially dangerous animals. Some species of nonnative animals may also be bred in captivity in North America.

The behavior of captive wildlife and wildlife hybrids cannot be predicted. The potential risks are enhanced when these animals are cared for by people who do not fully understand how the animals spread disease and how to prevent it, animal behavior, and how to maintain appropriate facilities, environment, and nutrition for captive animals.

How Do You Prevent Infections When Children Interact With Animals?

Infected animals often are asymptomatic carriers of germs that can cause disease in humans. Direct contact with animals (especially young animals), contamination of the environment or food or water sources, and inadequate hand hygiene facilities at animal exhibits have been responsible for infection of people who visit these settings. Pediatric health professionals, veterinarians, and other health professionals should be consulted about proper animal selection and care and how to minimize risks to infants and children. Pet size and temperament should be matched to the age and behavior of a child. Pet food should not be handled where human food is prepared. Food bowls should be carefully cleaned and disinfected after contact with pet foods. Be sure to practice the recommended steps for hand hygiene after handling animal foods or treats or touching anything in the animal's environment.

Acquisition and ownership of nontraditional pets should be discouraged in any setting with young children or other high-risk individuals. Information, in multiple languages, about guidelines for safe pet selection and appropriate handling is available from the CDC at www.cdc.gov/zoonotic/gi and www.cdc.gov/healthypets.

What Are the Roles of the Educator and the Family?

Young children should always be supervised closely when in contact with animals at home or in public settings, including early childhood education programs or schools. Children should be educated about appropriate human–animal interactions. Parents should be made aware of recommendations for preventing human diseases and injuries from exposure to pets, including nontraditional pets and animals in the home, animals in public settings, and pet products, including food and pet treats. Pets and other animals should receive appropriate veterinary care from a licensed veterinarian who can provide preventive care appropriate for the species.

Guidelines for Prevention of Human Diseases From Exposure to Pets, Nontraditional Pets, and Animals in Public Settings[a,b,c]

General
- Always supervise children, especially children younger than 5 years, during interaction with animals.
- Wash hands immediately after contact with animals, animal products, feed or treats, or animal environments and after taking off dirty clothes or shoes; hands should be washed even when direct contact with an animal did not occur.
- Closely supervise handwashing for children younger than 5 years.
- Do not allow children to kiss animals or to eat, drink, or put objects or hands into their mouths after handling animals or while in animal areas.
- Do not permit nontraditional pets to roam or fly freely indoors or in outdoor play areas of early childhood education (ECE) programs or allow domestic pets to have contact with wild animals.
- Do not permit animals in areas where food or drinks are stored, prepared, served, or consumed.
- Never bring wild animals into the ECE facility, and never adopt wild animals as pets.
- Teach children not to handle unfamiliar, wild, or domestic animals, even if animals appear friendly.
- Avoid rough play with animals to prevent scratches or bites.
- Pets and other animals should receive appropriate veterinary care from a licensed veterinarian who can provide preventive care, including vaccination and parasite control, appropriate for the species.
- Administer rabies vaccine to all dogs, cats, horses, and ferrets; livestock animals and horses with frequent human contact also should be up to date with all immunizations recommended for them.
- Keep animals clean and free of intestinal parasites, fleas, ticks, mites, and lice.
- People at increased risk of infection or serious complications of salmonellosis and other enteric infections should avoid contact with high-risk animals, animal-derived pet treats, and pet foods. This includes children younger than 5 years, people older than 65 years, and immunocompromised people. High-risk animals include turtles and other reptiles; poultry, including chicks, chickens, ducklings, and ducks in backyard flocks; aquatic frogs and other amphibians; and farm animals.
- People at increased risk of infection or serious complications of lymphocytic choriomeningitis virus infections (eg, pregnant women, immunocompromised people) should avoid contact with rodents, rodent housing, and rodent bedding.

Animals Visiting ECE Programs and Schools
- Designate specific areas for animal contact.
- Display animals in enclosed cages or under appropriate restraint.
- Do not allow food in animal-contact areas.
- Always closely supervise children, especially those younger than 5 years, during interaction with animals.
- Obtain a certificate of veterinary inspection for visiting animals and/or proof of rabies immunization according to local or state requirements.
- Properly clean and disinfect all areas where animals have been present.
- Consult with parents/legal guardians to determine special considerations needed for children who are immunocompromised or who have allergies or asthma.
- Animals not recommended in schools, ECE settings, hospitals, or nursing homes include nonhuman primates; inherently dangerous animals (eg, lions, tigers, cougars, bears, wolf/dog hybrids); mammals at high risk of transmitting rabies (eg, bats, raccoons, skunks, foxes, coyotes, mongooses); aggressive animals or animals with unpredictable behavior; stray animals with unknown health history; venomous or toxin-producing spiders, insects, reptiles, and amphibians; animals at higher risk for causing serious illness or injury, including reptiles and amphibians or chicks, ducks, or other live poultry; and ferrets. Additionally, children younger than 5 years should not be allowed to have direct contact with these animals.
- Farm animals are not appropriate in facilities with children younger than 5 years and should not be displayed to older children in school settings unless meticulous attention to personal hygiene and disinfection of areas the animals have occupied can be ensured.
- Ensure that people who provide animals for educational purposes are knowledgeable regarding animal handling and zoonotic disease issues.

Public Settings
- Venue operators must know about risks of disease and injury.
- Venue operators and staff must maintain a safe environment.
- Venue operators and staff must educate visitors about the risk of disease and injury and provide appropriate preventive measures.
- Venue operators and staff should be familiar with the recommendations detailed in the *Compendium of Measures to Prevent Diseases Associated with Animals in Public Settings.*[b]

Infections Caused by Interactions of Humans With Pets and Wild Animals (continued)

Guidelines for Prevention of Human Diseases From Exposure to Pets, Nontraditional Pets, and Animals in Public Settings[a,b,c]

Animal Specific

- Know that healthy animals can carry germs that can make people sick. People can become ill when they touch an animal, pick up an animal's dropping, or enter an animal environment even if they don't touch the animal.
- Children younger than 5 years, pregnant women, and immunocompromised people should avoid contact with reptiles, amphibians, rodents, ferrets, baby poultry (eg, chicks, ducklings), preweaned calves, and any items that have been in contact with these animals or their environments.
- Reptiles, amphibians, rodents, ferrets, and baby poultry (eg, chicks, ducklings) should be kept out of households and areas used by children younger than 5 years, pregnant women, immunocompromised people, people older than 65 years, or people with sickle cell disease. These animals should not be allowed in ECE facilities or other facilities that house high-risk individuals.
- Reptiles, amphibians, rodents, and baby poultry should not be permitted to roam freely in a facility occupied by humans. These animals should not be permitted in kitchens or other areas where food and drink are prepared, stored, served, or consumed.
- Animal cages or enclosures should not be cleaned in sinks or other areas used to store, prepare, serve, or consume food and drinks; these items should be cleaned outside the areas used by people, if possible.
- Mammals at high risk of transmitting rabies (ie, bats, raccoons, skunks, foxes, and coyotes) should not be touched. Disposable gloves should be used when cleaning fish aquariums. Aquarium water should not be disposed of in sinks used for food preparation or for obtaining drinking water.
- Pregnant women and immunocompromised people should avoid contact with cat feces or soil contaminated with cat feces.

[a] Pickering LK, Marano N, Bocchini JA, Angulo FJ; American Academy of Pediatrics Committee on Infectious Diseases. Exposure to nontraditional pets at home and to animals in public settings: risks to children. *Pediatrics*. 2008;122(4):876–886. Reaffirmed April 2020

[b] For complete recommendations, see *Compendium of Measures to Prevent Disease Associated with Animals in Public Settings*, 2017 by the National Association of State Public Health Veterinarians Animal Contact Compendium Committee (http://nasphv.org/Documents/AnimalContactCompendium2017.pdf).

[c] For practical guidelines related to contact with animals and infectious diseases, go to https://www.cdc.gov/onehealth/basics/zoonotic-diseases.html (reviewed July 1, 2021; accessed September 7 , 2022) and www.cdc.gov/healthypets (reviewed August 29, 2022; accessed September 7, 2022).

Symptom Record Form

Instructions: This form may be used by families or educators to document symptoms at home or while the child is in the program. Use the back of the form if more space is needed.

Name of facility/school: _____ _____

Child's first and last name: _____

Date: _____ Symptom(s): _____

When symptom began, how long it lasted, how severe, how often? _____

Any change in child's behavior? _____

Child's temperature if taken: _____ Time taken: _____ (Circle: axillary [armpit], oral, rectal, ear canal, other [specify]) _____

How much and what type of food and fluid did the child take in the past 12 hours? _____

_____

Number of times of urination: _____ and bowel movements: _____

How typical/normal for this child were urine and bowel movements in the past _____ hours? _____

_____

Circle or write in other symptoms:

Cough	Headache	Runny nose	Stomachache	Trouble urinating	Other pain (specify) _____
Diarrhea	Itching	Sore throat	Trouble breathing	Vomiting	_____
Earache	Rash	Stiff neck	Trouble sleeping	Wheezing	_____

Other symptoms: _____

Any medications in the past 12 hours (name, time, dose)? _____

Any exposure to animals, insects, or new foods, environments, or products? _____

Exposure to other people who were sick; who and what sickness? _____

Child's other chronic conditions or illnesses that might affect this illness (eg, asthma, allergy, anemia, diabetes, emotional trauma, seizures): _____

What has been done so far? _____

Advice from the child's health professional: _____

First and last name of person completing this form: _____

Relationship of person completing this form to the child: _____

Enrollment/Attendance/Symptom Record

Group _____

Month _____ 20 ___

For each child, each day: Code top box **+** = present, **O** = scheduled but absent, or **N** = not scheduled. Code bottom box **O** = well or choose from the symptom codes from the bottom of this chart.

(First and last) Legal Name	Age (mo)	Daily Hours in Care	1	2	3	4	5	6	7	8	9	10	11	12	13	14	15	16	17	18	19	20	21	22	23	24	25	26	27	28	29	30	31

SYMPTOM CODES

1 = Asthma, wheezing
2 = Behavior change with no other symptom
3 = Diarrhea

4 = Fever
5 = Headache
6 = Rash

7 = Respiratory (eg, cold, cough, runny nose, earache, sore throat, pinkeye)
8 = Stomachache

9 = Urine problem
10 = Vomiting
11 = Other (Specify on back.)

Child Emergency Information Form

To be completed by parent or guardian

CHILD'S INFORMATION			
CHILD'S FIRST AND LAST NAME		NICKNAME	DATE OF BIRTH
HOME ADDRESS			
HOME PHONE			
PARENT/GUARDIAN CONTACT INFORMATION			
FIRST AND LAST NAME			
WORK PHONE	HOME PHONE	CELL PHONE	EMAIL
FIRST AND LAST NAME			
WORK PHONE	HOME PHONE	CELL PHONE	EMAIL
EMERGENCY CONTACT INFORMATION (CHILD MAY BE RELEASED TO THE PERSONS BELOW IF PARENT/GUARDIAN IS UNAVAILABLE)			
FIRST AND LAST NAME		RELATIONSHIP TO CHILD	
ADDRESS		EMAIL	
HOME PHONE	CELL PHONE	WORK PHONE	
FIRST AND LAST NAME		RELATIONSHIP TO CHILD	
ADDRESS		EMAIL	
HOME PHONE	CELL PHONE	WORK PHONE	
FIRST AND LAST NAME		RELATIONSHIP TO CHILD	
ADDRESS		EMAIL	
HOME PHONE	CELL PHONE	WORK PHONE	
OUT-OF-AREA CONTACT (IN CASE LOCAL CALLS CANNOT BE MADE)			
FIRST AND LAST NAME		RELATIONSHIP TO CHILD	
ADDRESS		EMAIL	
HOME PHONE	CELL PHONE	WORK PHONE	
CHILD'S MEDICAL CARE			
PHYSICIAN'S NAME		PHONE NUMBER	
ADDRESS			
EMAIL		WEBSITE	
MEDICAL CONDITIONS, SPECIAL NEEDS, ALLERGIES, MEDICATIONS, ETC			
DENTIST'S NAME		PHONE NUMBER	
ADDRESS			
EMAIL		WEBSITE	
HOSPITAL NAME		PHONE NUMBER	
ADDRESS			

I grant permission for the early childhood education program to provide or arrange for medical treatment and/or transportation to an evacuation site and/or medical facility for my child during an emergency or disaster. I grant permission for my child to be released to any of the emergency contacts designated above if I am unable to pick them up in an emergency.

PARENT/GUARDIAN NAME (Please print)	SIGNATURE	DATE
PARENT/GUARDIAN NAME (Please print)	**SIGNATURE**	**DATE**

Child Care Resource Center, Emergency Preparedness Toolkit for Child Care Programs, funded by Los Angeles County Department of Public Health

Reprinted with permission from Child Care Resource Center. *Emergency Preparedness Toolkit for Child Care Programs*.

Situations That Require Medical Attention Right Away

In the following boxes, you will find lists of common medical emergencies or urgent situations you may encounter as an educator.

To prepare for a medical emergency, follow the procedures set forth in *Caring for Our Children*, Standard 9.2.4.1.

Call Emergency Medical Services (EMS) (911) Immediately If

- The child's life seems to be at risk or there is a risk of permanent injury.
- The child is acting strangely, much less alert, or much more withdrawn than usual.
- The child has difficulty breathing or is unable to speak.
- The child's skin or lips look blue, purple, or gray.
- The child has rapidly spreading raised red skin areas with throat-closing, tongue swelling, trouble breathing or wheezing, or decreased consciousness (severe allergic reaction—anaphylaxis).
- The child has rhythmic jerking of arms and legs and loss of consciousness (seizure).
- The child is unconscious.
- The child is becoming less and less responsive or confused.
- After a head injury, the child has any of the following conditions: decrease in level of alertness, confusion, headache, vomiting, irritability, difficulty walking.
- The child has increasing or severe pain anywhere.
- The child has a cut or burn that is large or deep or won't stop bleeding.
- The child is vomiting blood.
- The child has a severe stiff neck, headache, and fever.
- The child is significantly dehydrated (eg, sunken eyes, lethargic, not making tears, not urinating).
- Multiple children are affected by injury or serious illness at the same time.
- When in doubt about whether to call EMS (911), make the call.
- After calling EMS (911), call the child's parent/legal guardian.

Get Medical Attention Within 1 Hour

Some children may have urgent situations that do not necessarily require emergency medical services (EMS) (911) for ambulance transport but still need medical attention without delay. For the following conditions, the educator may first call the parent/legal guardian. If the parent/guardian is immediately available to pick up the child and take the child to a source of urgent pediatric health care within an hour, the parent/legal guardian should be instructed to do so. EMS (911) should be called to bring the child to a pediatric health professional if the parent/legal guardian cannot do so. When EMS is transporting the child, if possible, a staff member who knows the child should accompany the child until the parent/legal guardian can be present to provide information and reassure the child. Program policies should be clear about how such situations will be handled given local resources. Staff should develop contingency plans for emergencies or disaster situations when it may not be possible or feasible to follow standard or previously agreed on emergency procedures. The situations that require medical attention within an hour are

- Any infant or child older than 2 months who looks more than mildly ill with a temperature above 101 °F (38.3 °C) taken by any method (Note: Rectal temperatures in early childhood education programs or schools should be taken only by persons with specific health training in performing this procedure and with permission by parents/guardians. Never "correct" for an axillary temperature by adding 0.5 or 1 degree.)
- Temperature above 100.4 °F (38.0 °C) by any method in an infant younger than 2 months (8 weeks)
- A quickly spreading purple or red rash or a rapidly spreading rash that raises concern for an allergic reaction (eg, hives)
- A large volume of blood in stools
- A cut that may require stitches
- Any medical condition specifically outlined in a child's care plan that requires immediate action and/or notification of the child's parent/legal guardian

Sample Letter to Families About Exposure to Communicable Disease

See attached Quick Reference Sheet for information about this condition.

Name of Early Childhood Education Program: _____

Address of Early Childhood Education Program: _____

Telephone Number of Early Childhood Education Program: _____

Date: _____

Dear Parent/Legal Guardian:

A child in our program has or is suspected of having: _____

Information about this disease

The disease is spread by: _____

_____

_____

The symptoms are: _____

_____

The disease can be prevented by: _____

What the program is doing: _____

What you can do at home: _____

_____

_____

If your child has any symptoms of this disease, check the attached Quick Reference Sheet to determine whether you should consult a pediatric health professional by phone or office visit, and be sure to tell your health professional about this notice. If you do not have a regular pediatric health professional to care for your child, contact your local health department for instructions on how to find a pediatric health professional or ask other parents for names of and recommendations if they have contacted their children's health professionals for advice about this exposure. If you have any questions, please contact:

_____   (____)_____
EDUCATOR'S NAME   PHONE NUMBER

Glossary

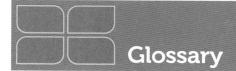
Glossary

AAP: American Academy of Pediatrics, a national organization of pediatricians founded in 1930 and dedicated to the improvement of child health and welfare.

Acute: Adjective describing an illness that has a sudden onset and is of short duration.

Adaptive equipment: Equipment (eg, eyeglasses, hearing aids, wheelchairs, standing aids, crutches, prostheses, oxygen tanks) that helps children with special health care needs adapt to and function within their surroundings (eg, equipment that allows children who cannot stand to wash their hands in a sink).

Antibiotic prophylaxis: Antibiotics that are prescribed to prevent infections in situations associated with an increased risk of serious infection with a specific disease.

Antibody: A protein substance produced by the body's immune defense system in response to something foreign to the body. Antibodies help protect against infections.

Antigen: Any substance that is foreign to the body. An antigen is capable of causing a response from the immune system.

Antiseptic: Antimicrobial substances that are applied to the skin or surfaces to reduce the number of microbial flora. Examples include alcohols, chlorhexidine, chlorine, hexachlorophene, iodine, chloroxylenol (PCMX), quaternary ammonium compounds, and triclosan.

APHA: Abbreviation for the American Public Health Association, a national organization of health professionals that protects and promotes the health of the public through education, research, advocacy, and policy development.

AQI: Abbreviation for Air Quality Index, a tool used by the US Environmental Protection Agency and other agencies to describe how clean the air is and whether members of the public should be concerned for their health. The AQI is focused on health effects that can happen within a few hours or days after breathing polluted air.

Assessment: An in-depth appraisal conducted to determine the health status or need for preventive health services of an individual, diagnose a condition, or evaluate the performance of a program or individual or the importance or value of a procedure.

Asymptomatic: Without symptoms. For example, children may not have symptoms of hepatitis infection but may still shed hepatitis A virus in their stool and may be able to infect others.

Bacteria: Plural of bacterium. Organisms that may be responsible for localized or generalized diseases and can survive in and out of the body. They are much larger than viruses and usually can be treated effectively with antibiotics.

BCG vaccine: Abbreviation for Bacille Calmette-Guérin vaccine, a tuberculosis vaccine used in other countries where tuberculosis is more common than in the United States.

Bleach solution: A chemical used to sanitize or disinfect environmental surfaces. See also *Disinfect* and *Sanitize.*

Blood-borne pathogens: Infectious gems present in blood that can cause disease in humans. These pathogens include, but are not limited to, hepatitis B virus; hepatitis C virus; HIV, the virus that causes AIDS; and cytomegalovirus, a common virus that infects young children, who then can infect a pregnant adult and damage the fetus.

Body fluids: Urine, feces, saliva, blood, nasal discharge, eye discharge, and injury or tissue discharge.

Bronchiolitis: An inflammation and swelling of the lining of the small air tubes (bronchioles) that connect the larger tubes (bronchi) with the smallest chambers within the lung (alveoli). Exchange of gases (eg, oxygen, carbon dioxide) with the blood occurs in the alveoli. Respiratory syncytial virus is the most common cause of bronchiolitis in young children. This illness is usually associated with runny nose and wheezing. Infection or inflammation of the larger tubes (bronchi) leads to swelling and increased mucus production in the large tubes that lead to the lungs, a condition called *bronchitis.*

Campylobacter: A type of bacterium that causes diarrhea.

Care plan: A document that provides specific health care information, including any medications, procedures, precautions, or adaptations to diet or environment that may be needed to care for a child with chronic medical conditions or special health care needs. Care plans also describe signs and symptoms of impending illness and outline the response needed to those signs and symptoms. A care plan is completed by a health professional and may be annotated by an educator to indicate specific actions to take, using the resources of the early childhood education program. The plan should be updated on a regular basis as determined by the child's health professional.

Carrier: A person or animal whose body carries a specific disease-causing organism without symptoms of disease and who can spread the disease to others. For example, some children may be carriers of group A streptococcus, which can cause strep throat; *Haemophilus influenzae*, which can cause infection of ears or other body tissues; or *Giardia*, which can cause diarrhea.

CCHA: Abbreviation for Child Care Health Advocate, also known as a *health advocate*. This staff person in an early childhood education program is responsible for implementation of policies and day-to-day practices related to the health, development, and safety of individual children, children as a group, staff, and parents/guardians. The CCHA works with the support of a health professional who fills the role of a Child Care Health Consultant. See also *CCHC*.

CCHC: Abbreviation for Child Care Health Consultant, a licensed or certified health professional with education and experience in child and community health and early childhood education; preferably someone with specialized training in child care health consultation.

CDC: Abbreviation for the Centers for Disease Control and Prevention, a federal government agency that is responsible for developing and applying activities for disease prevention and control, environmental health, health promotion, and health education to improve the health of the people of the United States. The CDC especially focuses its attention on infectious disease, foodborne pathogens, environmental health, occupational safety and health, health promotion, injury prevention, and educational activities. In addition, the CDC researches and provides information on noninfectious diseases such as obesity and diabetes. For more information about the CDC, go to www.cdc.gov.

Ceftriaxone: An antibiotic prescribed for some individuals with a bacterial infection.

Certification (as it relates to a form of licensing): Designation as having met the requirements to operate or practice in a specific sector. Permission from a state that is required to be allowed to carry out a specified function, such as operating an early childhood education program or certain types of professional activities. Some states use the term *licensing*; others use *certification* or *registration* to describe their regulatory process.

CFOC: Abbreviation for *Caring for Our Children: National Health and Safety Performance Standards; Guidelines for Early Care and Education Programs*.

Chikungunya: A mosquito-borne viral disease associated with fever and joint pain. Other symptoms may include headache, muscle pain, joint swelling, or rash. (See Mosquito-borne Diseases Quick Reference Sheet in Chapter 6.)

Child care center: A facility that provides care and education for any number of infants, toddlers, and preschool- or school-aged children in a nonresidential setting, or 13 or more children in any setting if the facility is open on a regular basis.

Child to staff ratio: The maximum number of children permitted per educator.

Children with special needs: Children who have or are at increased risk for a chronic physical, developmental, behavioral, or emotional condition and who also require more health and related services than required by children generally.

CHIP: Abbreviation for Children's Health Insurance Program, a program that provides free or low-cost health coverage for children in families that earn too much money to qualify for Medicaid. CHIP benefits are different in each state. The program covers US citizens and eligible immigrants. This insurance usually pays for routine recommended preventive health services such as immunization.

Chronic: Adjective describing an infection, illness, or condition that lasts a long time (months or years) or reoccurs frequently.

Ciprofloxacin: An antibiotic prescribed for some individuals with a bacterial infection.

Clean: *Adjective:* to be free of visible dirt; *verb:* to remove dirt and debris (eg, blood, urine, saliva, mucus, feces, soil) from skin by washing with soap and rinsing with water or from environmental surfaces with a detergent solution, and then rinsing with water.

CMV: Abbreviation for cytomegalovirus, a viral infection common to children. In most cases, cytomegalovirus causes no symptoms. When symptoms are experienced, they typically consist of fever, swollen glands, and fatigue. CMV can infect a pregnant woman who is not immune and damage her fetus, leading to developmental delay, hearing loss, and other problems in the fetus.

Cohort: Only the children and adults who are assigned to a specific group are kept together, even if it requires staff to care for smaller groups when children are arriving or departing.

Communicable disease: A disease caused by a microorganism (eg, bacterium, virus, fungus, parasite) that can be transmitted from person to person via an infected body fluid or respiratory spray, with or without an intermediary agent (eg, tick, mosquito, food or beverage) or environmental object (eg, table surface). Some communicable diseases are reportable to local health authorities.

Compliance: The act of carrying out a recommendation, policy, regulation, legal requirement, or procedure.

Congenital: Existing from the time of birth.

Conjunctivitis: Also known as *pinkeye*. Inflammation (redness and swelling) of thin tissue covering the white part of the eye and the inside of the eyelids. May be caused by infection or an irritant in the environment.

Contamination: The presence of infectious microorganisms in or on the body, environmental surfaces, articles of clothing, or food or water.

Contraindication: Something (eg, symptom, condition) that makes a particular treatment or procedure inadvisable.

Coronavirus: A family of viruses that cause upper respiratory infections. See *COVID-19* for a new member of that family that emerged in 2019.

COVID-19: Abbreviation for coronavirus disease 2019, the name of the disease caused by the virus, SARS-CoV-2, that started a global pandemic in late 2019/early 2020.

Croup: A respiratory infection, caused by various viruses, that results in swelling of the voice box (larynx) and area below the voice box that can cause difficult breathing, hoarse voice, and a cough sounding like a seal's bark. (See Croup Quick Reference Sheet in Chapter 6.)

Cryptosporidium: A parasite that causes cryptosporidiosis, a diarrheal illness.

Daily health check: Assessment of a child's health each day through observation of the child and talking with the parent/guardian and, if applicable, the child. (See *Caring for Our Children*, Standard 3.1.1.1 [https://nrckids.org/CFOC]).

DEET: An insect repellent (diethyltoluamide).

Delegation of medication administration: Personnel who are not licensed to administer medication may do so under the supervision of a licensed health professional or where regulations permit a delegated person who has received training and has demonstrated the skills required to administer specific types of medication.

Dengue: A mosquito-borne viral disease in some southern states, commonly occurring in Puerto Rico, the Virgin Islands, and American Samoa. Symptoms include fever, headache, muscle and joint pains, and a characteristic skin rash that is similar to measles. In a few, more serious illnesses with dengue, internal bleeding can occur. (See Mosquito-borne Diseases Quick Reference Sheet in Chapter 6.)

Dental caries: Damage to teeth as a result of decay-causing bacteria in the mouth that make acids that attack the tooth's surface or enamel. This can lead to a small hole in a tooth, called a cavity. If caries is not treated, it can cause pain, infection, and even tooth loss.

Dental sealants: Clear protective coatings that cover tooth surfaces and prevent bacteria and food particles from settling into the pits and grooves. Dental sealants are usually applied after a child reaches 6 years of age when the first permanent molars come in. Dental sealants last for 4 to 5 years and can be reapplied when they wear off. Application of sealants may be accompanied by application of fluoride varnish that hardens the enamel and reduces dental caries.

Dermatitis: An inflammation of the skin caused by irritation from an external exposure or internal reaction or by an infection.

Diarrhea: An illness in which an individual develops more watery and/or more frequent stools than is normal (typical) for that person.

Diphtheria: A serious infection of the nose and throat caused by the bacteria *Corynebacterium diphtheriae*, producing symptoms of sore throat, low fever, chills, and a grayish membrane in the throat. The membrane can make swallowing and breathing difficult and may cause suffocation. The bacteria produce a toxin (a type of poisonous substance) that can cause severe and permanent damage to the nervous system and heart. This infection has been eliminated almost entirely in areas where standard infant immunizations and boosters are performed.

Disease surveillance: Close observation for the occurrence of a disease, such as a type of infection. Surveillance is performed to discover a disease problem early, to understand a disease problem better, and to evaluate the methods used to control the disease.

Disinfect: To eliminate or inactivate virtually all germs from inanimate surfaces by using chemicals (eg, products registered with the US Environmental Protection Agency as "disinfectants") or physical agents (eg, heat). Disinfectants are used on nonporous surfaces, such as diaper- or soiled underwear-changing surfaces, doorknobs and cabinet handles, drinking fountains, and toilets and other toilet room surfaces.

Drop-in care facility: A program where children are cared for over short periods on a one-time, intermittent, unscheduled, and/or occasional basis. It is often operated in connection with a business (eg, health club, hotel, shopping center, recreation center).

E coli: Shortened form of *Escherichia coli*. A type of bacteria that can cause diarrhea. See also *STEC*.

Early childhood education: The education provided to children from birth through 8 years of age. For the purposes of this book, the term refers to all education that occurs before school entry.

Early childhood education program/setting/facility: Child care centers, family child care homes, elementary schools, religious centers, and others where children from more than one family gather for educational purposes.

Eastern equine encephalomyelitis: A mosquito-borne viral disease that usually causes mild disease with headache but can cause more serious illness. (See Mosquito-borne Diseases Quick Reference Sheet in Chapter 6.)

Educator: A person who is professionally responsible for the education of children and/or adults.

Emergency disaster plan: An action plan that specifies how to prepare for and what to do in particular disaster situations.

EMS: Abbreviation for emergency medical services, a system of care for individuals who are injured or have a sudden serious illness.

Encephalitis: Inflammation (redness and swelling) of the brain, which can be caused by a number of viruses, including measles, mumps, and varicella.

Endemic: A disease that is regularly found among people. An endemic infectious disease has been in a population for some time to allow a level of immunity to develop either from prior infection or immunization.

Enteric: Describes infections affecting the intestines (often with diarrhea) or liver.

Enterovirus: A common virus infection spread by fecal-oral and respiratory routes. A common enterovirus infection in young children is *hand-foot-and-mouth disease*, in which fever and blister-like eruptions in the mouth and/or a rash (usually on the palms and soles) may occur. (See Hand-Foot-and-Mouth Disease Quick Reference Sheet in Chapter 6.)

EPA: Abbreviation for the US Environmental Protection Agency, established in 1970, which administers federal programs and regulation related to air and water pollution, solid waste disposal, pesticides (agents that are intended to harm living pests, including microbes, insects, and any unwanted living thing), radiation, and noise.

Epidemic: The occurrence of more cases of disease than would be expected in a community or region during a given period that is not explained by normal seasonal variation.

Epiglottis: Tissue flap that closes during swallowing as a lid of the voice box. When this tissue becomes swollen and inflamed (a condition called *epiglottitis*), it can block breathing passages. *Haemophilus influenzae* type b commonly causes epiglottitis. This infection has been virtually eliminated in areas where standard infant immunizations and boosters are performed.

EpiPen: A registered trade name for an automatic epinephrine injector. Epinephrine is administered in response to some allergic reactions. Other trade names for this medicine are Adrenaclick, Adrenalin Chloride, Auvi-Q, EpiPen Jr, and Twinject.

EPSDT: Abbreviation for the Medicaid Early and Periodic Screening, Diagnostic, and Treatment program, which provides health assessments and follow-up services to income-eligible children.

Evaluation: A measurement of how well a person, program, or intervention is performing relative to goals and objectives.

Exclusion: Denying admission of an ill child or staff member to a facility or asking them to leave if they are already present.

Excretion: A process by which waste material that is formed and not used by the body (eg, feces, urine) is removed from the body.

Facility: A legal definition of the buildings, grounds, equipment, and program provided by people involved in early childhood education or schools of any type.

Facility for children who are mildly ill: A facility providing care for children, some or all of whom are mildly ill, to include up to 6 children who are mildly ill; a *special* facility cares only for children who are mildly ill or for more than 6 children who are mildly ill at a time.

Family child care home: A program in which early childhood education is provided in the home of the educator. *Small family child care* is a program that provides education and care for 1 to 6 children, including the educator's own children; family members or other helpers may be involved in assisting the educator, but often, only 1 educator is present at any time. *Large family child care* provides care and education for 7 to 12 children, including the educator's own children. In large family child care homes, 1 or more qualified adult assistants are present to meet child to staff ratio requirements.

Febrile: The condition of having an abnormally high body temperature (fever).

Fecal coliform: Bacteria in stool that normally inhabit the gastrointestinal tract and are used as indicators of fecal pollution. They denote the presence of intestinal material and the possibility of disease-causing organisms in water or food.

FERPA: Family Education Rights and Privacy Act. A federal law that protects the privacy of student education records.

Fever: An elevation of body temperature considered meaningfully above normal, although not necessarily an indication of a significant health problem. Body temperature can be elevated by overheating caused by overdressing or a hot environment, reactions to medications, inflammatory conditions (eg, arthritis, lupus), cancers, and response to infection. A temperature considered to be meaningfully above normal by any method is above 101 °F (38.3 °C) for infants and children older than 2 months and above 100.4 °F (38.0 °C) for infants younger than 2 months.

Fifth disease: A common viral infection with rash occurring 1 to 3 weeks after infection; caused by parvovirus B19.

Fluoride varnish: A topical fluoride product applied to the teeth by dental and medical professionals that prevents early childhood caries.

Foodborne illness/disease: An illness or disease transmitted through food products.

Fungi: Plural of fungus. Organisms, such as yeasts, molds, mildew, and mushrooms, that get their nutrition from other living organisms or dead organic matter.

Germ: Small particles (viruses) or organisms (bacteria, fungi, or parasites) that may cause infections. Some germs are helpful. For example, some types of germs in the stomach and intestine help properly digest food.

Giardia duodenalis: A parasite that causes giardiasis, an intestinal infection commonly referred to as *Giardia.*

Group A streptococcus: A bacterium commonly found in the throat and on the skin that can cause a range of infections, from relatively mild sore throats ("strep throat") and skin infections (eg, scarlet fever) to life-threatening disease.

HAV: Abbreviation for hepatitis A virus. See also *Hepatitis.*

HBV: Abbreviation for hepatitis B virus. See also *Hepatitis.*

HCV: Abbreviation for hepatitis C virus. See also *Hepatitis.*

Health advocate: See *CCHA.*

Health care provider: A health professional who provides direct health services to an individual.

Health consultant: A health professional who provides advice about some health-related issue. This advice is not necessarily provided on an ongoing basis. For the role of a health professional who collaborates with the early childhood educators on an ongoing basis, see *CCHC.*

Health professional: Someone who is certified by an established licensing body or accredited by a national organization generally recognized to use appropriate criteria to grant such recognition. Some types of health professionals with a potential to provide child care health consultation in early childhood education programs and schools include physicians, nurse practitioners, nurses, physician assistants, mental health professionals, oral health professionals (dentists, hygienists), environmental health professionals, and nutritionists.

Health supervision: Routine screening assessments, immunizations, and chronic or acute illness monitoring. For infants and children younger than 24 months, health supervision includes documentation and plotting of charts on standard sex-specific length, weight, weight for length, and head circumference; diet; activity; and fine and gross motor, language, and socioemotional development. For children 24 months and older, sex-specific height and weight graphs should be plotted and reviewed by the pediatric health professional in addition to body mass index. Ongoing assessment of development and coaching of family and others involved in the child's care continues throughout childhood.

Hepatitis: Inflammation of the liver caused by viral infection. Hepatitis can be caused by hepatitis A, B, non-A, non-B, C, and D viruses and many others.

Herpes simplex virus: A viral organism that causes a recurrent disease that is marked by blister-like sores on mucous membranes (eg, mouth, lips, genitals) that weep clear fluid and slowly crust over.

HHS: Abbreviation for the US Department of Health and Human Services.

HHV-6: Abbreviation for human herpesvirus 6. See also *Herpes simplex virus.*

Hib: Abbreviation for *Haemophilus influenzae* type b, a group of bacterial infections that can infect ears, eyes, sinuses, epiglottis (ie, the flap that covers the windpipe), skin, lungs, blood, joints, and coverings of the brain (meningitis). Hib should not be confused with "the flu," which is a disease caused by a virus. Hib infection is a vaccine-preventable disease.

HIPAA: Abbreviation for the Health Insurance Portability and Accountability Act of 1996, a federal act that provides protections for personal health information held by covered entities and gives patients an array of rights with respect to that information, including need for parents/legal guardians to give permission to health professionals to share health information with others involved in caring for their children.

HIV: Abbreviation for human immunodeficiency virus, which affects the body in a variety of ways. In the most severe infections, the virus progressively destroys the body's immune system, causing a condition called AIDS (acquired immunodeficiency syndrome).

HPV: Abbreviation for human papillomavirus, which causes a number of skin and mucous membrane infections; the most common infection is the skin wart.

HVAC: Abbreviation for heating, ventilation, and air-conditioning.

Hygiene: Protective measures taken by individuals to promote health and limit the spread of infectious diseases.

IEP: Abbreviation for Individualized Education Program, a written document, derived from Part B of the Individuals With Disabilities Education Act, that is designed to meet a child's individual educational program needs. The main purposes of an IEP are to set reasonable learning goals and to state the services (including a special care plan for the child's medical needs while in school) that a school district will provide for a child with special educational needs. Every child who qualifies for special educational services provided by the school is required to have an IEP.

IFSP: Abbreviation for Individualized Family Service Plan, a written document, derived from Part C of the Individuals With Disabilities Education Act, that is formulated in collaboration with the family to meet the needs of a child with a developmental disability or delay; to assist the family in its care for a child's educational, therapeutic, and health needs; and to deal with the family's needs to the extent to which the family wishes assistance.

IGRA: Abbreviation for interferon-gamma release assay, a blood test to detect whether a person has been infected by the tuberculosis bacterium. This is the screening test to use instead of the Mantoux intradermal tuberculosis skin test when the person has received BCG vaccine in the past. BCG vaccine usually makes the Mantoux test result unclear.

Immune globulin (gamma globulin, immunoglobulin): An antibody preparation made from human plasma that provides temporary protection against diseases such as hepatitis A. Health officials may wish to give immune globulin to children and staff members who have been exposed to hepatitis A.

Immunity: The body's ability to fight a particular infection. Immunity can come from antibodies (immune globulin), cells, or other factors. During the fetal period, antibodies from mothers are transferred to fetuses and provide some protection from infection for the first few months after birth while newborns and infants are making antibodies for themselves. Some antibodies are produced by the newborn. During the first months after birth, maternal antibodies steadily decrease in the infant's body and the infant's ability to make antibodies slowly increases. By 6 months of age, the healthy infant can make substantial amounts and types of antibodies from exposure to common infections and in response to immunizations. This ability usually reaches adult levels by 2 years of age.

Immunization: The process of providing immunity, usually using vaccines. Vaccines help children and adults develop protection (antibodies) against specific infections. Vaccines may contain an inactivated or killed agent, part of the agent, an inactivated toxin made by an agent (toxoid), or a weakened live organism.

Immunocompromised: The state of not having normal body defenses (immune responses) against diseases caused by germs.

Impervious: Not allowing entrance or passage of moisture or particles.

Impetigo: A common skin infection caused by streptococcal infection or staphylococcal bacteria.

Incubation period: Time between exposure to an infectious microorganism and beginning of symptoms.

Infant: A person between the time of birth and the age of ambulation, usually from birth through 12 months of age.

Infection: A condition caused by the multiplication of an infectious agent in the body.

Infectious: Capable of causing an infection. A disease is infectious when it is caused by a microorganism (bacterium, virus, fungus, or parasite) that can be transmitted from person to person via infected body fluids or respiratory spray, with or without an intermediary agent (eg, louse, mosquito) or environmental object (eg, table surface). Many infectious diseases are reportable to the local health authority.

Infestation: Common usage of this term refers to parasites (eg, lice, scabies) or pests (eg, ticks, bedbugs) living on or in the body or in the environment in places where they are troublesome to people.

Influenza ("flu"): An acute viral infection of the respiratory tract. Symptoms usually include fever, chills, headache, muscle aches, dry cough, and sore throat. Influenza should not be confused with *Haemophilus influenzae* infection, which is caused by bacteria, or with "stomach flu," which is usually an infection caused by a different type of virus.

Ingestion: The act of taking material (whether food or other substances) into the body through the mouth.

Integrated pest management: An approach to eliminating the causes of pest problems, providing safe and effective control of insects, weeds, rodents, and other pests while minimizing risks to human health and the environment.

Intradermal: Relating to areas between the layers of the skin (as in intradermal injections).

Isolation: The physical separation of a person from other persons. When an infection is the reason for separation, it is intended to prevent or lessen contact between the body fluids of an infected person and other persons who are thought not to have the infection.

Jaundice: Yellowish discoloration of the whites of the eyes, skin, and mucous membranes caused by deposition of bilirubin in these tissues. It occurs as a sign of certain diseases, such as hepatitis, that affect the processing of bile.

La Crosse encephalitis: A mosquito-borne viral disease that usually causes mild disease with headache but can cause more serious illness. (See Mosquito-borne Diseases Quick Reference Sheet in Chapter 6.)

Large family child care home: See *Family child care.*

Lethargy: Unusual sleepiness or low activity level.

Lice: Parasites that live on the surface of human heads, bodies, or pubic hair.

Licensing: Designation as having met the requirements to operate or practice in a specific sector. Permission from a state that is required to be allowed to carry out a specified function, such as operating an early childhood education program or certain types of professional activities. Some states use the term *licensing*; others use *certification* or *registration* to describe their regulatory process.

LTBI: Abbreviation for latent tuberculosis infection. The "latent" term is being phased out. Now called tuberculosis infection (TBI). See *TBI.*

Lyme disease: An infection caused by a type of bacteria known as spirochetes. The disease is transmitted when particular kinds of ticks attach to a person's skin and feed on that person's blood.

Lymphadenitis: An acute infection of one or more lymph nodes.

Malaria: A mosquito-borne disease caused by a parasite that occurs commonly in tropical areas of the world. It is extremely uncommon in the United States except among international travelers. (See Mosquito-borne Diseases Quick Reference Sheet in Chapter 6.)

Mantoux intradermal skin test: A type of tuberculin skin test. Involves the intradermal injection of a standardized amount of tuberculin antigen. The reaction to the antigen on the skin can be measured and the result used to assess the likelihood the person has had an infection with the bacteria that cause tuberculosis (*Mycobacterium tuberculosis*).

Measles (red measles, rubeola, hard measles, 8- to 10-day measles): A serious viral illness characterized by a red rash, high fever, light-sensitive eyes, cough, and cold symptoms.

Medicaid: A program that provides medical assistance for individuals and families with low incomes and resources. The program became law in 1965 as a jointly funded cooperative venture between the federal and state governments to assist states in the provision of adequate medical care to eligible needy persons.

Medical home: A site where medical care is provided that is accessible, continuous, comprehensive, family centered, coordinated, compassionate, and culturally effective. The pediatric health professional works in partnership with the family and patient to ensure that all the medical and nonmedical needs of the patient are met.

Medications: Any substances that are intended to diagnose, cure, treat, or prevent disease or affect the structure or function of the body of humans or other animals.

Meningitis: A swelling or inflammation of the tissue covering the spinal cord and brain. Meningitis is usually caused by a bacterial or viral infection.

Meningococcal disease: Pneumonia, arthritis, meningitis, or blood infection caused by the bacterium *Neisseria meningitidis*.

MIS-C: Abbreviation for multisystem inflammatory syndrome in children, a condition in which multiple body parts become inflamed in children infected with SARS-CoV-2, the virus that causes COVID-19.

MMR: Abbreviation for the vaccine against measles, mumps, and rubella.

MMRV: Abbreviation for the vaccine against measles, mumps, rubella, and varicella.

Mold: Fungi that are found virtually everywhere, indoors and outdoors. Mold can cause or worsen certain illnesses (eg, some allergic and occupation-related diseases and infections in health care settings).

Molluscum contagiosum: A common skin disease that is caused by a virus. Molluscum infection causes small white, pink, or flesh-colored bumps or growths with a dimple or pit in the center.

Morbidity: The incidence of a disease within a population.

MRSA: Abbreviation for methicillin-resistant *Staphylococcus aureus*, a potentially dangerous type of staphylococcal bacteria that is resistant to certain antibiotics and may cause skin and other infections.

Mucous membranes: The linings of body passages and cavities that make mucus and communicate directly or indirectly with the exterior of the body (eg, mouth, eyes, nose, ureters, urethra, urinary bladder, intestines, rectum, vagina).

Mumps: A viral infection with symptoms of fever, headache, and swelling and tenderness of the salivary glands, causing the cheeks and area under the jaw to swell.

Neisseria meningitidis (meningococcus): A bacterium that can cause meningitis, blood infections, pneumonia, and arthritis.

Nonprescription medications: Drugs that are available without a prescription. See also *Over-the-counter medication*.

Norovirus: Virus that causes diarrhea and vomiting. Noroviruses are very contagious. They usually are found in contaminated food or drinks, but they also can live on surfaces or be spread through contact with an infected person.

Organisms: Living things. Often used as a general term for germs (eg, bacteria, viruses, fungi, parasites).

OSHA: Abbreviation for the Occupational Safety and Health Administration of the US Department of Labor, which regulates health and safety in the workplace.

Otitis media: Inflammation or infection of the middle part of the ear, caused by viruses or bacteria.

Outbreak: An unusual rise in the incidence of a disease.

Over-the-counter medication: Medicine that can be purchased without a prescription.

Parasite: A multicellular organism that lives on or in another living organism (eg, ticks, tapeworm, louse, mite, pinworm).

Parent/legal guardian: The child's natural or adoptive mother or father, guardian, or other legally responsible person.

Pasteurized: The partial sterilization of a food substance and especially a liquid (as milk) at a temperature and for a period of exposure that destroys objectionable organisms without major chemical alteration of the substance.

Perishable foods: Foods, such as fruit, vegetables, meat, milk and dairy, and eggs, that are likely to spoil or decay.

Pertussis: A highly contagious bacterial respiratory infection, which begins with cold-like symptoms and cough and becomes progressively more severe, so that the person may experience vomiting, sweating, and exhaustion with the cough, also known as *whooping cough*.

Pesticides: Chemicals used to kill or control pests, particularly insects, rodents, and other troublesome living things. The US Environmental Protection Agency views germs as pests and germ-killing chemicals as pesticides.

Pneumonia: An acute or chronic disease marked by inflammation of the lungs and caused by viruses, bacteria, or other microorganisms and sometimes by physical and chemical irritants.

Poliomyelitis: A disease that is caused by the poliovirus with signs that may include paralysis and meningitis but often only include minor flu-like symptoms. This infection has been eliminated almost entirely in areas where standard infant immunizations and boosters are given.

Pooling: A practice in larger early childhood education settings in which children of various ages are brought together as they arrive at the beginning of the day or depart at the end of the day to consolidate the number of staff needed to meet child to staff ratios. The contrasting practice involves creating a *cohort*, in which only the children and adults who are assigned to a specific group are kept together, even if it requires staff to care for smaller groups when children are arriving or departing.

Prescription medications: Medications that can only be prescribed by a licensed health professional, such as a physician or nurse practitioner.

Primary health professional: A person who by education, training, certification, or licensure is qualified to and engaged in providing health care. A primary health professional coordinates the care of a child with the child's specialist and therapists.

Professional development: A continuum of learning and support opportunities designed to improve individuals' ability to work with and on behalf of young children and their families.

Pseudomonas aeruginosa: A type of organism that is commonly a contaminant of skin sores but occasionally causes infection in other parts of the body. It may be acquired during hospitalization.

Purulent: Containing pus, a thick white or yellow fluid.

Purulent conjunctivitis: Also known as *pinkeye*; a white or yellow eye discharge, often with matted eyelids after sleep, and including eye pain or redness of the eyelids or skin surrounding the eye. This type of conjunctivitis is more often caused by a bacterial infection, which may require antibiotic treatment.

QRIS: Abbreviation for Quality Rating and Improvement System, a systemic approach to assess, improve, and communicate the level of quality in early childhood education programs and schools. Similar to rating systems for restaurants and hotels, this system awards quality ratings to early childhood education programs and schools that meet a set of defined program standards.

Registration: Designation as having met the requirements to operate or practice in a specific sector. Permission from a state that is required to be allowed to carry out a specified function, such as operating an early childhood education program or certain types of professional activities. Some states use the term *licensing*; others use *certification* or *registration* to describe their regulatory process.

Respiratory etiquette: The process of coughing or sneezing into a tissue, shoulder, or elbow, followed by hand hygiene in an effort to reduce the spread of germ-containing droplets.

Respiratory tract: The nose, ears, sinuses, throat, windpipe, and lungs.

Rheumatic fever: An inflammatory disease that can develop as a complication of inadequately treated strep throat or scarlet fever caused by an infection with streptococcal bacteria. The symptoms include fever and painful inflammation of the joints. The disease can result in permanent damage to the valves of the heart.

Rhinorrhea: Excessive mucous secretion from the nose.

Rhinovirus: The virus that often causes the common cold.

Rifampin: An antibiotic often prescribed for those exposed to an infection caused by *Haemophilus influenzae* type b or *Neisseria meningitidis* (meningococcus) or given to treat an infection caused by tuberculosis.

Ringworm: A fungal infection that may affect the body, feet, or scalp.

Roseola: A viral infection causing rash in infants and children that primarily occurs between 6 and 24 months of age.

Rotavirus: A virus that causes diarrhea and vomiting.

RSV: Abbreviation for respiratory syncytial virus, which causes colds, bronchiolitis, and pneumonia.

Rubella: A mild viral illness, also known as *German measles*, that usually lasts 3 days, with symptoms of red rash, low-grade fever, swollen glands, and, sometimes, achy joints. The MMR vaccine, which is routinely administered in childhood, includes protection against rubella. Rubella can cause significant birth defects to the fetus of a woman infected with rubella.

Salmonella: A type of bacteria that causes food poisoning (salmonellosis) with symptoms of vomiting, diarrhea, and abdominal pain. *Salmonella* Paratyphi is the bacterium responsible for paratyphoid fever. This *Salmonella* serotype has 3 forms: A, B, and C. *Salmonella* Typhi is the bacterium responsible for causing the life-threatening illness typhoid fever.

Salmonellosis: A diarrheal infection caused by *Salmonella* bacteria.

Sanitize: To reduce germs on inanimate surfaces to levels considered safe by public health codes or regulations. For an inanimate surface to be considered sanitary, the surface must first be clean (see *Clean*) and the number of germs must be reduced to such a level that disease transmission by that surface is unlikely. Sanitization is less rigorous than disinfection (see *Disinfect*) and is applicable to a wide variety of routine housekeeping procedures involving, for example, plastic mouthed toys, mixed-use tables, high chair trays, food preparation surfaces, eating utensils, and computer keyboards.

SARS-CoV-2: See *COVID-19*.

Scabies: An infestation of the skin by small insects called mites.

Scarlet fever: A fine rash that makes the skin feel like sandpaper; caused by a streptococcal (bacterial) infection.

School-age child care facility: A facility offering activities to school-aged children before and after school, during vacations, and on nonschool days set aside for such activities as educators' in-service programs.

School-aged child: For the purposes of this book, a child at the entry into regular school, including kindergarten through sixth grade.

Screening: Examination of a population group or individual to detect the possible existence of a particular disease (eg, diabetes, tuberculosis) or to determine immunization status or other aspects of health status. Screening for a disease must be followed up by diagnostic testing to confirm the suspected condition is actually present.

Secretions: Wet materials, such as saliva, that are produced by cells or glands and have a specific purpose in the body.

Seizure: A sudden attack or convulsion caused by involuntary, uncontrolled bursts of electrical activity in the brain that can result in a wide variety of clinical manifestations, including muscle twitches, staring, tongue biting, loss of consciousness, and total body shaking.

Sepsis: An infection that involves having disease-causing germs or their toxins in the blood or other body tissues.

Serum: The clear liquid that separates in the clotting of blood.

Shigella: A type of bacterium that causes bacillary dysentery or shigellosis, a diarrheal infection.

Shigellosis: A diarrheal infection caused by the *Shigella* bacterium.

Shingles: A viral infection caused by the same virus that causes chickenpox. It is recognized as a painful rash, most often as a stripe of blisters that wraps around the body.

Small family child care home: See *Family child care*.

St Louis encephalitis: A mosquito-borne viral disease that usually causes mild disease with headache but can cause more serious illness. (See Mosquito-borne Diseases Quick Reference Sheet in Chapter 6.)

Staff members: Used in this book to indicate all personnel employed or serving as volunteers at an early childhood education program or school, including all caregivers, teachers, and personnel who do not provide direct care to children (eg, administrators, clerical workers, cooks, drivers, maintenance/housekeeping personnel).

Standard Precautions: Use of barriers (eg, gloves) to handle potential exposure to blood, including blood-containing body fluids and tissue discharges, and other potentially infectious fluids; proper hand hygiene and procedures to clean and disinfect contaminated surfaces. Although Standard Precautions were designed to apply to hospital settings, except for the use of masks and gowns, they also apply in early childhood education settings for children.

Standing orders: Orders written in advance by a health professional that describe the procedure to be followed in defined circumstances.

Staphylococcus: A common bacterium found on the skin that may cause skin infections or boils.

STEC: Abbreviation for Shiga toxin–producing *Escherichia coli*. Bacterial intestinal tract infection that causes diarrhea.

Streptococcal pharyngitis (strep throat)**:** A disease caused by a *Streptococcus* bacterium.

Streptococcus: A common bacterium that can cause sore throat, upper respiratory illnesses, pneumonia, skin rashes, skin infections, arthritis, heart disease (rheumatic fever), and kidney disease (glomerulonephritis).

Substitute staff members: Educators who are hired for 1 day or an extended period but are not considered to be permanent workers in their assigned positions.

SUID: Abbreviation for sudden unexplained infant death. The sudden death of an infant younger than 1 year that remains unexplained after a thorough case investigation, including performance of a complete autopsy, examination of the death scene, and review of the clinical history.

Systemic: Pertaining to a whole body rather than to one of its parts.

TB: Abbreviation for tuberculosis, a disease caused by a bacterium (*Mycobacterium tuberculosis*) that usually involves the lungs but can infect other parts of the body.

TBI: Abbreviation for tuberculosis infection. Formerly known as *latent tuberculosis infection*. See *LTBI*.

Tdap: Abbreviation for the vaccine given to older children and adults to protect against tetanus, diphtheria, and pertussis infections. This vaccine includes an acellular component to protect against pertussis, which is indicated by the "a" in the abbreviation.

Thrush: A yeast infection predominately produced by *Candida albicans* organisms, causing mouth infections in young infants.

Tick-borne diseases: Infections from ticks that bite people and transmit germs. Examples include Lyme disease and Rocky Mountain spotted fever.

Toddler: A child between the age of ambulation and toilet learning/training (usually between 13 and 35 months of age).

Toxoplasmosis: A parasitic disease that does not usually cause symptoms. If symptoms occur, they are swollen glands, fatigue, feeling sick, muscle pain, low fever, rash, headache, and sore throat. Toxoplasmosis can infect and damage a fetus even if the mother has no symptoms. This organism is commonly found in cat feces.

Transmission: The passing of an infectious organism or germ from person to person.

Under-immunized: A person who has not received the recommended number or types of vaccines for their age according to the current national and local immunization schedules.

Universal precautions: A term used by the US Occupational Safety and Health Administration that applies to blood and other body fluids that contain blood, semen, and vaginal secretions but not to feces, nasal secretions, sputum, sweat, tears, urine, saliva, and vomitus, unless they contain visible blood or are likely to contain blood. Universal precautions include avoiding injuries that are caused by sharp instruments or devices and the use of protective barriers, such as gloves, gowns, aprons, masks, or protective eyewear, that can reduce the risk of exposure of the worker's skin or mucous membranes that could come in contact with materials that may contain bloodborne pathogens while the worker is providing first aid or care.

Varicella zoster: The virus that causes chickenpox and shingles.

Vector-borne diseases: Diseases in which the germ is spread from one infected individual or animal to another by an arthropod (eg, insect) or other agent.

Virus: A microscopic organism, smaller than a bacterium, containing DNA or RNA but not both, that may cause disease. Viruses can grow or reproduce only in living cells. Examples include respiratory syncytial virus, influenza, measles, and hepatitis B.

West Nile virus: A mosquito-borne viral disease that is usually associated with mild symptoms. (See Mosquito-borne Diseases Quick Reference Sheet in Chapter 6.)

Western equine encephalomyelitis: A mosquito-borne viral disease that usually causes mild disease with headache but can cause more serious illness. (See Mosquito-borne Diseases Quick Reference Sheet in Chapter 6.)

Zika: A mosquito-borne viral disease that usually causes mild illness but may damage the fetus of a pregnant woman who is infected. (See Mosquito-borne Diseases Quick Reference Sheet in Chapter 6.)

Index

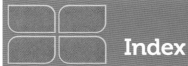

Index

Green Seal, 28–29, 228
Group A streptococcus, 253
Group size, 10

H

H1N1 influenza, 199
Haemophilus influenzae type b (Hib), 42, 111–112, 137, 254
Hand-foot-and-mouth disease, 49, 113–114, 147–148, 200
Hand hygiene, 5, 11
    after diapering, 235
    alcohol-based hand sanitizers for, 5, 11, 20–21, 22–23
    assisting children with, 21–22
    effective, 21
    handwashing method for, 22
    importance of, 20–21
    premoistened cleansing towelettes, 22
    sinks for routine handwashing, 21
    staff members, 38
    when to practice, 21
Hand sanitizers, 11, 20–21, 22–23
HAV. *See* Hepatitis A virus
HBV. *See* Hepatitis B virus
HCV. *See* Hepatitis C virus
HDV. *See* Hepatitis D virus
Headache, 63
Head lice. *See* Lice (pediculosis capitis)
Head Start Early Childhood Learning & Knowledge Center (ECLKC), 10, 14, 200
Health advocate, 250, 253
    qualifications and specific responsibilities of, 13
    role of, 13
    staff member education to perform role of, 13–14
Health and Human Services (HHS), US Department of, 254
Health assessments
    for adults who work in early childhood education programs, 7–8
    for children, 6–7
Health care provider, 253
Health check, 47
Health consultants, 253
Health education, 10
Healthful actions, 6–13
    changing areas for diapers, disposable training pants, or soiled underwear, 11
    daily practices, 11
    exclusion, 12–13
    hand hygiene, 11
    health education, 10
    healthful environment, 12
    HVAC systems and, 12
    immunizations for adults who work in early childhood education programs, 7–8
    immunizations for children, 6–7
    infection control and prevention by structuring and managing the environment, 10–12
    integrated pest management, 12
    nutrition, 10
    roles of families, staff members, and health professionals in managing, 13–15

    routine health assessments for adults who work in early childhood education programs, 7–8
    routine health assessments for children, 6–7
    safe activities, 10
    safe food preparation and service, 11
    sleep and exercise, 10
    space, 10
    special needs care, 10
    Standard Precautions, 11
    surface hygiene, 11
    surfaces, 11
    toilets and sinks, 11
    toothbrushing, 11–12
    vaccine refusal and, 8–10
Health Information Consent Form, Sample, 231
Health Insurance Portability and Accountability Act of 1996 (HIPAA), 254
Health policies. *See* Policies and procedures
Health professional, 253
Health supervision, 253
HealthyChildren.org, 10
Healthy Kids, Healthy Future, 10
Healthy Young Children: A Manual for Programs, 14
Hearing screening for staff members, 37
Heating, ventilation, and air-conditioning (HVAC) systems, 12, 33, 254
Hepatitis, 253
Hepatitis A virus, 51, 115–116
    return-to-work after, 42
Hepatitis B virus, 6, 117–118
    chronic, 50
    vaccine for, 39–40
Hepatitis C virus, 6
Hepatitis D virus, 6
Herpes simplex (cold sores), 42, 119–120, 147–148, 254
Herpes zoster (shingles), 175–176, 258
    return-to-work after, 42
HHS. *See* Health and Human Services (HHS), US Department of
HHV-6. *See* Human herpesvirus 6 and 7 (roseola)
Hib. *See* Haemophilus influenzae type b (Hib)
HIPAA. *See* Health Insurance Portability and Accountability Act of 1996 (HIPAA)
HIV. *See* Human immunodeficiency virus (HIV)
Hospital-grade germicides, 30
HPV. *See* Human papillomavirus (HPV)
Human bites, 75–76
Human herpesvirus 6 and 7 (roseola), 163–164, 254
Human immunodeficiency virus (HIV), 6, 50, 121–122, 254. *See also* Acquired immunodeficiency syndrome (AIDS)
Human milk, 10
Human papillomavirus (HPV), 193, 254
Human parvovirus B19, 38, 107–108
HVAC. *See* Heating, ventilation, and air-conditioning (HVAC) systems
Hygiene, 254

I

Ibuprofen, 104, 105, 147
Icaridin. *See* Picaridin
IEP. *See* Individualized Education Program (IEP)